☆CRACK
THE CORE EXAM

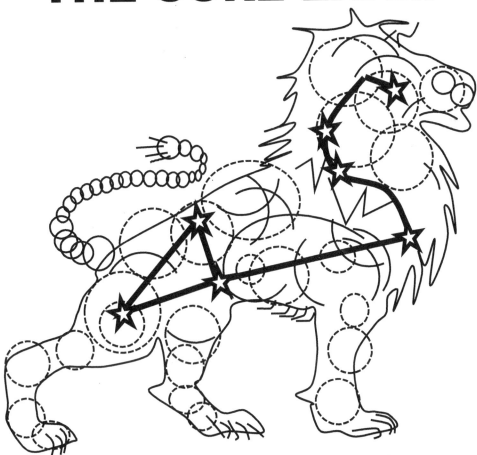

7th (2020) EDITION
VOLUME 2

WRITTEN & ILLUSTRATED BY:

PROMETHEUS LIONHART, M.D.

CRACK THE CORE EXAM - VOL 2

SEVENTH ED. - VERSION 1.0

DISCLAIMER:

READERS ARE ADVISED - THIS BOOK IS NOT TO BE USED FOR CLINICAL DECISION MAKING. HUMAN ERROR DOES OCCUR, AND IT IS YOUR RESPONSIBILITY TO DOUBLE CHECK ALL FACTS PROVIDED. TO THE FULLEST EXTENT OF THE LAW, THE AUTHOR ASSUMES NO RESPONSIBILITY FOR ANY INJURY AND/OR DAMAGE TO PERSONS OR PROPERTY ARISING OUT OF OR RELATED TO ANY USE OF THE MATERIAL CONTAINED IN THIS BOOK.

ISBN: 9781673777888

INDEPENDENTLY PUBLISHED — PROMETHEUS LIONHART (EARTH DIMENSION C-137)

NO SLAVE LABOR (RESIDENT OR FELLOW) WAS USED IN THE CREATION OF THIS TEXT

VOLUME 2

WRITTEN & ILLUSTRATED BY
PROMETHEUS LIONHART, M.D.

- -

VOLUME 1:

TOPICS: PEDS, GI, GU, REPRODUCTIVE, ENDOCRINE, THORACIC, CARDIAC, NUKES

WAR MACHINE:

TOPICS: PHYSICS, NON INTERPRETIVE SKILLS, BIOSTATS

LEGAL STUFF

READERS ARE ADVISED - THIS BOOK IS NOT TO BE USED FOR CLINICAL DECISION MAKING. HUMAN ERROR DOES OCCUR, AND IT IS YOUR RESPONSIBILITY TO DOUBLE CHECK ALL FACTS PROVIDED. TO THE FULLEST EXTENT OF THE LAW, THE AUTHOR ASSUMES NO RESPONSIBILITY FOR ANY INJURY AND/OR DAMAGE TO PERSONS OR PROPERTY ARISING OUT OF OR RELATED TO ANY USE OF THE MATERIAL CONTAINED IN THIS BOOK.

ARE RECALLS IN THIS BOOK? ABSOLUTELY NOT.

THE AUTHOR HAS MADE A CONSIDERABLE EFFORT (IT'S THE OUTRIGHT PURPOSE OF THE TEXT), TO SPECULATE HOW QUESTIONS MIGHT BE ASKED. A PHD IN BIOCHEMISTRY CAN FAIL A MED SCHOOL BIOCHEMISTRY TEST OR BIOCHEM SECTION ON THE USMLE, IN SPITE OF CLEARLY KNOWING MORE BIOCHEM THAN A MEDICAL STUDENT. THIS IS BECAUSE THEY ARE NOT USED TO MEDICINE STYLE QUESTIONS. THE AIM OF THIS TEXT IS TO EXPLORE THE LIKELY STYLE OF BOARD QUESTIONS AND INCLUDE MATERIAL LIKELY TO BE COVERED, INFORMED BY THE ABR'S STUDY GUIDE.

THROUGHOUT THE TEXT THE AUTHOR WILL ATTEMPT TO FATHOM THE MANNER OF QUESTIONING AND INCLUDE THE CORRESPONDING HIGH YIELD MATERIAL. A CORRECT ESTIMATION WILL BE WHOLLY COINCIDENTAL.

HUMOR / PROFANITY WARNING

I USE PROFANITY IN THIS BOOK. I MAKE "GROWN UP" JOKES. PROBABLY NOT A GOOD IDEA TO READ THE BOOK OUT LOUD TO SMALL CHILDREN OR ELDERLY MEMBERS OF YOUR CHURCH / TEMPLE / MOSQUE. NOW IS NOT THE OPTIMAL TIME TO BE RECREATIONALLY OUTRAGED - I'M JUST TRYING TO MAKE THE BOOK READABLE AND FUN.

I ALSO TALK A MESS OF SHIT ABOUT DIFFERENT MEDICAL SPECIALTIES. I DO THIS BECAUSE RADIOLOGISTS ARE TRIBAL, AND STROKING THAT URGE TENDS TO CALM PEOPLE. PROBABLY NOT A GOOD IDEA TO READ THE BOOK OUT LOUD TO MEMBERS OF YOUR FAMILY THAT ARE IN SPECIALTIES OTHER THAN RADIOLOGY. THE TRUTH IS I RESPECT ALL THE OTHER SUB-SPECIALTIES OF MEDICINE (EVEN FAMILY MEDICINE) - THOSE ARE DIRTY JOBS (POOP, PUS, & NOTE WRITING) BUT SOMEONE NEEDS TO DO THEM.

IF YOU STILL FEEL THE DESIRE TO EMAIL ME ABOUT HOW I HURT YOUR FEELINGS AND RUINED YOUR LIFE, CONSIDER THAT "MAYBE PEOPLE THAT CREATE THINGS AREN'T CONCERNED WITH YOUR DELICATE SENSIBILITIES."

What Makes This Book Unique?

SHORT ANSWER — FUCKING EVERYTHING

HOW ? — WELL FOR STARTERS, THESE BOOKS WEREN'T WRITTEN BY 30 RESIDENTS, 20 FELLOWS, AND 10 TURBO NERD ATTENDINGS.

INSTEAD THE BOOKS WERE WRITTEN BY A RELENTLESSLY SELF IMPROVING MANIAC, DRIVEN TO PURGE THE HERETICS (ORC SCUM), LAUNCH VENGEANCE UPON THIS PLANET, AND DELIVER MERCILESS JUSTICE UPON THE ENEMIES OF FREEDOM AND LIBERTY.

THE IMPETUS FOR THIS BOOK WAS NOT TO WRITE A REFERENCE TEXT OR STANDARD REVIEW BOOK, BUT INSTEAD, A STRATEGY MANUAL FOR SOLVING MULTIPLE CHOICE QUESTIONS FOR RADIOLOGY. THE AUTHOR WISHES TO CONVEY THAT THE MULTIPLE CHOICE TEST IS DIFFERENT THAN ORAL BOARDS IN THAT YOU CAN'T ASK THE SAME KINDS OF OPEN-ENDED ESSAY-TYPE QUESTIONS. "WHAT'S YOUR DIFFERENTIAL?"

QUESTIONING THE CONTENTS OF ONE'S DIFFERENTIAL WAS THE ONLY REAL QUESTION ON ORAL BOARDS. NOW THAT SIMPLE QUESTION BECOMES NEARLY IMPOSSIBLE TO FORMAT INTO A MULTIPLE CHOICE TEST. INSTEAD, THE FOCUS FOR TRAINING FOR SUCH A TEST SHOULD BE ON THINGS THAT CAN BE ASKED. FOR EXAMPLE, ANATOMY FACTS - WHAT IS IT? ... OR... TRIVIA FACTS - WHAT IS THE MOST COMMON LOCATION, OR AGE, OR ASSOCIATION, OR SYNDROME? ... OR... WHAT'S THE NEXT STEP IN MANAGEMENT? THINK BACK TO MEDICAL SCHOOL USMLE STYLE, THAT IS WHAT YOU ARE DEALING WITH ONCE AGAIN. IN THIS BOOK, THE AUTHOR TRIED TO COVER ALL THE MATERIAL THAT COULD BE ASKED (REASONABLY), AND THEN APPROXIMATE HOW QUESTIONS MIGHT BE ASKED ABOUT THE VARIOUS TOPICS. THROUGHOUT THE BOOK, THE AUTHOR WILL INTIMATE, "THIS COULD BE ASKED LIKE THIS," AND "THIS FACT LENDS ITSELF WELL TO A QUESTION." INCLUDED IN THE SECOND VOLUME OF THE SET IS A STRATEGY CHAPTER FOCUSING ON HIGH YIELD "BUZZWORDS" THAT LEND WELL TO CERTAIN QUESTIONS.

THIS IS NOT A REFERENCE BOOK.
THIS BOOK IS NOT DESIGNED FOR PATIENT CARE.
THIS BOOK IS DESIGNED FOR STUDYING SPECIFICALLY FOR MULTIPLE CHOICE TESTS, CASE CONFERENCE, AND VIEW-BOX PIMPING/QUIZING.

Radiology Master of Sport - National Champion
Americans love to fight. Americans love the champion.

This right here is about recognizing a commitment to being the best. Being the best, standing on the top stand - and more importantly <u>the quest</u> to stand on the top stand and wear the yellow medal is what I want to recognize.

The quest is very lonely. They say it is lonely at the top - that is not true. When I started to become recognized internationally as the top educator in the field I suddenly had alot of people who wanted to be my friend. I didn't have any friends on the way there - nobody was getting up at 4am with me to write… nobody, not one person. It was just me - alone. It is lonely getting to the top and that is where most people fall off. It's Friday and everyone else is going out, or there is a party or whatever - I'm tired and I want to sleep in. I was on call last night- it is just not worth it. What I'm hoping to share is that for me that is not what life is. Life is about being the best person you can be in whatever it is you are doing. That does not have to be Radiology, but because you are reading this book well that is what it means for you now.

You make the quest. If you get the top score on the exam - I'll be putting your name in this book next year and you can motivate the next legend of tomorrow. Plus, I'll give you some money and have an enormous lion trophy made for you.

The most important thing is not actually winning. People think I only care about winning because I rant and rave about how only the gold medals count - but the quest is what I really value. I'm not training for silver. I'm training for gold. The quest for gold is more important than someone handing you a gold medal. The katana sword of the black dragon society cannot be stolen - it can only be earned. Outcomes really don't matter, because the truth is in this life you can do everything 100% perfect and still fail and you can do almost everything wrong and still win. If you don't focus on outcomes and instead the quest itself you will get something much greater — besides a high probability of passing the test - what you can gain from the quest, the ability to really dedicate yourself to something 100% - it is a skill you can use for the rest of your life. This is *the way* to always achieve victory. Once you know *the way*, you can see it in all things - as the samurai say.

HALL OF CHAMPIONS

2017 Champion	2018 Champion	2019 Champion	2020 Champion
Dr. Gary Dellacerra, D.O.	Dr. Thomas Pendergrast, M.D.	Dr. Nick Broadbent, D.O.	
- Hofstra (formerly North Shore -LIJ)	—Wake Forrest	- University of Illinois in Peoria	May the Mightiest Warrior Prevail

I FIGHT FOR THE USERS

-TRON 1982

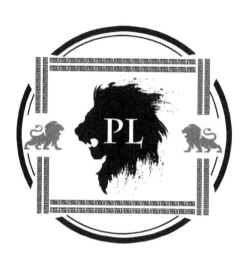

10

NEURORADIOLOGY

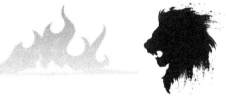

PROMETHEUS LIONHART, M.D.

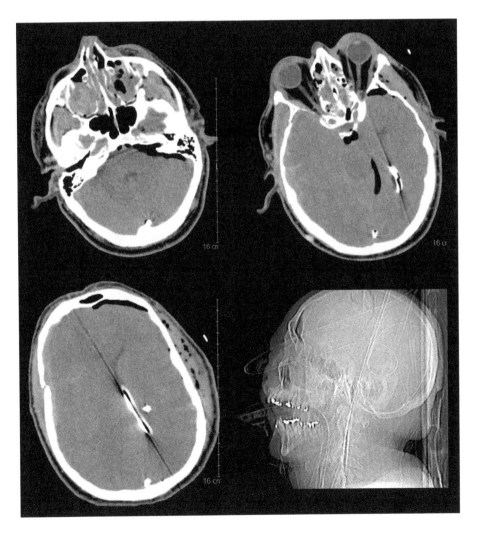

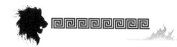 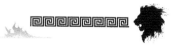
There is a ton of anatomy that can be asked on a multiple choice test. My idea is to break it down into three categories: (1) soft tissue – brain parenchyma (*including normal development*), (2) bony anatomy – which is basically foramina, and (3) vascular anatomy.

Soft Tissue Brain Anatomy:

Central Sulcus - This anatomic landmark separates the frontal lobe from the parietal lobe, and is useful to find if you haven't learned the lazy Neuroradiolgist's go to descriptor "fronto-parietal region." Old school grey bearded Radiologists (likely the ones who are important enough to write test questions) love to ask how you find this important structure. There are about 10 ways to do this, which brings me to the main reason this is a great pimping question. Even if you can name 9 ways to do it, they can still correct you by naming the 10th way. I noticed during my time as a "trainee" that Attendings tend to be excellent at knowing the answers to the questions they are asking.

Practically speaking, this is the strategy I use for finding the central sulcus:

Pretty high up on the brain, maybe the 3rd or 4th cut, I <u>find the pars marginalis</u>. This is called the **"pars bracket sign"** - because the bi-hemispheric symmetric pars marginalis form an anteriorly open bracket. The bracket is immediately behind the central sulcus. This is *present about 95% of the time* - it's actually pretty reliable.

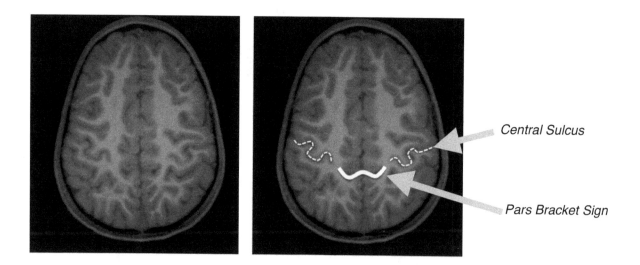

Central Sulcus

Pars Bracket Sign

Central Sulcus Trivia - Here are the other less practical ways to do it.

- Superior frontal sulcus / Pre-central sulcus sign: The posterior end of the superior frontal sulcus joins the pre-central sulcus
- Inverted omega (sigmoid hook) corresponds to the motor hand
- Bifid posterior central sulcus: Posterior CS has a bifid appearance about 85%
- *Thin post-central gyrus sign* – The precentral gyrus is thicker than the post-central gyrus (ratio 1.5 : 1).
- *Intersection* – The intraparietal sulcus intersects the post-central sulcus (works almost always)
- *Midline sulcus sign* – The most prominent sulcus that reaches the midline is the central sulcus (works about 70%).

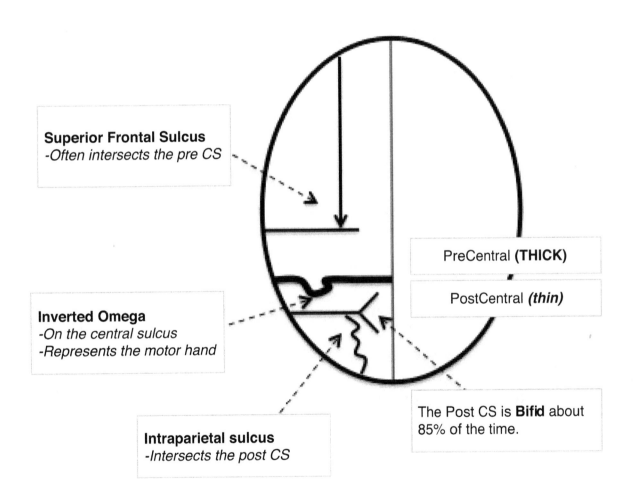

Superior Frontal Sulcus
-Often intersects the pre CS

PreCentral **(THICK)**

PostCentral *(thin)*

Inverted Omega
-On the central sulcus
-Represents the motor hand

The Post CS is **Bifid** about 85% of the time.

Intraparietal sulcus
-Intersects the post CS

Homunculous Trivia:

- The inverted omega (posteriorly directed knob) on the central sulcus / gyrus designates the motor cortex controlling hand function.

- ACA territory gets legs,

- MCA territory hits the rest.

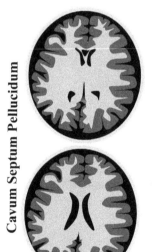

Normal Cerebral Cortex: As a point of trivia, the cortex is normally 6 layers thick, and the hippocampus is normally 3 layers thick. I only mention this because the hippocampus can look slightly brighter on FLAIR compared to other cortical areas, and this is the reason why (supposedly).

Dilated Perivascular Spaces (Virchow-Robins): These are fluid filled spaces that accompany perforating vessels. They are a normal variant and very common. They can be enlarged and associated with multiple pathologies; mucopolysaccharidoses (Hurlers and Hunters) ,"gelatinous pseudocysts" in cryptococcal meningitis, and atrophy with advancing age. They don't contain CSF, but instead have interstitial fluid. The common locations for these are: around the lenticulostriate arteries in the lower third of the basal ganglia, in the centrum semiovale, and in the midbrain.

Cavum Variants:

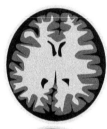

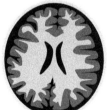

Normal

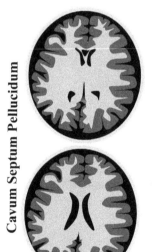

Cavum Septum Pellucidum

-100% of preterm infants,
-15% of adults.
-Rarely, can cause hydrocephalus
-Anterior to the foramen of Monroe
-Between frontal horns

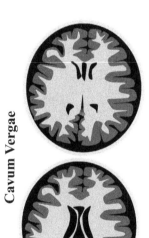

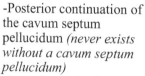

Cavum Vergae

-Posterior continuation of the cavum septum pellucidum *(never exists without a cavum septum pellucidum)*
-Posterior to the foramen of Monroe
-Between bodies of lateral ventricles

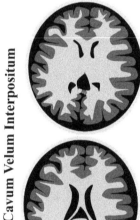

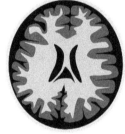

Cavum Velum Interpositum

-Extension of the quadrigeminal plate cistern to foramen of Monro.
-Seen above the 3rd ventricle and below the fornices.

Ventricular Anatomy:

Just a quick refresher on this.

You have two lateral ventricles that communicate with the third ventricle via the interventricular foramen (of Monro), which in turn communicates with the fourth ventricle via the cerebral aqueduct.

> **Arachnoid Granulations:** These are regions where the arachnoid projects into the venous system allowing for CSF to be reabsorbed. They are hypodense on CT (similar to CSF), and usually round or oval. This round shape helps distinguish them from clot in a venous sinus (which is going to be linear). On MR they are typically T2 bright (iso to CSF), but can be bright on FLAIR (although this varies a lot and therefore probably won't be tested). These things can scallop the inner table (probably from CSF pulsation)

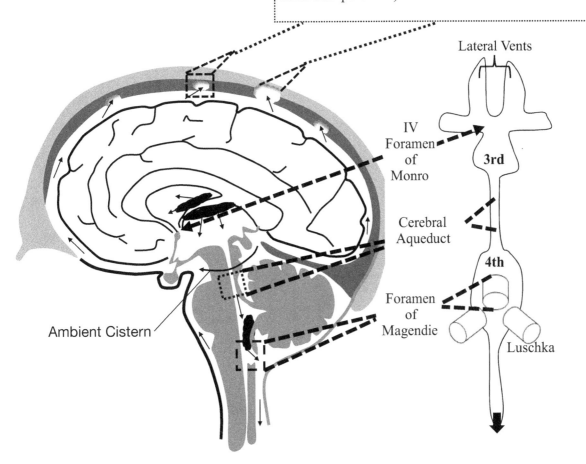

The fluid in the fourth ventricle escapes via the median aperture (foramen of Magendie), and the lateral apertures (foramen of Luschka). A small amount of fluid will pass downward into the spinal subarachnoid spaces, but most will rise through the tentorial notch and over the surface of the brain where it is reabsorbed by the arachnoid villi and granulations into the venous sinus system.

Blockage at any site will cause a noncommunicating hydrocephalus. Blockage of reabsorption at the villi / granulation will also cause a noncommunicating hydrocephalus.

Basal Cisterns: The basal cisterns are good for (1) evaluating mass effect, and (2) anatomy questions.

People say the suprasellar cisterns look like a star, with the five corners lending themselves nicely to multiple choice questions. So let us do a quick review; the top of the star is the interhemispheric fissure, the anterior points are the sylvian cisterns, and the posterior points are the ambient cisterns.

The quadrigeminal plate looks like a smile, or … I guess it looks like a sideways moon, if you don't like smiles.

No Time for Smiles. Training for Domination.
Snarls Not Smiles.

Smile later… once you've passed the test.

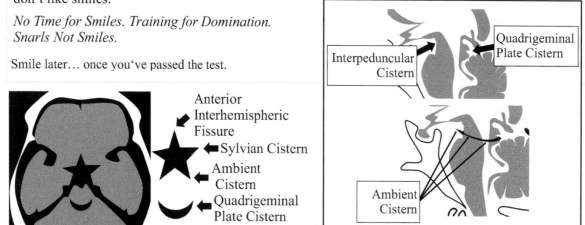

Anterior Interhemispheric Fissure
Sylvian Cistern
Ambient Cistern
Quadrigeminal Plate Cistern

Interpeduncular Cistern
Quadrigeminal Plate Cistern
Ambient Cistern

The Ambient Cistern is a bridge between the Interpeduncular C. ◄──► Quadrigeminal C.

Midbrain Tectum vs Tegmentum :

Atrophy patterns of the midbrain will become important when we start talking about some of the more obscure neurodegenerative disorders. So it's good to review the vocab words.

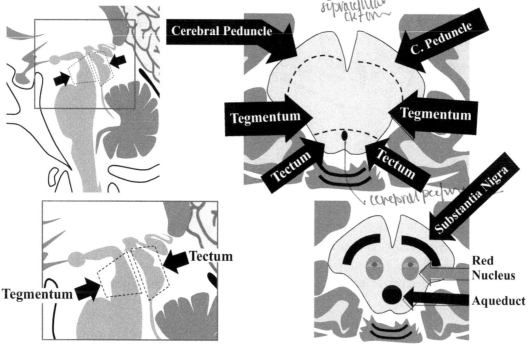

Cerebral Peduncle
C. Peduncle
Tegmentum
Tegmentum
Tectum
Tectum
Substantia Nigra
Red Nucleus
Aqueduct
Tectum
Tegmentum

When I was in medical school my anatomy teacher told me the midbrain looks like a monkey face.
I said "Please don't confuse me. Last week you said the monkey face was a penis cut in cross section."
I always thought the midbrain looked more like a stoner dog that just got higher than a giraffe's vagina.

Bony Anatomy: Skull Base Foramina (Rotundum, Oval, Spinosum, Hypoglossal)

First let us review the where - then we will do the what. Remember, they don't have to show you the hole in the axial plane. They can be sneaky and show it in the coronal or sagittal plane. In fact, showing **Foramen Rotundum (FR)** in the coronal and sagittal planes is a very common sneaky trick.

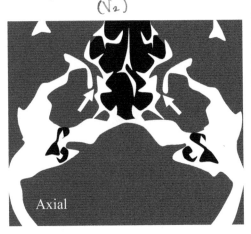

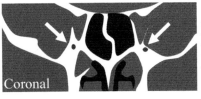

On the coronal view, FR looks like you are staring into a gun barrel.

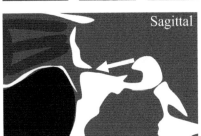

On the sagittal view, think about FR as being totally level or horizontal.

cribriform plate (1)
optic
sup. orb. fissure
lacerum
spinosum
rotundum
ovale
int. acoustic meatus
magnum
jugular
hypoglossal

With regard to the relationship between **Spinosum and Ovale**, I like to think of this as the footprint a woman's high heeled shoe might make in the snow, with the oval part being Ovale, and the pointy heel as Spinosum.

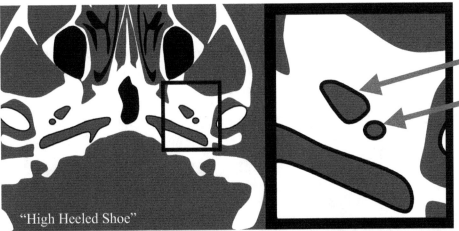

"High Heeled Shoe"

Foramen Ovale

Foramen Spinosum

cribriform: olfactory (I)
optic: optic (II)
sup. orbit.: III, IV, V₁, VI
rotundum: V₂
ovale: V₃
int. acoustic: VII, VIII
jugular: IX, X, XI
hypoglossal: XII

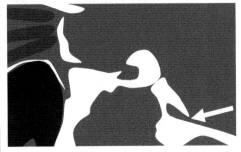

The **Hypoglossal Canal** is very posterior and inferior.

This makes it unique as a skull base foramen.

Trigeminal n
V₁: opthalmic
V₂: ~~trigeminal~~ maxillary
V₃: mandibular.

Bony Anatomy: Skull Base Foramina (Jugular Foramen)

The jugular foramen has two parts which are separated by a bony "jugular spine."

Pars Nervosa - The nervous guy in the front. This contains the Glossopharyngeal nerve (CN 9), along with it's tympanic brach - the "Jacobson's Nerve"

Pars Vascularis - This is the "vascular part" which actually contains the jugular bulb, along with the Vagus nerve (CN 10), Auricular branch "Arnold's Nerve," and the Spinal Accessory Nerve (CN 11)

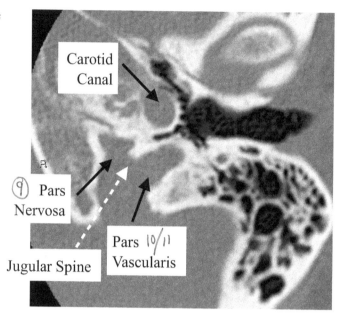

Bony Anatomy: Orbital Fissures and the PPF

The relationship between the Superior Orbital Fissure (SOF), the Inferior Orbital Fissure (IOF), Foramen Rotundum (FR), and the Pterygopalatine Fossa (PPF) is an important one, that can really lead to some sneaky multiple choice questions (mainly what goes through what - *see chart on page 18*).
I've attempted to outline this relationship on both sagittal and coronal views.

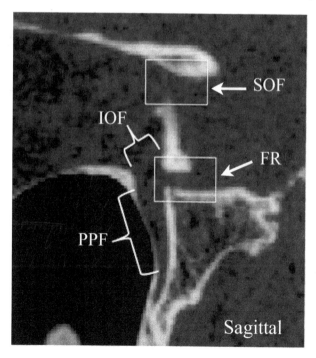

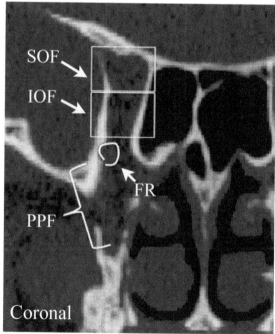

Anatomy: Cavernous Sinus

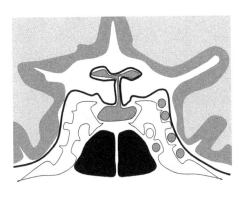

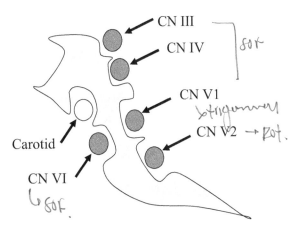

The question is most likely, what's in it (or asked as what is NOT in it).

- CN 3, CN 4, CN V1, CN V2, CN 6, and the carotid - run through it.

- CN 2 and CN V3 - do **NOT** run through it.

The only other anatomy trivia I can think of is that CN6 runs next to the carotid, the rest of the nerves are along the wall. This is why you can get lateral rectus palsy earlier with cavernous sinus pathologies.

Anatomy: Internal Auditory Canal - "IAC"

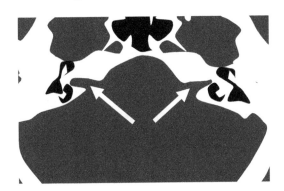

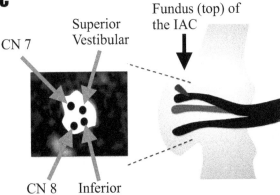

The thing to remember is "7UP, and COKE Down" - with the 7th cranial nerve superior to the 8th cranial nerve (the cochlear nerve component).

As you might guess, the superior vestibular branch is superior to the inferior one.

If it is shown, it is always shown in this orientation.

The ideal sequence to find it is a heavily T2 weighted sequence with super thin cuts through the IAC.

Anatomy - What's in It ?

Considering multiple choice questions regarding the skull base anatomy.
"What goes where?" questions essentially write themselves.

Hole / Compartment	Contents
Foramen Ovale	CN V3, and Accessory Meningeal Artery
Foramen Rotundum	CN V2 ("**R2V2**"),
Superior Orbital Fissure	CN 3, CN 4, CN V1, CN6
Inferior Orbital Fissure	CN V2
Foramen Spinosum	Middle Meningeal Artery
Jugular Foramen	*Pars Nervosa:* CN 9, *Pars Vascularis:* CN 10, CN 11
Hypoglossal Canal	CN 12
Optic Canal	CN 2 , and Opthalmic Artery
Cavernous Sinus	CN 3, CN 4, CN V1, CN V2, CN 6, and the carotid
Internal Auditory Canal	CN 7, CN 8 (Cochlear, Inferior Vestibular and Superior Vestibular components). "7 Up - Coke Down"
Meckel Cave	Trigeminal Ganglion
Dorello's Canal	Abducens Nerve (CN 6), Inferior petrosal sinus

Vascular Anatomy -

Arterial vascular anatomy can be thought of in four sections. (1) The branches of the external carotid (commonly tested as the order in which they arise from the common carotid). (2) Segments of the internal carotid, with pathology at each level and variants. (3) Posterior circulation, (4) Venous anatomy

(1) Branches of the External Carotid

Some **A**dministrative assistants **L**ove **F**ucking **O**ver **P**oor **M**edical **S**tudents

Superior Thyroid
Ascending Pharyngeal
Lingual
Facial
Occipital
Posterior Auricular
Maxillary
Superficial Temporal

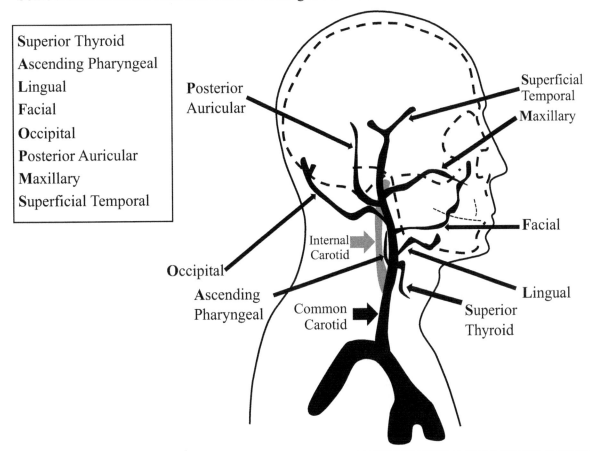

THIS vs THAT: External vs Internal Carotid via Ultrasound		
	Internal	**External**
Branches	Nope	Yup
Orientation	Posterior	Anterior
Resistance	Low (continuous diastolic)	High
Temporal Tap (poking the head)	No Change in Waveform	Waveform Reacts

[2] Segments of the Internal Carotid

Internal Carotid	• The bifurcation of the IAC and ECA usually occurs at C3-C4 • Cervical ICA has no branches in the neck - if you see branches either (a) they are anomalous or more likely (b) you are a dumb ass and actually looking at the external carotid. *Remember finding branches is a way you can tell ICA from ECA on ultrasound. • Low resistance waveform with continuous forward flow during diastole • Flow reversal in the carotid bulb is common	
C1 (Cervical)	• *Atherosclerosis:* The origin is a very common location • *Dissection:* Can be spontaneous (women), and in Marfans or Ehlers-Danlos, and result in a partial Horner's (ptosis and miosis), followed by MCA territory stroke. • Can have a retropharyngeal course and get "drained" by ENT accidentally. • Pharyngeal infection may cause pseudoaneurysm at this level.	
C2 (Petrous)	Not much goes on at this level.	Aneurysms here can be surprisingly big (thats what she said).
C3 (Lacerum)	Not much here as far as vascular pathology. The anatomic location is important to neurosurgeons for exposing Meckel's cave via a transfacial approach.	
C4 (Cavernous)	This segment is affected by multiple pathologies including the development of cavernous – carotid fistula.	Aneurysms here are strongly associated with hypertension.
C5 (Clinoid)		Aneurysm here could compress the optic nerve and cause blindness.
C6 (Ophthalmic - Supraclinoid):	Origin at the "dural ring" is a buzzword for this artery.	Common site for aneurysm formation.
C7 (Communicating)		Aneurysm here may compress CN III and present with a palsy.

Schematic ICA Angiographic Runs

You don't need to know every branch, but you should be able to recognize the main vessels.

Lateral ICA Runs:

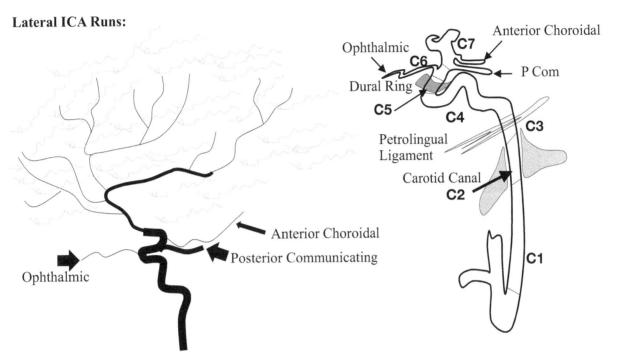

AP ICA Run:

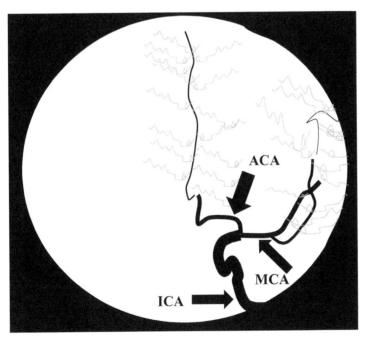

This is a pretty good look for an AP ICA run.

Notice that half the image is relatively blank. This is because you have 2 ICAs (right and left), only one of which is getting injected. For the total neuro angiography novice (most residents), this is a helpful thing to notice when deciding AP vs Lateral.

Also notice the MCA is lateral, and the ACA is medial.

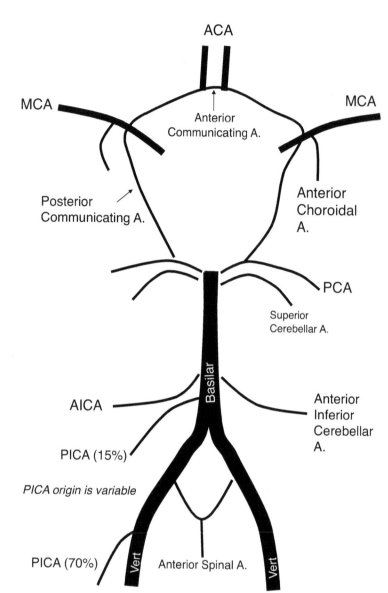

ACA

MCA

MCA

Anterior Communicating A.

Posterior Communicating A.

Anterior Choroidal A.

PCA

Superior Cerebellar A.

Basilar

AICA

Anterior Inferior Cerebellar A.

PICA (15%)

PICA origin is variable

PICA (70%)

Vert

Anterior Spinal A.

Vert

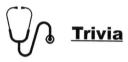
Trivia

Acute CN3 Palsy (unilateral pupil dilation) a classic neurology boards question - *grab a relax hammer STAT!*

The answer is <u>PCOM aneurysm</u> until proven otherwise (although it can also be caused by an aneurysm at the apex of the basilar artery or its junction with the superior cerebellar / posterior cerebral arteries).

The reason is the relationship between the CN3 and vessels (arrows).

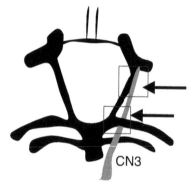

CN3

AP Vertebral Run

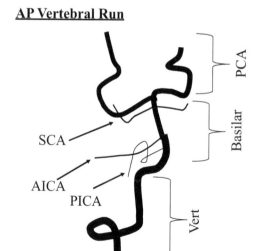

PCA

Basilar

SCA

AICA

PICA

Vert

Lateral Vertebral Run

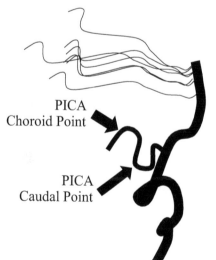

PICA Choroid Point

PICA Caudal Point

Vascular Variants:

Fetal Origin of the PCA: Most common vascular variant (probably) - seen in up to 30% of general population.

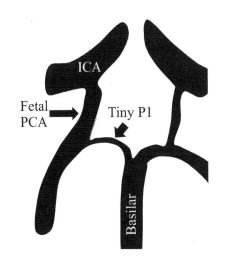

Definitions vary on what a fetal PCA is. Just think of this as a situation where the PCA is feed primarily as an anterior circulation artery (occipital lobe is feed by the ICA).

Therefore, <u>the PCOM is large</u> (some people define this vessel as PCOM larger than P1).

Another piece of trivia is that *anatomy with a fetal PCA has the PCOM superior / lateral to CN3 (instead of superior / medial - in normal anatomy).*

Persistent Trigeminal Artery:

Persistent fetal connection between the cavernous ICA to the basilar.

A characteristic *"tau sign"* on Sagittal MRI has been described.

It **increases the risk of aneurysm** (anytime you have branch points).

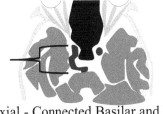

Axial - Connected Basilar and IC

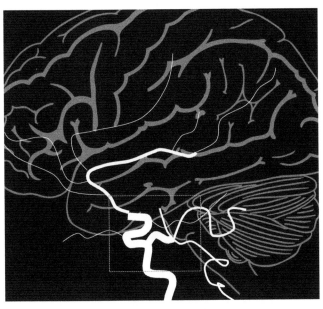

Sag - Connected Basilar and ICA
-Looks like a "T"au

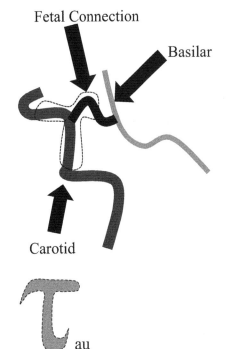

Aberrant Carotid Artery: Discussed later with T-Bone pathology.

(4) Venous:

You can ask questions about the venous anatomy in roughly three ways (1) what is it – on a picture, (2) what is a deep vein vs what is a superficial vein, (3) trivia.

What is it?

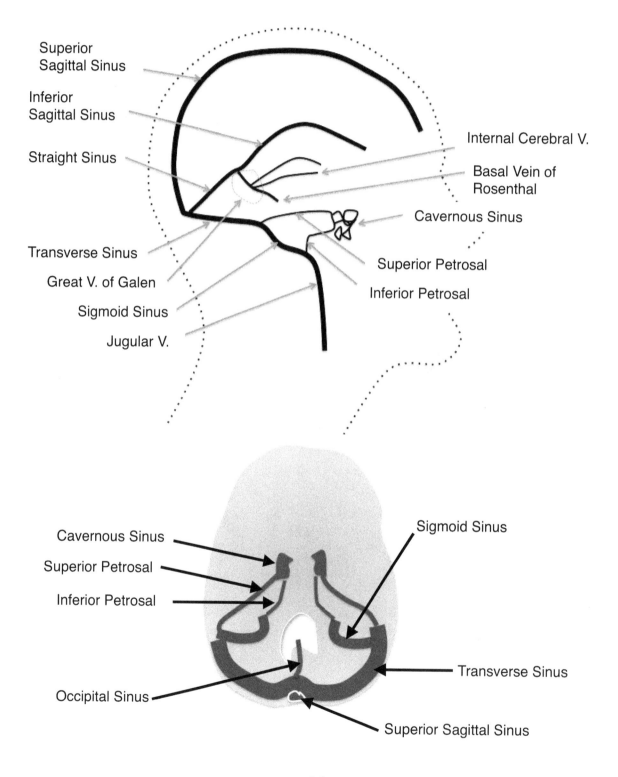

24

Anastomotic Superficial Veins:

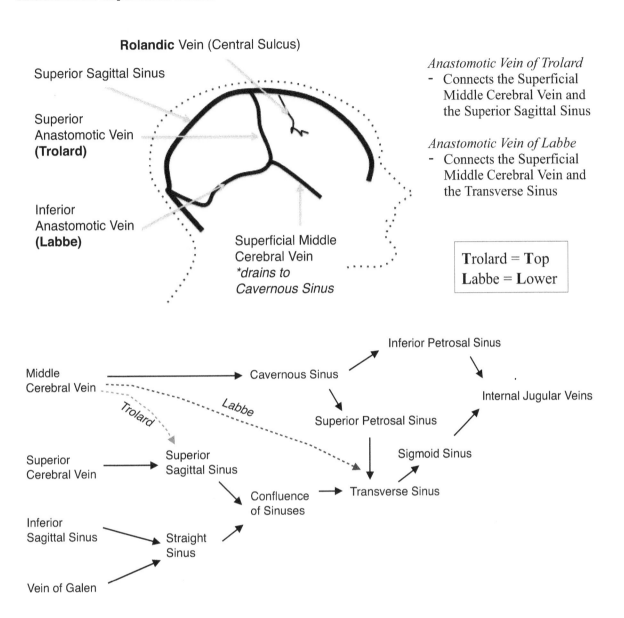

Rolandic Vein (Central Sulcus)

Superior Sagittal Sinus

Superior
Anastomotic Vein
(Trolard)

Inferior
Anastomotic Vein
(Labbe)

Superficial Middle
Cerebral Vein
*drains to
Cavernous Sinus*

Anastomotic Vein of Trolard
- Connects the Superficial
  Middle Cerebral Vein and
  the Superior Sagittal Sinus

Anastomotic Vein of Labbe
- Connects the Superficial
  Middle Cerebral Vein and
  the Transverse Sinus

Trolard = Top
Labbe = Lower

Middle Cerebral Vein → Cavernous Sinus
Trolard / Labbe
Inferior Petrosal Sinus
Superior Petrosal Sinus
Internal Jugular Veins
Superior Cerebral Vein → Superior Sagittal Sinus
Sigmoid Sinus
Confluence of Sinuses → Transverse Sinus
Inferior Sagittal Sinus → Straight Sinus
Vein of Galen

⚖ THIS vs THAT: Superficial vs Deep:

There is a superficial venous system and a deep
venous system. The easiest way to test material
like this is your *"which of the following is not?"*
or *"which of the following is ?"* type question.

The big ones to remember are in the chart.

Superficial	Deep
Superior Cerebral Veins	Basal Vein of Rosenthal
Superior Anastomotic Vein of Trolard	Vein of Galen
Inferior Anastomotic Vein of Labbe	Inferior Petrosal Sinus
Superficial Middle Cerebral Veins	

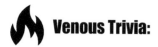 **Venous Trivia:**

Collateral Pathways: The dural sinuses have accessory drainage pathways (other than the jugular veins) that allow for connection to extracranial veins. These are good because they can help regulate temperature, and equalize pressure. These are bad because they allow for passage of sinus infection / inflammation, which can result in venous sinus thrombosis.

Inverse Relationship: There is a relationship between the Vein of Labbe, and the Anastomotic Vein of Trolard. Since these dudes share drainage of the same territory, as one gets large the other get small.

Sounds Latin or French: As a general rule, anything that sounds Latin or French has an increased chance of being on the test.

- *Vein of Labbe:* Large draining vein, connecting the superficial middle vein and the transverse sinus

- *Vein of Trolard:* Smaller (usually) vein, connecting the superficial middle vein and sagittal sinus

- *Basal veins of Rosenthal:* Deep veins that passes lateral to the midbrain through the ambient cistern and drains into the vein of Galen. Their course is similar to the PCA.

- *Vein of Galen:* Big vein ("great") formed by the union of the two internal cerebral veins.

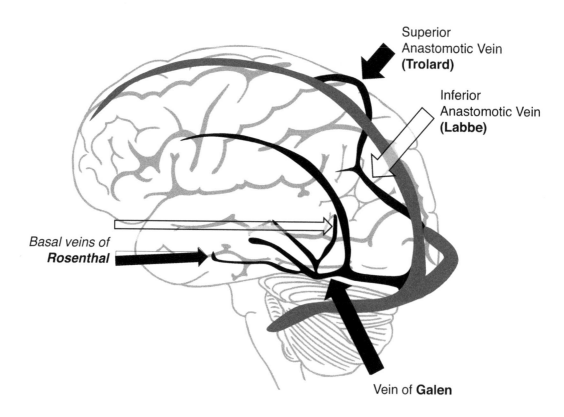

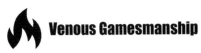 **Venous Gamesmanship**

An embolus of venous gas is common and often not even noticed. The classic location is the cavernous sinus (which is venous), but if the volume is large enough, air can also be seen in the orbital veins, superficial temporal veins, frontal venous sinus, and petrosal sinus.

Why does this happen?

Peripheral (or central IV) had some air in the tubing. Thats right, you can blame it on the nurse (which is always satisfying). *"Nurse Induced Retrograde Venous Air Embolus"*

Significance?

Don't mean shit. It pretty much always goes away in 48 hours with no issues.

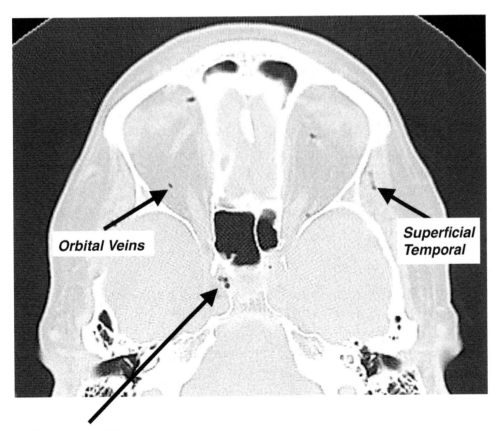

Orbital Veins

Superficial Temporal

Cavernous Sinus
-The most common
spot to see this

Sinus Trivial Anatomy Bonus - The Concha Bullosa

This is a common variant where the middle concha is pneumatized. It's pretty much of no consequence clinically unless it's fucking huge - then (rarely) it can cause obstructive symptoms.

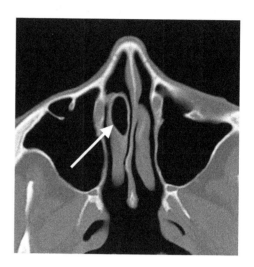

In my private practice, an ENT told me he wanted these mentioned in all his CT sinus reports.

That way he can justify doing FESS...

He drives a nice car.

 # Gamesmanship for Neuro Anatomy

- *First Order Trivia:*
    - *"What is it?"* Style questions are most likely; with possibilities including CTA, MRA, or Angiograms. Considering when the people writing the questions trained, angiograms are probably the most likely.
    - *"What goes through there?"* Neuro foramina
    - *"What doesn't?"* Style questions - CN 2 and CN V3 don't go through the cavernous sinus.

- *Second Order Trivia:*
    - CN 3 Palsy - Think Posterior Communicating Artery Aneurysm
    - CN 6 Palsy - Think increased ICP

    Increased ICP ⟶ Brain Stem Herniates Interiorly ⟶ CN 6 Gets Stretched

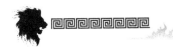
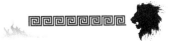

SECTION 2:
BRAIN DEVELOPMENT

Brain Myelination:

The baby brain has essentially the opposite signal characteristics as the adult brain. **The T1 pattern of a baby is similar to the T2 pattern of an adult.** The T2 pattern of a baby is similar to the T1 pattern of an adult. This appearance is the result of myelination changes.

The process of myelination occurs in a predetermined order, and therefore lends itself easily to multiple choice testing. The basic concept to understand first is that immature myelin has a higher water content relative to mature myelin and therefore is brighter on T2 and darker on T1. During the maturation process, water will decrease and fat (brain cholesterol and glycolipids) will increase. Therefore mature white matter will be brighter on T1 and darker on T2.

Immature Myelin	*Mature Myelin*
High Water, Low Fat	Low Water, High Fat
T1 dark, T2 bright	T1 bright, T2 dark

Testable Trivia: the T1 changes precede the T2 changes (adult T1 pattern seen around age 1, adult T2 pattern seen around age 2). Should be easy to remember *(1 for T1, 2 for T2)*.

Take Home Point: T1 is most useful for assessing myelination in the first year (especially 0-6 months), T2 is most useful for assessing myelination in the second year (especially 6 months to 18 months).

Order of progression: Just remember, inferior to superior, posterior to anterior, central to peripheral, and sensory fibers prior to motor fibers. The testable trivia is that **the subcortical white matter is the last part of the brain to myelinate**, with the occipital white matter around 12 months, and the frontal regions finishing around 18 months. The "terminal zones" of myelination occur in the subcortical frontotemporoparietal regions – finishing around 40 months.

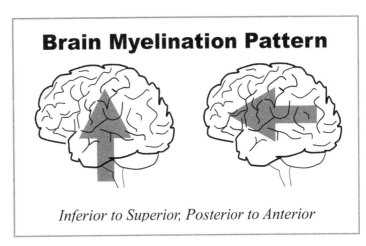

Brain Myelination Pattern

Inferior to Superior, Posterior to Anterior

Another high yield piece of testable trivia is that the **brainstem, and posterior limb of the internal capsule are normally myelinated at birth.**

Additional Brain / Skull Development Trivia:

Pituitary: Both the Anterior and Posterior Pituitary are T1 Bright at Birth *(anterior only T1 bright until 2 months)*.

	Birth	**Adult**
Ant Pituitary	T1 Hyper	T1 Iso, T2 Iso
Posterior Pituitary	T1 Hyper	T1 Hyper, T2 Hypo

Brain Iron: Brain Iron increases with age (globus pallidus darkens up).

Bone Marrow Signal: Calvarial Bone Marrow will be active (T1 hypointense) in young kids and fatty (T1 hyperintense) in older kids

Sinus Development:

The sinuses form in the following order:

1- Maxillary,
2- Ethmoid,
3- Sphenoid,
4- Frontal

Most are finished forming by around 15 years.

	Order	Visible on CT	
Maxillary	1	Present at Birth	5 month
Ethmoid	2	Present at Birth	1 year
Frontal	4	NOT Present at Birth	6 year
Sphenoid	3	NOT Present at Birth	4 year

Congenital Malformations:

This is a very confusing and complicated topic, full of lots of long Latin and French sounding words. If we want to keep it simple and somewhat high yield you can look at it in 5 basic categories: (1) Failure to Form, (2) Failure to Cleave, (3) Failure to Migrate, (4) Development Failure Mimics, and (5) Herniation Syndromes.

Failure to Form - Dysgenesis / Agenesis of the Corpus Callosum

A classic point of trivia is that the corpus callosum forms front to back (then **rostrum last**).

Therefore hypoplasia of the corpus callosum is usually absence of the splenium (with the genu intact).

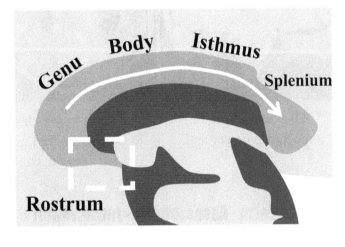

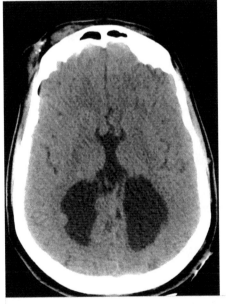

Colpocephaly
(asymmetric dilation of the occipital horns).

🔥 **GAMESMANSHIP:**

With agenesis of the corpus callosum, a common trick is to show colpocephaly (asymmetric dilation of the occipital horns).

When you see this picture you should think:

(1) **Corpus Callosum Agenesis**

(2) **Pericallosal Lipoma**
   * Discussed on next page

Failure to Form - Dysgenesis / Agenesis of the Corpus Callosum Continued

Other common ways to show this include:

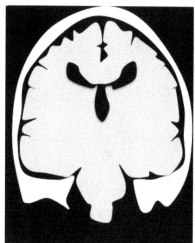 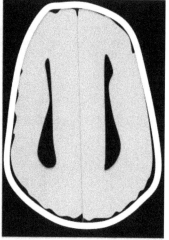

The "**steer horn**" appearance on coronal.

"**Vertical Ventricles**" widely spaced (*racing car*) on axial.

Why are the lateral ventricles widely spaced when you have no corpus callosum ?

There are these things called **"Probst bundles"** which are densely packed WM tracts - destined to cross the CC - but can't (because it isn't there).

So instead they run parallel to the interhemispheric fissure - making the vents look widely spaced.

Failure to Form - Associations - Intracranial Lipoma

Dysgenesis / Agenesis of the Corpus Callosum is associated with lots of other syndromes/ malformations (Lipoma, Heterotopias, Schizencephaly, Lissencephaly, etc…). Some sources will even say it is the *"most common anomaly seen with other CNS malformations."* — whatever the fuck that means.

Intracranial Lipoma:

The most classic association with CC Agenesis. 50% are found in the interhemispheric fissure, as shown here. The 2nd most common location is the quadrigeminal cistern (25%).

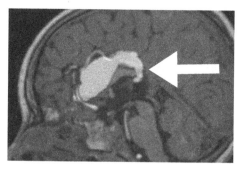

Trivia • CNS Lipomas are congenital malformations, not true neoplasms.

• *"Maldifferenitation of the Meninx Primitiva"* - is a meaningless French sounding explanation for the frequent pericollasal location.

• Non Fat Sat T1 is probably the most helpful sequence (most non-bleeding things in the brain are not T1 bright).

• These things don't cause symptoms (usually) are rarely treated.

Failure to Form - Open Neural Tube Defects

Anencephaly	Iniencephaly

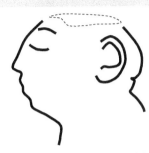

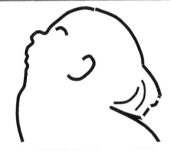

Neuro Tube Defect
(Defect at the top of head)

The Top of the Head is Absent
(Above the Eyes)

Reduced /Absent cerebrum and cerebellum.
The hindbrain will be present.

Mercifully, not compatible with life.
Potential to be awful at Jeopardy

Classic Image Appearance:
Incredibly creepy **"Frog Eye" appearance** on
the coronal plane (due to absent cranial bone /
brain with bulging orbits).

Secondary Signs / Gamesmanship:

• Antenatal Ultrasound With Polyhydramnios
  (hard to swallow without a brain)

• AFP will be elevated
  (true with all open neural tube defects)

Neural Tube Defect
(Defect at the level of the cervical spine)

Deficient Occipital Bone with Defect in the
Cervical Region. Inion = Back of Head / Neck

Extreme Retroflexion of the Head.
Enlarged foramen magnum.
Jacked up spines.
Often visceral problems.

Usually, not compatible with life.
*When they do survive, they tend to have a
natural talent for amateur astronomy*

Classic Image Appearance:
"Star Gazing Fetus" - contorted in a way that
makes their face turn upward (hyper-extended
cervical spine, short neck, and upturned face).

It's every bit as horrible as the Frog Eye thing
(both would make incredible Halloween costumes.)

AFP will be elevated
(true with all open neural tube defects)

Failure to Form - Open Neural Tube Defects - Encephalocele (meningoencephalocele)

Neural tube defect where <u>*brain + meninges*</u> herniate through a defect
in the cranium. There are lots of different types and locations — but
most are midline in the occipital region.

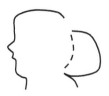

There are numerous associations: - most classic = **Chiari III**

Failure to Form - Cerebellar Vermis

Rhombencephalosynapsis	Joubert Syndrome:

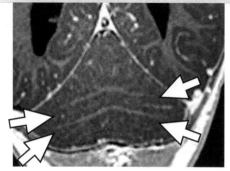

-Note the Vertical Lines Across the Cerebellum-

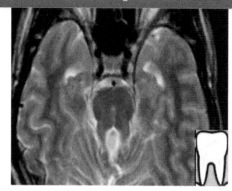

Vermis is Absent.	Vermis is Absent (or Small)
<u>Classic Image Appearance:</u> Transversely oriented single lobed cerebellum as shown above (this is an Aunt Minnie).	<u>Classic Image Appearance:</u> **"Molar Tooth"** appearance of the superior cerebellar peduncles (elongated like the roots of a tooth).
Absence of the vermis results in an abnormal fusion of the cerebellum.	Small Cerebellum
	Absence of pyramidal decussation *(whatever the fuck the means)*
Small 4th Ventricle	Large 4th Ventricle *"Batwing Shaped"*
Rounded Fastigial Point, Absent Primary Fissure	Absent Fastigial Point, Absent Primary Fissure
Associations: Holoprosencephaly Spectrum	*Associations:* Retinal dysplasia (50%), Multicystic dysplastic kidneys (30%). Liver Fibrosis ("COACH" Syndrome)

 Gamesmanship: This stuff is tricky. Let me suggest the following tactics.

If you are faced with this level of trivia (on an intermediate level exam), first start by looking for the two markers of normal vermian development: (1) the primary fissure and (2) fastigial point - both of which are best seen mid sagittal. The *"fastigial point"* is normal angular contour (not round) along the ventral surface of the cerebellum. The *primary cerebellar fissure* is a deep trapezoid shaped cleft along the posterior cerebellum. Absence or abnormal morphology of these landmarks should trigger a multiple choice brain reflex indicating the vermis is not normal.

Normal Primary Fissure

Normal Point

Point should be located just below the mid pons.

Absent Fissure

Abnormal Ventral Contour Absent Vermis

Failure to Form - <u>Dandy Walker</u> and Friends

Radiologists love to nitpick and obsess over details. The more meaningless the details the more intense and emotional the debate. Along those lines, Dandy Walker malformations are typically described along a spectrum. The arbitrary stops along this spectrum often lead to ferocious beta male nerd confrontations amongst Academics - filled with ferocious exchanges of gossip, innuendo, finger nail scratching / pinching, biting, hair pulling, and empty threats of reputation destruction.

Despite the very real threat of being scratched and pinched by an enraged Academic - I now offer my simplified strategy for dealing with this complex pathology.

"Classic" Dandy Walker:

There are **3 key findings** which are consistently present and reliable to make the diagnosis.

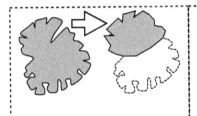

1 Hypoplasia of the Vermis *(usually the inferior part)*

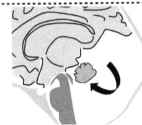

2 Hypoplastic Vermis is Elevated and Rotated

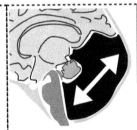

3 Dilated Cystic 4th Ventricle

Normal for Comparison

On axial, there is the nonspecific appearance of an enlarged posterior fossa CSF space. It can look like a retrocerebellar cyst on axial only (although <u>it's not a cyst</u> - it's the expanded 4th ventricle).

The cerebellar hemispheres will be displaced forward and laterally but their overall volume and morphologic characteristics should be preserved.

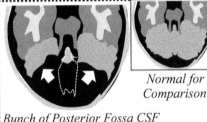

Normal for Comparison

Bunch of Posterior Fossa CSF Cerebellum Displaced Anterolaterally

"TORCULAR-LAMBDOID INVERSION"

This classic buzzword(s) describes the torcula *(confluence of venous sinuses)* above the level of the lambdoid suture, secondary to elevation of the tentorium.

It's worth mentioning that this inversion is often NOT seen in the "variant" version of Dandy Walker.

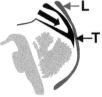

- Normal -
Lambdoid Above Torcula

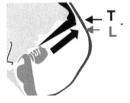

- Dandy Walker -
Torcula Above Lambdoid
"High-Inserting Venous Confluence"

Trivia

- Often identified on OB screening US.
- Otherwise, presents with symptoms of increased intracranial pressure (prior to month 1)
- Most Common Manifestation = Macrocephaly (nearly all cases with the first month)
- Associations: Hydrocephalus (90%), Additional CNS malformations (~ 40%)
  (agenesis of the corpus callosum, encephaloceles, heterotopia, polymicrogyria, etc...).

Failure to Form - Dandy Walker and Friends

As I mentioned on the prior page, Dandy Walker malformations are typically described along a spectrum. We covered the "*classic*" subtype in depth on the prior page. The stragglers (presumed to be of lower yield) and classic type are contrasted on the chart below.

	Least Severe ⟶ Most Severe			
Name	Mega Cisterna Magna	Blake Pouch	"Variant" DWM	"Classic" DWM
Alternative Term Used To Trick You			*"Hypoplastic Rotated Vermis"*	
Mid Sagittal Doodle				
Overview	*Normal Variant:* Focal enlargement of the retrocerebellar CSF space.	Sac like cystic protrusion through the foramen of Magendie into the infra / retro cerebellar region.	Hypoplastic vermis with dilation of the 4th ventricle.	Hypoplastic, elevated, rotated vermis with cystic dilation of the 4th ventricle.
Vermis	Normal	Normally Formed But Upwardly Displaced	Hypoplastic (less severe)	Hypoplastic & Rotated
4th Ventricle	Normal	Dilated	Dilated	Markedly Dilated
Cerebellar Hemispheres	Normal	Normal	Hypoplastic	- Normal In Size - Displaced Anterolaterally
Posterior Fossa	Normal	Normal	Normal	Expanded
Torcula	Normal	Normal	Normal	High Insertion
Hydrocephalus	Nope	Yes	25 % of Cases	90% of Cases
Trivia	• No supratentorial abnormalities	• Choroid from the 4th ventricle swinging into the pouch is classic (but not always present). • The pouch only communicates with the 4th ventricle. NOT the cisternal CSF.		• Diagnosis on antenatal ultrasound must be done <u>after 18 weeks</u> *(prior to 18 weeks the vermis hasn't finished forming).*

Now, let us switch gears from fusion to cleaving problems.

Failure to Cleave - Holoprosencephaly (HPE)

This entity also occurs along a spectrum with the common theme being some element of abnormal central fusion. Although, it isn't actually a fusion problem. Instead, it is a failure to perform the normal midline cleaving. In the normal embryology, the fancy latin word *"P-lon"* starts out like a peanut butter sandwich, then mom cuts the bread into two perfect halves (separate lateral hemispheres). The sandwich cutting (cleavage) always occurs back to front (opposite of the formation of the corpus callosum), so in milder forms the posterior cortex is normal and the anterior cortex is fused.

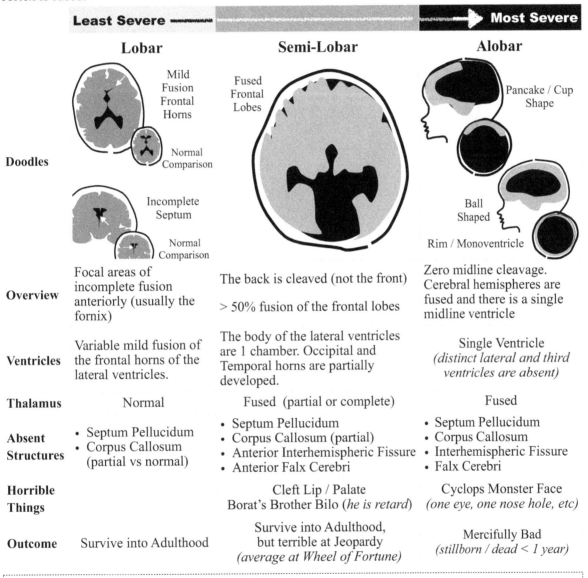

	Lobar	Semi-Lobar	Alobar
Overview	Focal areas of incomplete fusion anteriorly (usually the fornix)	The back is cleaved (not the front) > 50% fusion of the frontal lobes	Zero midline cleavage. Cerebral hemispheres are fused and there is a single midline ventricle
Ventricles	Variable mild fusion of the frontal horns of the lateral ventricles.	The body of the lateral ventricles are 1 chamber. Occipital and Temporal horns are partially developed.	Single Ventricle *(distinct lateral and third ventricles are absent)*
Thalamus	Normal	Fused (partial or complete)	Fused
Absent Structures	• Septum Pellucidum • Corpus Callosum (partial vs normal)	• Septum Pellucidum • Corpus Callosum (partial) • Anterior Interhemispheric Fissure • Anterior Falx Cerebri	• Septum Pellucidum • Corpus Callosum • Interhemispheric Fissure • Falx Cerebri
Horrible Things		Cleft Lip / Palate Borat's Brother Bilo (*he is retard*)	Cyclops Monster Face *(one eye, one nose hole, etc)*
Outcome	Survive into Adulthood	Survive into Adulthood, but terrible at Jeopardy *(average at Wheel of Fortune)*	Mercifully Bad *(stillborn / dead < 1 year)*

Face predicts Brain, BUT Brain doesn't predict Face
Possible BUZZWORDS for HPE spectrum.

Monster Cyclops Eyes
Cleft lips / Palates
Pyriform Aperture Stenosis (*from nasal process overgrowth*)
Solitary Median Maxillary Incisor (MEGA-Incisor)

Arhinencephaly:

- "Minor" HPE expression.
- Midline olfactory bulbs / tracts are absent.
- *"Can't Smell"* - is the clinical buzzword.
- Could be tested as **Kallmann Syndrome** (which also has hypogonadism, & mental retardation).

Meckel-Gruber Syndrome:

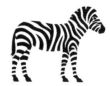

Classic triad:
1. Occipital Encephalocoele
2. Multiple Renal Cysts
3. Polydactyly

Also strongly associated with **Holoprosencephaly**

Septo Optic Dysplasia:

This "Minor" HPE expression could be referred to by its French sounding name, for the sole purpose of fucking with you — *"de Morsier Syndrome"*

The classic findings are inferred by the name.

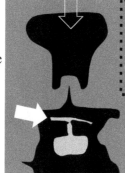
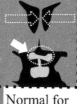
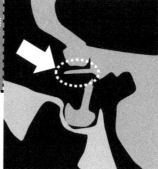
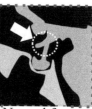

Normal for comparison

Normal for comparison

Absent Septum Pellucidum "*Septo*" and
Hypoplastic "*Optic*" structures such as the Optic Chiasma (circle) and Optic Nerves

 Trivia - Associated with Schizencephaly

 Gamesmanship - The other thing they can show is an ***azygos anterior cerebral artery*** - which is basically a common trunk of the ACAs. This is rare , but associated with SOD and lobar HPE.

Normal Comparison

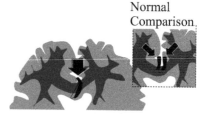

Azygos ACA (1 trunk)

Now… switching gears to failures in migration / proliferation.

Failure to Migrate / Proliferate: Lissencephaly-Pachygyria Spectrum and Friends

An understanding of this complex pathology requires a rapid review of embryologic neuronal cortex formation. Unfortunately, my medical school embryology professor was Dr. Eleanor Abernathy, M.D. (youtube her if you aren't familiar). Anytime I read embryology I can't help but think of her and wonder "can anyone who loves animals so much, really be crazy?" The answer to that… is yes. Yes they can. They can be a drunken lunatic. So much so, that I was convinced that anyone who understood embryology risked ending up just like her. Then I accepted the truth. You either die a hero or live long enough to see yourself become the villain. *Many more Batman references coming up in the next few pages.*

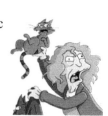

Dr. Abernathy as I remember her.

Prologue: The brain is said to form *"inside-out,"* as neurons that will eventually make up the cortex are originally birthed from a thick slurry surrounding the fetal ventricles. Sleep inducing texts will refer to this as the "proliferative neuroepithelium." I prefer the term "Lazarus Pit," or just the "Pit." It is from this Periventricular Pit, where cells will make "the climb" to the cortex.

Act 1 - Proliferation: Before making "the climb" to the cortex the neuronal-glial stem cells are born into (and molded by) the darkness of the periventricular Lazarus Pit. It is there that they learn the truth about despair, first by dividing into additional stem cells in a symmetric fashion (1 stem cell splits into 2 stem cells). Later this process will change to asymmetric proliferation (1 stem cell splits into 1 stem cell and 1 differentiated cell - glial cell or neuron). This process continues for several cycles until the stem cells receive the signal to undergo apoptosis - *they expect one of us in the wreckage brother*.

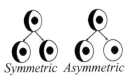
Symmetric Asymmetric

The number of neurons in the cortex is determined by the frequency and number of symmetric / asymmetric divisions by these stem cells. Disturbance in this process will therefore result in either too many, too few, or improperly differentiated neurons.

Act 2 - Migration (*RISE*): From the periventricular proliferative pit of despair, cells will make the climb. As they climb to freedom, they are guided by structural cells, chemical signals, and the chant "Deshi, Deshi, Basara, Basara." They make the climb in 6 waves, with the first generation forming the "pre-plate" and the second generation forming the more permanent "cortical plate."

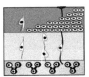

In other words, the younger cells always moving past the older ones becoming more superficial in their final position, (hence the idea - "inside out" or "outside last"). Disturbance in this mechanism (guidance, timing of detachment etc...) will result in under-migration, over-migration, or ectopic neurons.

Act 3 - Organization: At this point you may think the cells have given everything to the cortex, and they don't owe them anymore. But, they haven't given everything... not yet. There is still the process of cortical folding (gyrification).

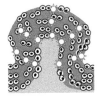

The process actually occurs simultaneously with and depends heavily on the first two steps. The differential speed of cortex expansion (relative to the deeper white matter) is probably the key mechanism for brain folding. For this expansion to occur properly there needs to be the right number of cells (act 1) migrated in the right order (act 2). There is the additional mechanism of continued differentiation into structural cell types which organize into horizontal / vertical columns creating an underlying cytoarchitecture need for structure and function. Disturbance in these mechanisms will result in an absence of or excessive number of folds.

Failure to Migrate / Proliferate: Lissencephaly-Pachygyria Spectrum and Friends

Now, we are going to discuss the testable pathologies associated with how this process can fuck up.

I'm going to try and group them according to the stage of disturbance (although they don't always fit nicely into a single stage).

Failure to Proliferate: Hemimegalencephaly:

Rare, but unique (Aunt Minnie), malformation characterized by **enlargement** (from hamartomatous overgrowth) **of all or part/s of one cerebral hemisphere**. The presumed cause is a failure in the normal neuronal differentiation in the involved hemisphere - resulting in an "abnormal mixture of normal tissues" - which defines a hamartoma. This process is often mixed with other errors in migration resulting in associated polymicrogyria, pachygyria, and heterotopia.

The combo of (1) dilated ventricle and (2) mismatched hemisphere size can be confused with destructive pathologies. So lets do a quick comparison to negate any potential fuckery.

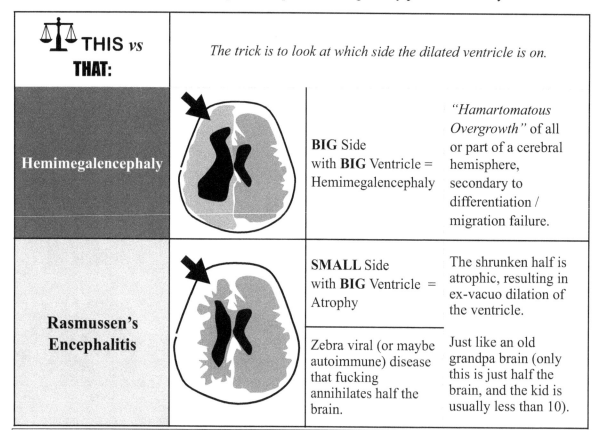

⚖ THIS vs THAT:	*The trick is to look at which side the dilated ventricle is on.*		
Hemimegalencephaly		**BIG** Side with **BIG** Ventricle = Hemimegalencephaly	*"Hamartomatous Overgrowth"* of all or part of a cerebral hemisphere, secondary to differentiation / migration failure.
Rasmussen's Encephalitis		**SMALL** Side with **BIG** Ventricle = Atrophy	The shrunken half is atrophic, resulting in ex-vacuo dilation of the ventricle.
		Zebra viral (or maybe autoimmune) disease that fucking annihilates half the brain.	Just like an old grandpa brain (only this is just half the brain, and the kid is usually less than 10).

Dyke-Davidoff-Masson (Cerebral Hemi-Atrophy):

This is another zebra that can look a lot like Rasmussen encephalitis - but also has weird unilateral skull thickening and expanded sinuses.
The superior sagittal sinus and fissure are moved across the midline.
It is supposedly caused by an in utero or childhood stroke (supposedly).

Since literally anything is fair game on this exam, I'm including it for completeness (it's probably low yield).

Failure to Migrate / Proliferate: Lissencephaly-Pachygyria Spectrum and Friends

The pathologies related to abnormal migration are best though of along a spectrum ranging from agyria (no gyri) to pachygyria (flat gyri) to band heterotopias.

Lissencephaly "Classic" Type 1	Double Cortex Band Heterotopia	Lissencephaly "Cobblestone" Type 2	Periventricular Nodular Heterotopia
Smooth Surface Thick Cortex Colpocephaly Figure 8 Shape			
Undermigration	**Undermigration**	**Overmigration**	**Failed Migration**
Failure to migrate both in amount an in order - with a reverse outside-in pattern. Large numbers of neurons do not even reaching the cortical plate, depositing diffusely between the ventricular and pial surfaces. The distribution is fucked with 4 thick layers formed instead of 6.	Considered the mildest form of Classic Lissencephaly Disorganized migration results in a second layer of cortical neurons deep to the more superficial cortex. This creates the classic *"double cortex"* appearance.	Instead of failing to migrate an adequate number of neurons to the cortical surface (as is the case in the classic type of lissencephaly), this pathology is the result of an over migration. This over migration results in an additional layer of cortex composed on gray matter nodules. These nodules come in a variety of shapes and sizes (unilateral, bilateral, small, large, symmetric or asymmetric).	Neurons in the periventricular (subependymal) region were too lazy to migrate to the cortex. The result is nodular grey matter deposition along the ventricle borders. Most common location for grey matter heterotopia. Associated with seizure disorders.
Normal 6 Layers / *Lissencephaly 4 Layers*			
As a result of this disorganized / inadequate migration the process of cortical folding does not take place. Smooth Surface, Thick Cortex Colpocephaly is Common. "Figure 8" shaped brain on axial -due to shallow, vertical Sylvan fissures Autosomal Inheritance (M=F) Associated with CMV (maybe)	Associated with seizure disorders. Gyral pattern is normal (or mildly simplified). Subcortical band of heterotopic gray matter X-Linked Inheritance (F>M)	Most commonly It is commonly located adjacent to the Sylvian fissures Cobblestoned Cortex (variable in size / location) Associated with <u>congenital muscular dystrophy</u>, and retinal detachment - *"muscle- eye-brain disease"*	THIS VS THAT: **Heterotopias** follow grey matter on all sequences and NOT enhance. **Subependymal tubers of TS** are usually brighter on T2 relative to grey matter and may also be calcified.

Failure to Organize: Polymicrogyria "PMG"

I've heard people blame this on TORCH infections, toxic exposure, chromosomal issues, God's wrath for "stuff the Democrats do." There are likely many causes. I wouldn't expect someone to ask for "the cause," other than perhaps the broad category of failed organization.

Having said that, I've read some PhD papers saying that layer 5 gets obliterated (by infection, toxins, wrath, etc..) after completion of normal migration. With layer 5 gone the other more superficial layers overfold and fuse resulting in an excessive number of small folds - the hallmark finding.

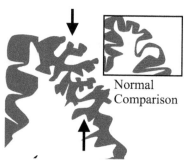

Normal Comparison

Fine Undulations / Bumps

Classic Look: **Fine undulating / bumpy cortex**.
This anomaly come in a variety of shapes and sizes (unilateral, bilateral, small, large, symmetric or asymmetric). Most common location is adjacent to the Sylvian fissure bilaterally.

 Trivia: Zika Virus is the most common cause of PMG in Brazil and South America

Failure to Organize: Schizencephaly — "Split Brain"

Just like polymicrogyria there are likely many causes and I wouldn't expect someone to ask for "the cause," other than perhaps the broad category of failed organization.

Having said that, one popular theory is the idea of a vascular insult. What is this vascular insult ? Well, you could say it's the cortex's reckoning (it damages the radial glial fibers). These radial glial fibers are in charge (or at least they "feel in charge") of the ropes used by neurons to "make the climb." Although, I've head it's best to make the climb as the child did - without the rope. I mention this because about 30% of patient's with schizencephaly also have non-CNS vascular stigmata (example = gastroschisis - which supposedly occurs from a vascular insult to the abdominal wall).

Classic Look: Schizencephaly literally means "split brain" with the defining feature being a cleft (lined with grey matter) connecting the CSF spaces with the ventricular system. How wide this cleft is depends on the flavor; Closed Lip (20%) or (2) Open Lip (80%), although in both cases the cleft should span the full thickness of the involved hemisphere. The clefts can be unilateral or bilateral.

Closed Lip (20%) - *Less Common, Less Severe*

In this form, the "Lip" will appear closed without a CSF filled cleft. To make the call you want to look for is the grey matter running across the normally uniform corona radiata.

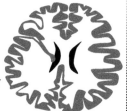

Sometimes you can see a "nipple" of grey mater pouching at the ependymal (ventricular) surface.

Open Lip (80%) - *More Common, More Severe*

This one is more obvious.

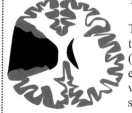

To make the call you want to see a CSF-filled cleft (lined with grey matter) extending from the ventricle to the pial surface.

The gray matter lining is often weird looking (kinda nodular like a heterotopia).

Associations: Absent Septum Pellucidum (70%), Focally Thinned Corpus Callosum, Optic Nerve Hypoplasia (30%), Epilepsy (demonic possession)

Developmental Failure Mimics — Hydranencephaly and the Porencephalic Cyst

These can be thought of along a spectrum of severity.	Least Severe ➤ More Severe	
	Porencephalic Cyst	**Hydranencephaly**
These things may look like a severe developmental anomaly but the underlying mechanism is different. They are "acquired." Classically by a vascular insult - but really from anything that can cause encephalomalacia (focal necrosis of both the gray matter and white matter with eventual cystic degeneration). This would include a trauma after birth (this doesn't have to happen in utero). Understanding that the brain develops normally first - then gets crushed, helps to remember the key findings. In particular, the <u>absence of a gray matter lining</u> along the defect. It's almost like someone took an ice-cream scoop to the brain. In the case of Porenchephaly, they just took one scoop. In the case of Hydranencephaly, the glutinous pig took pretty much the entire brain - leaving only the cerebellum, midbrain, and the falx.	*External* / *Internal*	*Cortical Mantle is Gone*
	Brain cleft / hole from a prior ischemic event resulting in encephalomalacia. Cyst/Cleft can communicated with the Subarachnoid Space ("external") mimicking an open lip Schizencephaly or communicated only with the ventricular system ("internal").	Bilateral ICA occlusion causes massive destruction of both cerebral hemispheres. only the cerebellum, midbrain, and the falx (usually) remain. / <u>Herpes is the most classic</u>, but in utero infection with toxo or CMV are also described causes.

THIS vs THAT:	*The trick is to look for gray matter lining the cleft.*		
Open Lip Schizencephaly	Brain cleft / hole from a prior event (maybe ischemic) resulting in damage to the structural cells needed to properly organize the cortex. Not Normally Formed	CSF-filled cleft extending from the ventricle to the pial surface.	Cleft is **Lined with Gray Matter**
Porencephalic Cyst	Brain cleft / hole from a prior ischemic / traumatic event resulting in encephalomalacia. Normally formed - but massive insult make it look developmental.	CSF-filled cleft extending from the ventricle and/or the pial surface.	Cleft is **<u>NOT</u> Lined with Gray Matter**

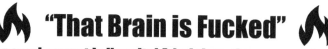

"That Brain is Fucked"

His only hope for employment is Hospital Administration... or maybe QA Officer.

Unless *"Brain is Fucked"* is a choice on the exam, you'll need to narrow down your choices. I suggest the following strategic algorithm, simplified essentially into 2 questions.

(1) Is the Cortical Mantle (outside of brain) present or gone fishing ?
(2) If the Mantle is still there (even if it's very thin), look for the falx cerebri.

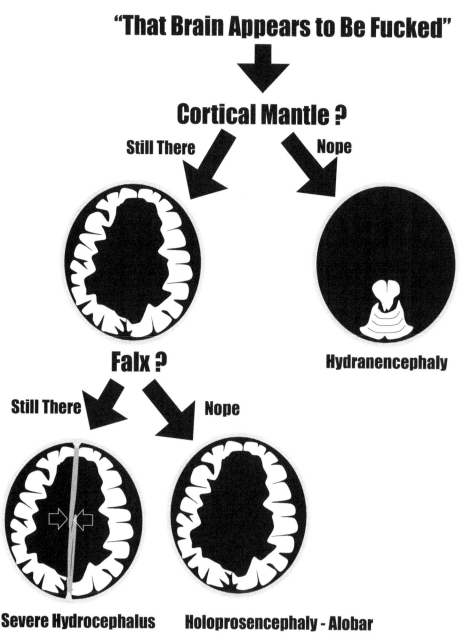

"That Brain Appears to Be Fucked"

Cortical Mantle ?

Still There   **Nope**

Hydranencephaly

Falx ?

Still There   **Nope**

Severe Hydrocephalus
-Still Got a Falx

Holoprosencephaly - Alobar
—Anterior falx usually missing in the semi-lobar form
—Lobar (mild) subtype should still have the flax

Herniation Syndromes - Testable Vocab and Chiari Malformations

Testable Vocab: Cephaloceles

"**Cephalocele**" is an umbrella term for a herniation of the cranial contents through a defect in the skull. While retaining the suffix "cele" they are then sub-classified based on (1) location, and (2) what is in the herniation sac.

(1) LOCATION

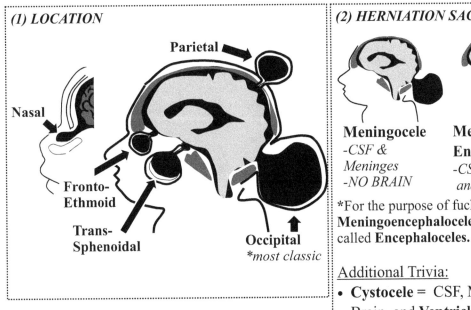

Parietal

Nasal

Fronto-Ethmoid

Trans-Sphenoidal

Occipital
most classic

(2) HERNIATION SAC CONTENTS

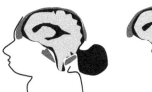

Meningocele
-*CSF & Meninges*
-*NO BRAIN*

Meningo-Encephalocele
-*CSF, Meninges, and **BRAIN***

*For the purpose of fucking with you, **Meningoencephaloceles** are sometimes called **Encephaloceles**.

Additional Trivia:
- **Cystocele** = CSF, Meninges, Brain, and **Ventricle**
- **Myelocele** = **Spinal Cord**

Herniation Syndromes: Chiari Malformations

This topic is incredibly complicated. There are literally entire books written on the individual subtypes. The following is my best effort to distill the potentially testable trivia down to about 1.5 pages.

There are several numbered sub-types of Chiari malformations, with the shared finding of a downward displacement of the cerebellum. Here is a quick overview of the subtypes.

Type I	Type II	Type III	Type IV
Herniation of cerebellar tonsils (more than 5 mm)	Relatively less tonsillar herniation. Relatively more cerebellar vermian displacement	Features of Chiari 2 AND Occipital Encephalocele	Historically used to describe severe cerebellar hypoplasia without herniation. The term has fallen out of favor with the powerful men and women who control the Chiari nomenclature. We shall not speak of it again.
Classic Association *(not always present):* • Syrinx (cervical cord)	Classic Features: -Low lying torcula -Tectal beaking -Hydrocephalus -Clival hypoplasia	**Type 1.5**	
		Hybrid term used to describe conditions that have features of both type 1 and type 2. Not associated with neural tube defects, despite the significant downward movement of the tonsils and brain stem.	

Chiari Type I	Chiari Type II	Chiari Type III

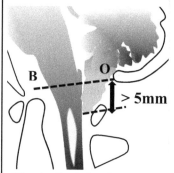

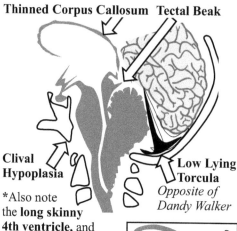

Thinned Corpus Callosum **Tectal Beak**

Clival Hypoplasia

Low Lying Torcula
Opposite of Dandy Walker

*Also note the **long skinny 4th ventricle,** and the **"towering cerebellum."**

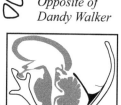

Normal for Comparison

Occipital Encephalocele, (meningoencephalocele) containing cerebellum and/ or the brainstem, occipital lobe, and sometimes even the fourth ventricle. PLUS features of of Chiari 2

Classically defined as 1 or both tonsils > 5mm below the level of the **B**asion - - - **O**pisthion.

Note the commonly associated Syrinx.

Classic Mechanism: Congenital underdevelopment of the posterior fossa, leading to overcrowding, and downward displacement.

Non-Classic: Post traumatic deformity - acquired later in life.

Clinical Symptoms are produce in two flavors: (1) Occipital headache from pressure of the cerebellar tonsils - worse with sneezing (2) Weakness, spasticity, and loss of proprioception from pressure on the cord

Classic Association (not always present):

• Syrinx of the cervical cord

Less Classic (but still highly testable) association: -Klippel-Feil Syndrome (congenital C-spine fusion).

NOT associated with a neural tube defect

Compared to Type 1, there is relatively less tonsillar herniation, but more cerebellar vermian displacement

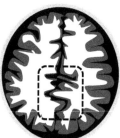

Interdigitated Cerebral Gyri *(most classically demonstrated on axial CT)*

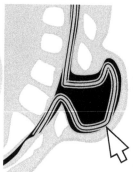

Myelomeningocele– Lumbar Spine

Classic Mechanism: Neural Tube Defect "sucks" the cerebellum downward prior to full development of the cerebellar tonsils.

Classic Association:

-Lumbar myelomeningocele / Spina Bifida

Only seen in patients <u>with a neural tube defect</u>

Classic Associations:

• Syrinx (cervical)

• Tethered cord

• Hydrocephalus

• Agenesis of the corpus callosum

Only seen in patients <u>with a neural tube defect</u> (NTD). Encephalocele = NTD

Special Topic - Mesial Temporal Sclerosis

This is a pattern of findings (hippocampal volume loss + gliosis / scar), which classically result in intractable seizures.   The etiology is not certain, but it is most likely developmental (hence the inclusion in this section).

Clinical Trivia: This is the most common cause of partial complex epilepsy.

Clinical Trivia: Surgical removal can "cure" the seizures / demon. Alternatively, perfect intracranial positioning of a tooth (from a red haired woman) has been described as therapeutic in the Kazakhstani literature.

The hippocampal region represents the medial portion of the temporal lobe (black box).

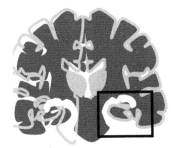 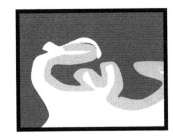 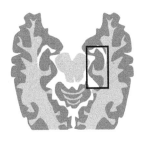

For the purpose of multiple choice, the primary imaging findings are:

- **Reduced Hippocampal Volume** (best seen when compared to the opposite site).
  10% of the time volume loss is bilateral - other findings are necessary to exclude fuckery
- **Increased T2 Signal** (from gliosis / scar)
- **Loss of Normal Morphology** (loss of normal interdigitations)

*Note the compensatory enlargement of the temporal horn of the lateral ventricle
white arrow

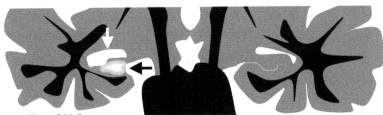

*Reduced Volume, Increased T2 Signal
black arrow

Normal Side for Comparison

Additional described findings - less likely to be shown (more likely to be asked)

- Atrophy of the ipsilateral fornix and maxillary body
- Contralateral amygdala <u>enlargement</u>

MRI Epilepsy Protocol Trivia:
- T1 - Superior for Cortical Thickness, Eval of Grey / White
- FLAIR - Superior for Cortical / Subcortical Hight Signal (Gliosis)
- T2* / SWI - Superior for Blood Breakdown Products (for other things that can cause seizures; calcifications of tuberous sclerosis, Sturge-Weber, Cavernomas, Gangliogliomas etc..)

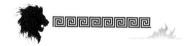 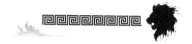

Monro-Kellie Hypothesis:

The Monro-Kellie Hypothesis is the idea that the head is a closed shell, and that the three major components: (1) brain, (2) blood – both arterial and venous, and (3) CSF, are in a state of dynamic equilibrium. As the volume of one goes up, the volume of another must go down.

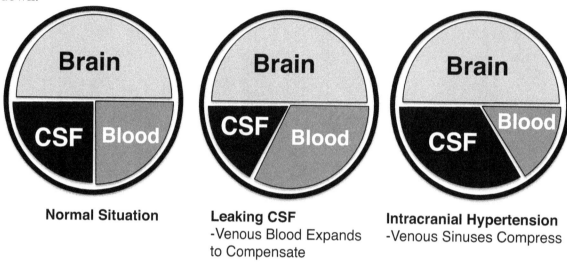

Normal Situation

Leaking CSF
-Venous Blood Expands
to Compensate

Intracranial Hypertension
-Venous Sinuses Compress

Intracranial Hypotension: If you are leaking CSF, this will decrease the overall fixed volume, and the volume of venous blood will increase to maintain the equilibrium. The result is meningeal engorgement (enhancement), distention of the dural venous sinuses, prominence of the intracranial vessels, and engorgement of the pituitary ("pituitary pseudo-mass"). The development of subdural hematoma and hygromas is also a classic look (again, compensating for lost volume).

Idiopathic Intracranial Hypertension (Pseudotumor Cerebri): Classic scenario of a fat middle-aged women with a headache. Etiology is not well understood (making too much CSF, or not absorbing it correctly). It has a lot of associations (hypothyroid, cushings, vitamin A toxicity). The findings follow the equilibrium idea. With increased CSF the ventricles become slit-like, the pituitary shrinks (partially empty sella), and the venous sinuses appear compressed. You can also have the appearance of vertical tortuosity of the optic nerves and flattening of the posterior sclera.

Changes in intracranial pressure can create a downward displacement of the brainstem stretching the 6th cranial nerve - it is said that 1/3 of patients with pseudotumor cerebri have sixth nerve paresis as their only neurologic deficit

Hydrocephalus — "Too Much CSF"

Questions on this topic are most likely to be centered on the sub-type, location of obstruction, and cause. So, let us now review the vocab.

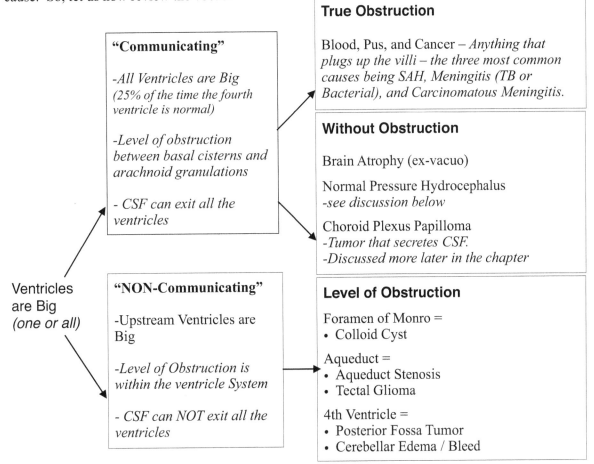

Ventricles are Big *(one or all)*

"Communicating"

-All Ventricles are Big (25% of the time the fourth ventricle is normal)

-Level of obstruction between basal cisterns and arachnoid granulations

- CSF can exit all the ventricles

"NON-Communicating"

-Upstream Ventricles are Big

-Level of Obstruction is within the ventricle System

- CSF can NOT exit all the ventricles

True Obstruction

Blood, Pus, and Cancer – *Anything that plugs up the villi – the three most common causes being SAH, Meningitis (TB or Bacterial), and Carcinomatous Meningitis.*

Without Obstruction

Brain Atrophy (ex-vacuo)

Normal Pressure Hydrocephalus
-*see discussion below*

Choroid Plexus Papilloma
-*Tumor that secretes CSF.*
-*Discussed more later in the chapter*

Level of Obstruction

Foramen of Monro =
• Colloid Cyst

Aqueduct =
• Aqueduct Stenosis
• Tectal Glioma

4th Ventricle =
• Posterior Fossa Tumor
• Cerebellar Edema / Bleed

Normal Pressure Hydrocephalus: It's not well understood – and idiopathic. The step 1 trivia is "wet, wacky, and wobbly" – describing the clinical triad of urinary incontinence, confusion, and ataxia. The key points clinically are the patient is **elderly (60s)**, and the **ataxia comes first** and is most pronounced.

The buzz-phrase is "ventricular size out of proportion to atrophy." The frontal and temporal horns of the lateral ventricles are the most affected. "Upward bowing of the corpus callosum" is another catch phrase. On MRI you may see transependymal flow and/or a flow void in the aqueduct and 3rd ventricle. This is treated with surgical shunting.

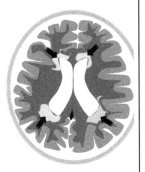

Quiz: Is transependymal flow seem more with acute hydrocephalus or chronic hydrocephalus?

Answer: Acute.

Communicating Hydrocephalus + Elderly + Ataxia = NPH.

Syndrome of **H**ydrocephalus in the **Y**oung and **M**iddle-aged **A**dult (**SHYMA**): Similar to NPH but in a middle aged population - and more headaches less peeing of the pants (HA+Wacky+Wobbly). Communicating Hydrocephalus + Middle Aged + Headache = SHYMA.

Congenital Hydrocephalus

There are several causes of hydrocephalus that can be present at birth or be related to fetal development. These conditions are typically diagnosed prior to birth via routine ultrasound (discussed partially in the reproductive chapter in volume 1).

The big 4 are: (1) Aqueductal stenosis, (2) Neural tube defect - usually Chiari II, (3) Arachnoid cysts, and (4) Dandy-Walker. I've discussed Chiari II and Dandy-Walker already.

So, let us turn our attention to Aqueductal Stenosis and Arachnoid Cysts.

Aqueductal Stenosis:

This is the most common cause of congenital obstructive hydrocephalus. Classically from a web or diaphragm at the aqueduct (hence the name). Because of the location you get a "non-communicating" pattern with a dilation of the lateral ventricles and 3rd ventricle with a normal sized 4th ventricle. You can have a big noggin (macrocephaly) with thinning of the cortical mantle.

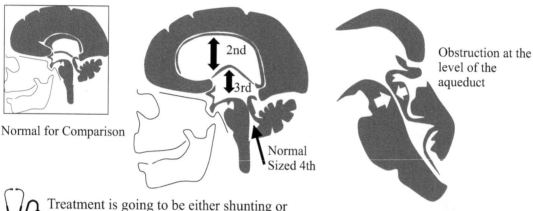

Normal for Comparison

2nd

3rd

Normal Sized 4th

Obstruction at the level of the aqueduct

Treatment is going to be either shunting or poking a hole in the 3rd ventricle (third ventriculostomy).

Clinical Trivia: Question header may describe "sunset eyes" or an upward gaze paralysis.

Clinical Trivia: A male with *"flexed thumbs"* should make you think about the x-linked variant. (Bickers Adams Edwards syndrome).

Arachnoid Cysts:

As the name implies, these are cysts located in the subarachnoid space. They are CSF density, without any solid components, or abnormal restricted diffusion. You wouldn't even notice them expect that they can exert mass effect on the adjacent brain, or in the context of this discussion block a CSF pathway (obstructive type).

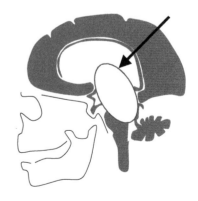

CSF Shunt Malfunction

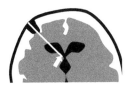

Normal: The most basic shunt consists of a proximal tube (usually placed in the frontal horn of the lateral ventricle just anterior to the foramen of Monro), a valve to control flow, and a distal tip (usually dumped in the peritoneum, but can be placed in the pleural space or right atrium).

Shunt Evaluation Options: Your first line options for shunt evaluation are going to be (a) non-con CT or (b) rapid single shot T2 sequence - mainly looking at catheter position and ventricle size. *May need to verify shunt settings with a plain film post magnet. If the ventricles are big (shunt is not working) you might follow that up with a radiograph series (neck, chest, abd) to make sure the catheter is intact. Ultrasound or CT can be used to inspect the distal tip for a fluid collection. Alternatively (if you are a weirdo) you can inject < 0.4ml pertechnetate into the shunt reservoir and take images to look for leakage or blockage (remember to not aspirate when you inject).

Under-Shunting	Obstruction (proximal)	-Proximal > Distal -Most common cause = ingrowth of choroid plexus and particulate debris / blood products -Can also be from catheter migration	Prior Comparison
	Obstruction (distal)	-Pseudocyst *(loculated fluid along the distal tip)* -Catheter migration *(more common in children)*	Loculated fluid around the tip of the catheter
Over-Shunting		-*"Slit Like Ventricles"* - can be meaningless or suggest too much shunting. - The big fear is that not enough CSF will cause subdural hygroma or hematoma formation via Monroe Kelly mechanics (less CSF - more blood).	Slit Ventricles Extra-Axial Fluid Collections (subdural hygroma)
Infection		-Usually within 6 months of placement -Blood cultures are usually negative (fluid from the shunt should be cultured instead). -Mild enhancement after catheter placement can be normal - be on guard for fuckery. -The best sign is <u>debris within the ventricles</u>, ideally shown with <u>DWI</u> - this is the weapon of choice for diagnosis of ventriculitis.	T1+C: ventricular / ependymal enhancement DWI: Debris / Pus Restricts Diffusion
		-Late stigmata may include <u>ventricular loculations</u> - which can cause restricted flow / obstruction and in some case isolate or "*trap*" the 4th ventricle — as shown in diagrams.	
Hydrothorax		Either deliberately or via migration the catheter can end up in the pleural space. A little bit of pleural fluid doesn't mean shit. But, if the volume gets large enough and the patient becomes symptomatic - then revision might be needed.	
Ascites		Usually the ascites from a VP shunt isn't symptomatic, although there are reports of inguinal hernias and hydroceles forming secondary to the increased abdominal pressure.	

Edema:

Cytotoxic: This type of edema can be thought about as intracellular swelling secondary to malfunction of the Na/K pump. It tends to favor the gray matter, and **looks like loss of the gray-white differentiation**. This is classically **seen with stroke** (or trauma), and is why EARLY signs of stroke involve loss of the GM-WM interface.

Vasogenic: This type of edema is extracellular, secondary to disruption of the blood-brain barrier. It looks like **edema tracking through the white matter** (which is less tightly packed than the gray matter). This is classically **seen with tumor and infection**. You can also see this type of edema as a LATE stage of cerebral ischemia. A response to steroids is characteristic of vasogenic edema.

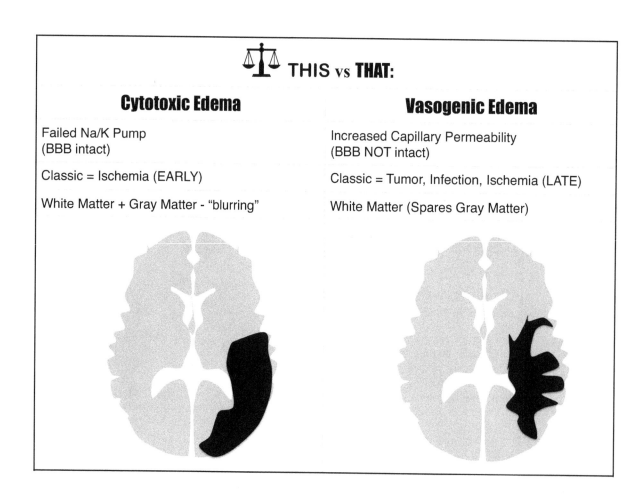

⚖️ THIS vs THAT:

Cytotoxic Edema

Failed Na/K Pump
(BBB intact)

Classic = Ischemia (EARLY)

White Matter + Gray Matter - "blurring"

Vasogenic Edema

Increased Capillary Permeability
(BBB NOT intact)

Classic = Tumor, Infection, Ischemia (LATE)

White Matter (Spares Gray Matter)

Brain Herniation:

Subfalcine (*Cingulate*) **Herniation:** This is just a fancy way of saying midline shift (deviation of ipsilateral ventricle and bowing of the falx). The trivia to know is that the ACA may be compressed, and can result in infarct.

Descending Transtentorial *(Uncal)* **Herniation:** The uncus and hippocampus herniate through the tentorial incisura. Effacement of the ipsilateral suprasellar cistern occurs first.

Things to know:

- Perforating basilar artery branches get compressed resulting in *"Duret Hemorrhages"*- classically located in the midline at the pontomesencephalic junction (in reality they can also affect cerebellar peduncles).

- CN 3 gets compressed between the PCA and Superior Cerebellar Artery causing ipsilateral pupil dilation and ptosis

- "Kernohan's Notch / Phenomenon" – The midbrain on the tentorium forming an indentation (notch) and the physical exam finding of ipsilateral hemiparesis – which Neurologists call a *"false localizing sign."* Of course, localization on physical exam is stupid in the age of MRI, but it gives Neurologists a reason to carry a reflex hammer and how can one fault them for that.

Ascending Transtentorial Herniation: Think about this in the setting of a posterior fossa mass. The vermis will herniate upward through the tentorial incisura, often resulting in severe obstructive hydrocephalus.

Things to know
- The "Smile" of the quadrigeminal cistern will be flattened or reversed
- *"Spinning Top"* is a buzzword, for the appearance of the midbrain from bilateral compression along its posterior aspect
- Severe hydrocephalus (at the level of the aqueduct).

Cerebellar Tonsil Herniation:
Can be from severe herniation after downward transtentorial herniation. Alternatively, if in isolation you are thinking more along the lines of Chiari (Chiari I = 1 tonsil - 5 mm).

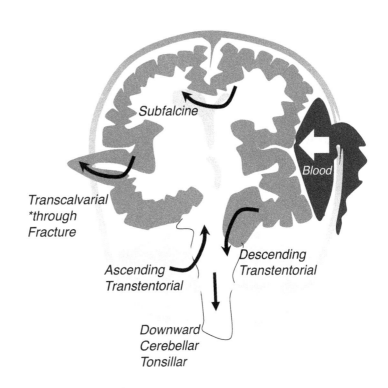

Subfalcine

Blood

Transcalvarial
*through
Fracture

Ascending
Transtentorial

Descending
Transtentorial

Downward
Cerebellar
Tonsillar

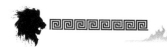 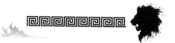

Metabolic Plagues on the Alcoholic Urban Outdoorsman - part 1

Osmotic Demyelination or Central Pontine Myelinolysis

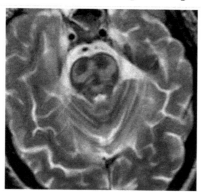

T2 Bright Central Pons (spares the periphery)

Most Classic Scenario: Asshole drunk Hobo shows up to the ER with a low Na. Like most asshole drunks in the ER, he starts out demanding a cheeseburger and a Sprite (not a fucking Sierra Mist!), then threatens to leave against medical advice. …after finishing the burger.

Family Medicine Resident begs him to stay (a decision he will soon regret). The Resident eventually tires of his bullshit and decides to correct his hyponatremia as rapidly as possible - with the goal of expediting discharge.

2 days later the guy is still in house, acting like a massive prick - acutely encephalopathic with spastic quadriparesis.

Neurology gets consulted and writes *"pseudobulbar palsy"* in the chart. Family Medicine Resident doesn't know what the fuck that means, but is humble enough to ask. A below average 2nd year medical student explains to him that it is slurred speech, sensitive gag reflex, and being an even bigger cry baby than normal- "labile emotional response".

Coma, the above MRI, death, then a lawsuit follow (in that order).

- T2 bright in the central pons (spares periphery)
- Earliest change: restricted diffusion in lower pons
- Trivia: Can also have an extra-pontine presentation involving the basal ganglia, external capsule, amygdala, and cerebellum.

Wernicke Encephalopathy

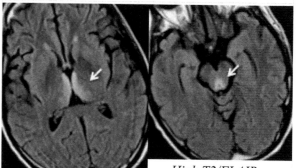

High T2/FLAIR Signal in the Medial Thalamus

High T2/FLAIR Signal in the Periaqueductal Gray

Most Classic Scenario: Very friendly Hobo - known for singing songs from the 70s (mostly Supertramp's goodbye stranger) - starts acting squirrelly. "His tempo seems off" - notes the feminine male nurse.

An above average medical student suggests he is exhibiting the clinical triad of (1) acute confusion, (2) ataxia, and (3) ophthalmoplegia, but is dismissed by the Medicine Intern who talks non-stop about going into Cardiology ("Cards" - he calls it).

Only moments later the same Intern will suggest to his Attending the same triad of findings before stating "my medical student" seems disinterested and may benefit from more call.

Still desperate to honor the clerkship, the student suggests **thiamine (vitamin B1) deficiency** as the etiology, and says the symptoms could progress to chronic memory loss and confabulation (Korsakoff psychosis) or even death.

The cycle repeats - additional call is assigned, and a formal letter of reprimand is issued to the student.

- T2/FLAIR bright classically seen in medial/dorsal thalamus (around the 3rd ventricle), periaqueductal gray, mamillary bodies, and the tectal plate.
- Enhancement is classic in the mamillary bodies
- MR Spect = Lactate
- Treatment = Thiamine replacement.

Metabolic Plagues on the Alcoholic Urban Outdoorsman - part 2

Marchiafava-Bignami

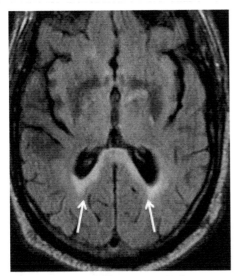

-High T2/FLAIR in the Corpus Callosum-

Most Classic Scenario: A middle aged (50s) man is stumbles into the ER. On the pre-assessment forms he has described himself as a "semi-professional red wine taster." He seems to exhibit variable degrees of mental confusion, and his gait appears altered.

His chief complaint is seizure and muscle rigidity.

He interrupts the H&P stating that he needs to urinate ("drain his hog" - he says). A nurse hands him a urinal but his muscle rigidity seems to be impair his coordination. It looks like the floor is about to get very wet, when his the nurse (a shy, but aggressively religious, elderly women) tries to assist him. The patient barks at the nurse "Not now woman! Leave the dick alone!" Her face blushes with embarrassment. The ER Attending can't help but laugh. The medical student shadowing him also laughs (but only after the Attending does so first).

Later the Attending will reprimand the medical student for laughing. In a formal letter, the Attending says the student's lack of professionalism is shocking - additional call is assigned.

- Swelling / T2 bright signal at the **corpus callosum** *(represents an acute demyelination)*
- Order is progressive - typically **beginning in the body**, then genu, and lastly splenium
- "**Sandwich sign**" on sagittal imaging - describes the pattern of preference for **central fibers** with relative sparing of the dorsal and ventrals fibers
- Chronic Phase: **Thinned corpus callosum + cystic cavities favoring** in the **genu and splenium**

Misc

Direct Alcoholic Injury:

Most Common / Classic Finding(s):

Brain **Atrophy**. Particularly the cerebellum and especially the cerebellar vermis

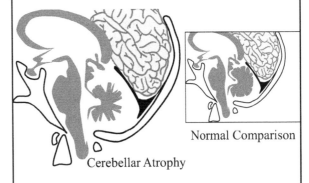

Normal Comparison

Cerebellar Atrophy

Copper & Manganese Deposition:

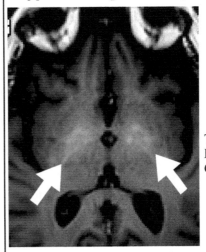

T1 Bright Basal Ganglia

-Non-Specific and related To Liver Disease.
-Can be seen without hepatic encephalopathy
-Also seen in TPN, Wilson's Disease,
-Also seen in Non-Ketotic Hyperglycemia (HNK) in which it's often unilateral

Methanol Toxicity:

"Drinking Windshield Wiper Fluid" as an idiotic attempt to get drunk. Can also be seen from consuming "poorly adulterer moonshine" - or "West Virginia Budweiser."

Classic Findings: *Optic nerve atrophy*, hemorrhagic **putaminal** and subcortical white matter necrosis

⚖ THIS vs THAT: Carbon Monoxide vs Methanol:

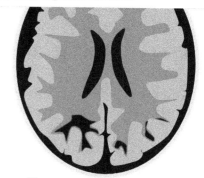

| **Carbon Monoxide** | CT Hypodensity / T2 Bright: **Globus Pallidus** (*carbon monoxide causes "globus" warming*). |
| **Methanol** | T2 Bright: **Putaminal** - which may be *hemorrhagic*, and thus CT Hyperdense. |

PRES (Posterior Reversible Encephalopathy Syndrome):

Classic Features:

- Asymmetric cortical and subcortical white matter edema (usually in parietal and occipital regions *but doesn't have to be - superior frontal sulcus is also common).

- <u>Does NOT restrict</u> on diffusion (helps tell you it's not a stroke).

Etiology: Poorly understood auto regulation fuck up.

Classic History: <u>Acute</u> <u>Hypertension</u> or <u>Chemotherapy</u>.

Vasogenic Edema Pattern
Bilateral, Posterior, Mildly Asymmetric

Post Chemotherapy:

It is fairly common. There are lots of named offenders. <u>Methotrexate</u> seems to be the one people write the most papers about (especially in kids with ALL)

There are two main looks:

(1) **PRES** - As above, chemo is a classic cause. BUT! It tends to have a "<u>non-classic</u>" look relative to the hypertension type. It will <u>often spare the occipital lobes</u>, and instead target the basal ganglia, brainstem, and cerebellum.

(2) **Leukoencephalopathy** (treatment induced): The classic look would be centered in the <u>periventricular white matter</u> - bilateral, symmetric, confluent, T2/FLAIR bright changes (history is obviously key to the diagnosis).

Other Misc Trivia:
- Can progress to brain atrophy.

- *"Mineralizing Microangiopathy"* - the vocab word to use if there are calcifications

- *"Disseminated necrotizing leukoencephalopathy"* - severe white matter changes, which <u>demonstrate ring enhancement</u> , classically seen with leukemia patients undergoing radiation and chemotherapy. It is bad news and can be fatal (it believes in nothing Lebowski).

Post Radiation:

The quick and dirty version is that after radiation therapy to the brain you can see T2 bright areas and atrophy corresponding to the radiation portal. You can also see hemosiderin deposition and mineralizing microangiopathy (calcifications involving the basal ganglia and subcortical white matter). There is a latent period, so imaging findings don't typically show up for about two months post therapy. Now… if you want to get crazy, you can discuss changes at different time periods.

Acute (Days-Weeks):	Too rare to give a fuck about (at least for the test)	
Early Delayed (1-6 months):	The classic look is similar to chemo - high T2/FLAIR signal in the periventricular white matter.	This is reversible change (usually).
Late Delayed (6 months):	Described as a "mosaic" pattern with high WM signal changes again favoring the deep white matter. Can appear "mass-like" and expansile. Classically sparing of the U-Fibers & Corpus Callosum.	Progressive… but reversible (mostly)
Long Term Sequela	*Radiation-Induced Vasculopathy:* Strokes and Moya-Moya type of look. *Mineralizing Microangiopathy* - I mentioned this on the previous page. This is a delayed finding — like two years following treatment. Think calcifications (basal ganglia and subcortical white matter) - hence the term "mineralizing." *Radiation-Induced Vascular Malformations:* The most classic types are **capillary telangiectasias / cavernous malformations**. The most classic scenario is a kid getting whole brain radiation for ALL. Remember the key finding is <u>blooming on GRE/SWI sequences.</u> *Radiation-induced Brain Cancer:* • XRT is the "most important risk factor" for primary CNS neoplasm. • Most common type is a meningiomas (70%) - usually seen ~ 15 years post XRT • More aggressive types Gliomas, Sarcomas, etc, have a shorter window < 10 years	

🐉 "Chasing the Dragon" - Heroin Inhalational Leukoencephalopathy

Most toxic leukoencephalopathies (either from chemotherapy, immunosuppressives, antibiotics, or the aristocratic art of paint thinner huffing) all create a similar non-specific pattern of widespread high T2/FLAIR signal in the supra and infratentorial white matter. The "Chasing the Dragon" pattern is also not specific - but it does have a catchy name, so people love collecting cases of it to show in conference ("catchy name" = high yield for boards).

The most classic look (diagrams are FLAIR sequences):

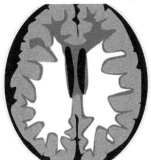

Symmetric "Butterfly" in the Centrum Semiovale

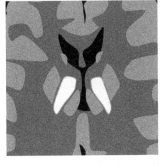

High Signal in the Posterior Limb of the Internal Capsule

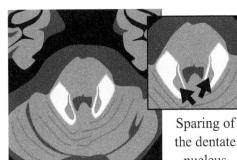

High Signal in the Deep Cerebellar White Matter

Sparing of the dentate nucleus (arrows)

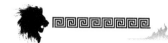
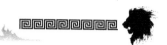
Multiple Sclerosis:

White matter patterns can be confusing as there are tons of overlapping non-specific features. To help understand this (and avoid being tricked) let me introduce a few concepts. White matter lesions come in a few patterns. MS is the poster child of the "perivascular pattern." This pattern favors involvement of the juxtacortical and periventricular regions with lesions that have ovoid and/or fusiform morphology.

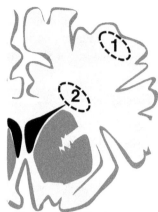

(1) Juxtacortical
(2) Periventricular

 Ovoid, Fusiform

Size can be helpful. A single lesion > 15 mm in size suggests the underlying etiology is not vascular.

Certain locations will also make you think "not vascular." When you think "not vascular pattern" you should think demyelinating. When you think demyelinating you should think MS first (it's by far the most common).

	Vascular Pattern	Perivascular Pattern (MS)
Corpus Callosum	RARE	COMMON
Juxtacortical	RARE	COMMON
Infratentorial	RARE	COMMON
Basal Ganglai	COMMON	RARE

McDonald Diagnostic Criteria for MS:

This was last revised in 2010, so it's kind of an old McDonald's Diagnostic Criteria.

• And on his criteria he had a section of lesions <u>disseminated in space</u> (periventricular, juxtacortical, infratentorial, spinal cord) - more than 1 in at least 2 of these locations.

• And on his criteria he had a section on <u>dissemination in time</u>: best shown as a T2 bright lesion that does enhance (active) and a T2 bright lesion that does not enhance (in-active) — lesions are in different phases of the disease and therefore separated by time.

Epidemiological trivia:

• Usually targets women 20-40 (in children there is no gender difference).
• There are multiple sub-types with the *relapsing-remitting* form being the most common (85%).
• Clinical history of *"separated by time and space"* is critical.

Additional MS Related Trivia:

- Most Classic Finding: T2/FLAIR oval and periventricular perpendicularly oriented lesions.
- Involvement of the calloso-septal interface is 98% specific for MS (and helps differentiate it from vascular lesions and ADEM).
- In children the posterior fossa is more commonly involved.
- Brain atrophy is accelerated in MS.
- Solitary spinal cord involvement can occur but it is typically seen in addition to brain lesions.
- The cervical spine is the most common location in the spine (65%).
- Spinal cord lesions tend to be peripherally located.
- FLAIR is more sensitive than T2 in detection of juxtacortical and periventricular plaques.
- T2 is more sensitive than FLAIR for detecting infratentorial lesions
- MR spectroscopy (discussed later in the chapter) will show reduced NAA peaks within the plaques.

Active vs Not Active : Acute demyelinating plaques should enhance and restrict diffusion (on multiple choice tests and occasionally in the real world).

Tumor vs MS: You can sometimes get a big MS plaque that looks like a tumor. **It will ring enhance but classically incomplete (*like a horseshoe*),** with a leading demyelinating edge.

Tumor = Complete Ring   Demyelination = Incomplete Ring

—

Multiple Sclerosis Variants:

ADEM (Acute Disseminated Encephalomyelitis): Typically presents in childhood or adolescents, after a viral illness or vaccination. Classically has multiple LARGE T2 bright lesions, which enhance in a nodular or ring pattern (open ring). Lesions **do NOT involve the calloso-septal interface.**

Acute Hemorrhagic Leukoencephalitis (Hurst Disease): This a fulminant form of ADEM with massive brain swelling and death. The hemorrhagic part is only seen on autopsy (not imaging).

Devics (neuromyelitis optica): Transverse Myelitis + Optic Neuritis.
Lesions in the Cord and the Optic Nerve

Marburg Variant: Childhood variant that is fulminant and terrible leading to rapid death. It usually has a febrile prodrome. "MARBURG!!!" = DEATH

Subcortical Arteriosclerotic Encephalopathy (SAE)

Also referred to as Binswanger Disease - for the purpose of fucking with you.

It's best thought of as a multi-infarct dementia that ONLY involves the white matter.

Trivia:

- It favors the white matter of the centrum semiovale (white matter superior to the lateral ventricles / corpus callosum).

- Classically spares the subcortical U fibers.

- Strong association with Hypertension.

- It's seen in older people - 55 and up

- If they show you a case that looks exactly like SAE but that patient is 40 and has migraines they are leading you to the genetically transmitted form of this disease called CADASIL.

WTF are "U Fibers" ?

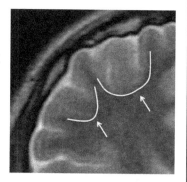

They are the fibers under the cortex, that look like "U"s.

They come up a lot, as being spared or not spared.

CADASIL *(Cerebral Autosomal Dominant Arteriopathy with Subcortical Infarcts & Leukoencephalopathy)*

Basically it is SAE in a slightly younger person (40), with migraines.

Classic Scenario: 40 year old **presenting with migraine headaches**, strokes, then eventually dementia. CADASIL is actually the most common hereditary stroke disorder.

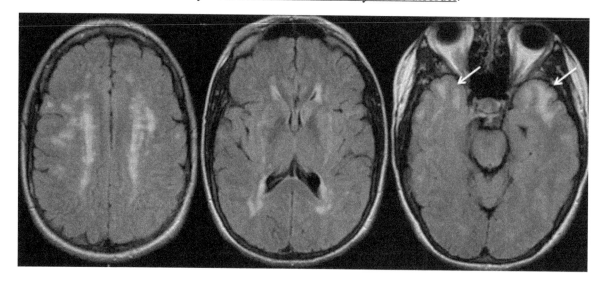

Step 1 Trivia: NOTCH3 mutations on chromosome 19

Classic Imaging Findings: Severe white matter disease (high T2/FLAIR signal) involving multiple vascular territories, in the frontal and **temporal lobe**. The occipital lobes are often spared. Temporal lobe involvement is classic.

Dementia Disorders:

This topic was split up in prior editions on the text, with half in neuro and half in nukes. The reason I did that was because these disorders are often evaluated with FDG PET. To keep you from having to hop around I decided to consolidate it this time around.

FDG PET for dementia is a worthless and expensive component of the workup. Like most imaging exams it is ordered with no regard to the impending collapse of the health care system under crippling rising costs (with inevitable progression into a Mad Max style dystopian future or even better Mega-City 1). As such, it is standard practice in most academic centers to obtain the study.

The idea is that "demented brain" will have less perfusion and will have less metabolism relative to "not demented brain." PET can assess perfusion (^{15}O-H_2O) but typically it uses ^{18}FDG to assess metabolism (which is analogous to perfusion). Renal clearance of ^{18}FDG is excellent, giving good target to background pictures. Resolution of PET is superior to SPECT.

HMPAO, and ECD (tracers that are discussed in more depth in the nukes chapter) can also be used for dementia imaging and the patterns of pathology are the same.

It's important to remember that external factors can affect the results; bright lights stimulating the occipital lobes, high glucose (>200) causes more competition for the tracer and therefore less uptake, etc...etc... so on and so forth.

Before we begin with the subtypes, a quick pearl: *On FDG PET the motor strip is always preserved in a _degenerative type_ of dementia.*

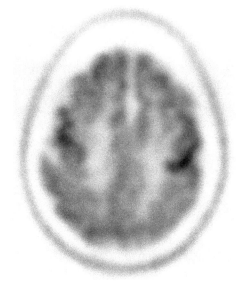

Preserved Motor Strip
—Seen in degenerative dementias

Dementia - The Primary Tribes

Alzheimer Disease	Multi-infarct Dementia	Dementia with Lewy Bodies
Most common cause	2nd most common	3rd most common
Tauopathy, Amyloid Cascade, and Neurofibrillary Tangles are all buzzwords people use when they pretend to understand the pathophysiology.	Also called "Vascular Dementia" - for the purpose of fucking with you.	Alpha synuclein and syncleinopathy are buzzwords people use when they pretend to understand the pathophysiology.
Risk Factor(s): The biggest one is <u>Age</u>. A more obscure one (but certainly testable) is <u>Downs Syndrome.</u> Downs patients nearly always get AD, and they get it earlier than normal - that extra 21st isn't doing them any favors.	Risk Factor(s): • McDonalds, Burger King, Taco Bell, Pizza Hut • Hypertension, • Smoking (tobacco), and • <u>CADASIL</u>	Clinical Scenario: There is a triad of classic features. (1) <u>Visual hallucinations</u> (2) Spontaneous parkinsonism, (3) Fluctuating ability to concentrate / stay alert Clinical picture can be similar to Parkinson's dementia - the major difference <u>in DLB, the dementia comes before the Parkinsonism</u>
Most Classic Feature(s): **hippocampal atrophy** (which is first and out of proportion to the rest of the brain atrophy). They could ask temporal horn atrophy > 3 mm , which is seen in more than 65% of cases.	*Most Classic Feature(s):* Cortical infarcts and lacunar infarcts are seen on MRI. Brain atrophy (generalized) is usually advanced for the patients age.	*Most Classic Feature(s):* Mild generalized atrophy without lobar predominance (unlike multi-infarct). Hippocampi will be normal in size (unlike AD)
FDG Pattern: **Low posterior temporoparietal uptake -** *"headphones"* or *"ear muffs."* **11C PiB (Pittsburgh compound B)** is an even better way to waste money making this diagnosis. It works as an *Amyloid Binding Tracer.*	*FDG Pattern:* Multiple scattered areas of decreased activity. No specific lobar predominance. Unlike the neurodegenerative dementias - this one <u>could knock out the motor strip</u> (if the strokes happen to involve that region). This is different that AD and DLB.	*FDG Pattern:* decreased FDG uptake in the lateral occipital cortex, with sparing of the mid posterior cingulate gyrus (**Cingulate Island Sign**).

Picks: Also be referred to a *"frontotemporal dementia"* - for the purpose of fucking with you.

Clinical: Onset is earlier than AD (like 40s-50s). Classic presentation is described as "compulsive or inappropriate behaviors." In other words, acting like an asshole (fucking prostitutes, and buying miracle weight loss potions from Dr. Oz - when you aren't even going to the gym or trying to eat right). Just being a real **Prick.**

Classic Feature(s): Severe symmetric <u>atrophy of the</u> <u>frontal lobes</u> (milder volume loss in the temporal lobes).

FDG Pattern: Low uptake in the frontal and temporal lobes.

FDG PET - Brain

Alzheimers	Low posterior temporoparietal cortical activity	-Identical to Parkinson Dementia -Posterior Cingulate gyrus is the first area abnormal
Multi Infarct	Scattered areas of decreased activity	
Dementia with Lewy Bodies	Low in lateral occipital cortex	Preservation of the mid posterior cingulate gyrus **(Cingulate Island Sign)**
Picks / Frontotemporal	Low frontal lobe	

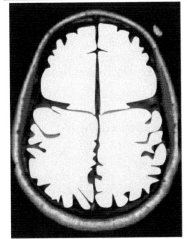 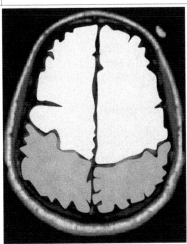 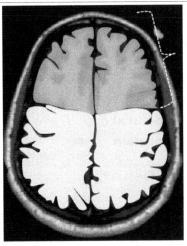

Normal

Alzheimers
-Low posterior temporoparietal

Frontotemporal
-Low Frontal Lobe

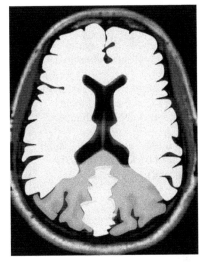 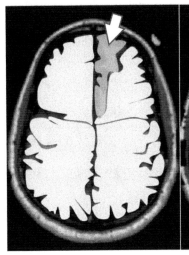

Lew Body Dementia
-Low Lateral Occipital with sparing of the cingulate gyrus

Multi-Infarct
-Scattered Areas of Low Uptake

The Defias Brotherhood of Neurodegeneration - Part 1

Fahr Disease (syndrome)	Also called *"Bilateral Striatopallidodentate Calcinosis"*, and sometimes *"Primary Familial Brain Calcification"* for the sole purpose of fucking with you on the exam. Many are asymptomatic. Others go insane and start stumbling around	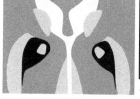 ***Extensive Calcification*** *in the Basal Ganglia and Thalami.* **Globus is typically involved first*
Hallervorden Spatz	Also called **PKAN** (pantothenate kinase-associated neuropathy) for the sole purpose of fucking with you on the exam. Etiology: Iron in the Globus Pallidus **T2 Dark Globus** with central bright area of necrosis **"Eye of the Tiger"**. No enhancement. No Restricted Diffusion.	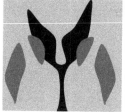 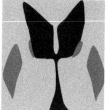 *Normal Comparison* ***T2: Dark Medial Basal Ganglia*** *(Globus), with central high signal dot (necrosis)*
Amyotrophic Lateral Sclerosis	Upper motor neuro loss in the brain and spine. Most people die within 5 years (unless you are really good at physics).	• Does NOT show gross volume loss. • T2/FLAIR tends to be Normal (rarely can be bright in the posterior internal capsule).
Cortico-basal Degeneration	Tauopathy (whatever the F that means). Awesome clinical manifestations like the *"Alien limb phenomenon"* -50% of cases.	• Asymmetric frontoparietal atrophy.
Huntington Disease	One of those AD repeat sequence things. *What Sequence ?* 38 CAGs Mother Fuckers. Yes, I still remember that worthless factoid from Step 1. *Why?* It's a curse. My mind is like a bear trap, you gotta chew your leg off to get out. So, between Step 1 & the CORE exam, I've got tons of worthless bullshit up there. Remember these poor guys turn into huge assholes - then start flopping around.	**Caudate Atrophy** and reduced FDG uptake. The frontal horns will become enlarged and outwardly convex (from the atrophy pattern)  *Normal Comparison* *Huntington*
Leigh Disease	*Mitochondrial Disorder* Elevated Lactate peak at 1.3 ppm	• T2/FLAIR bright lesions in the Brainstem, Basal Ganglia , and Cerebral Peduncles. • They can restrict, but do NOT enhance.
MELAS Syndrome	*Mitochondrial Disorder* Lactic Acidosis, Seizures, and Strokes Elevated Lactate "doublet" at 1.3 ppm	• Atypical strokes in the cortical gray matter with a <u>nonvascular</u> distribution (usually occipital and parietal). • Underlying WM is normal
Hurler Syndrome	Lysosomal Storage Disease / Mucopolysaccharidoses (1) Macrocephaly with Metopic "beak" (2) Enlarged Perivascular Spaces (3) Beaked Inferior L1 Vertebral Body	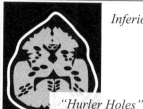 *Inferior Anterior Beak* *"Hurler Holes"*

The Defias Brotherhood of Neurodegeneration - Part 2

Parkinson Disease (PD)

Classic Clinical Hx: Resting tremor, Rigid / Slow movements (shuffling gate, etc..).

Etiology: Reduced dopaminergic input to striatum (whatever the fuck that means).

DAT Scan - Ioflupane 123 - This exotic Nukes study is certainly fair game for an "intermediate level" exam.

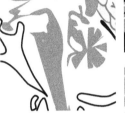

Normal (Commas)

ABnormal (Periods)

Possible Parkinsonian Syndrome (PD, MSA or PSP)

Impossible to diagnose on CT or MR alone - but supposedly has mild midbrain volume loss with a "butterfly" pattern (this would have to be stated, it is too subtle to show).

Worth noting in the *sparing of the midbrain and superior cerebellar peduncles*. This is a fairly high yield piece of trivia as it helps distinction Parkinsons from multi-system atrophy.

"Parkinson-Plus"

Multi-System Atrophy (MSA)

This is a monstrously complex entity, that is actually 3 separate renamed entities ("P", "C", and "A").

The highest yield pearl is the appearance of the **C**erebellar subtype *MSA-C* ➡

Trivia: <u>I-123 MIBG</u> can be used to differentiate PD from MSA, by looking at the cardiac/mediastinal ratio (which is normal in MSA, and abnormal in PD)

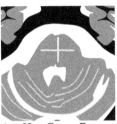

Cerebellar Hemisphere / **Peduncle Atrophy** with a **Shrunken Flat Pons** & an enlarged 4th vent.

Hot Cross Bun Sign (loss of the transverse fibers)

"Parkinson-Plus"

Progressive Supra-nuclear Palsy (PSP)

- Also called *Steele-Richardson-Olszewski* for the purpose of fucking with you.
- PSP = Most Common Parkinson Plus
- Unlike PD & MSA, PSP is a Tauopathy (whatever the fuck that means).

Micky Mouse Sign: Tegmentum Atrophy with Sparing of the Tectum & Peduncles.

*If needed anatomy refresher - page 14

Hummingbird Sign: Midbrain volume loss with a concave upper surface + relative sparing of the Pons.

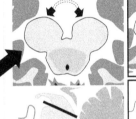

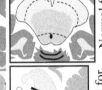

Normal for Comparison

Normal for Comparison

Selective Midbrain Atrophy, with Sparing of Pons (divided by line)

Wilson Disease

AR copper metabolism malfunction. Once the liver fills up with copper it starts spilling over into other organs including the brain.

Trivia: "Kayser-Fleischer Rings" - seen in 95% of patients. Prepare the Slit Lamp.

Trivia: Cortical Atrophy is the most common CT finding (although obviously very non-specific).

Trivia: T1 Bright BG is the most common initial MR findings (supposedly).

Trivia: Copper has been suggested to be Metro Man's only vulnerability (this is controversial). Since literally anything is fair game for the exam, I figured I better mention that for completeness.

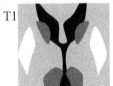

T1

T2

T1 and T2 Bright Basal Ganglia
T2 Bright Dorsal Medial Thalamus

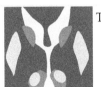

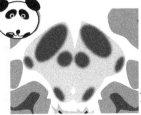

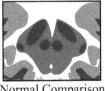

Normal Comparison

Panda Sign: <u>T2 Bright Tegmentum</u> with normal dark red nuclei & substantial nigra

Deep Brain Stimulators

I want to quickly touch on deep brain stimulators. These things are used in the treatment of Parkinson disease, essential tremor, and chronic pain.

It is common to get a CT immediately after DBS placement to evaluate for correct positioning of the electrode or any obvious complications (bleeding, etc...). Knowing the "correct" position is the most useful piece of trivia.

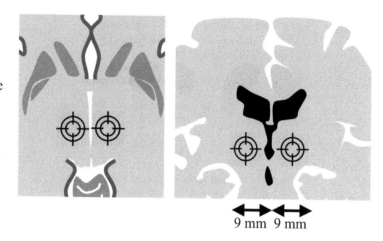

For Parkinson Disease, the electrodes are <u>typically positioned in the sub thalamic nucleus with the tips of the electrons located 9 mm from the midline</u> (just inside the upper most margin of the cerebral peduncle).

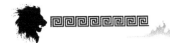 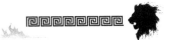

Introduction to MRI Spectroscopy

The old joke in Neuroradiology is if you need to use MRS to figure something out, then you need to go back and read the book again - starting at page 1. Someone told me that's Yousem's joke, but I don't see how that is possible - because it's actually a little funny. Regardless of who made the joke first, there is near universal acceptance that MRS is "of limited clinical utility" (a worthless turd). Therefore, it is fair game for an intermediate level exam and we should at least talk about it a little. I'm not going to get into the physics much here (there will be a write up in the new 3rd Edition of the War Machine covering that). For now, I'm going to give a very basic overview and emphasize the pathology / clinical trivia. Then I'll be sprinkling more MRS in sporadically throughout the chapter.

Overview: The general idea is that the various metabolites which exist on the cellular level (choline, lactate, N-acetylaspartate "NAA," etc... etc..., so on and so forth...) occur in different concentrations depending on the pathology. For example, "NAA" is a neuronal marker. Things that destroy neurons (like tumors) will decrease NAA. So, in general the lower the NAA the higher the grade tumor.

You will see a graph like this one, with "PPM" on the X-Axis, and "Intensity" on the Y-Axis.

Intensity is going to tell you "how much" of a thing there is.

It's not a raw number, and better thought of as a ratio.

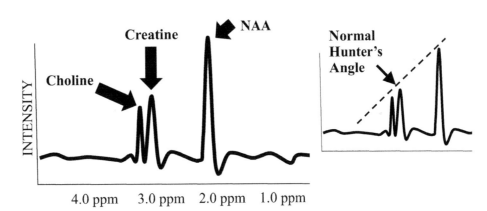

PPM stands for parts per million. Better understood as a percent of the Larmor Frequency (1 ppm = 1 millionth of the Larmor frequency). This is important because each metabolite will have a unique frequency distribution. For example NAA is at 2.0 ppm.

Why are the numbers counting backwards on the scale ? I'm going to answer this with the same explanation I received as a small child when I asked why I couldn't just eat my dessert first, and my vegetables last —- "because I'm your mother that's why!"

Hunter's Angle: This is a method to quickly decide if the MRS is normal or not. Under normal conditions Choline, Creatine, and NAA should ascending in that order. Using a line to connect the tips gives you a 45 degree~ish angle. If it slopes the other way (as shown) then it is not normal.

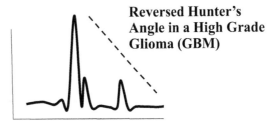

Reversed Hunter's Angle in a High Grade Glioma (GBM)

MRI Spectroscopy High Yield Pearls

Lipid	0.9-1.4	Product of brain destruction - lipids are present in necrotic brain tissue (necrosis marker).	Necrotic Tissue (spilling of membrane lipids). Elevated with high grade tumors, brain infarcts, and brain abscess.	
Lactate	1.3	Product of anaerobic metabolism. Absent under normal conditions.	Brain tumor has outgrown its blood supply - is forced into anaerobic pathways for metabolism. Also elevated with cerebral abscess.	*Classic Trivia:* It's normal to see lactate elevated in the first hours of life *Classic Trivia:* Lactate and Lipid peaks superimpose - you need to use an intermediate TE (around 140) to causes an "inversion" of the lactate peak (so you can see it)
Alanine	1.48	Amino Acid	Found in Meningiomas	
N-acetylaspartate "NAA"	2.0	Neuronal Marker (Neuron Viability). Usually the tallest peak.	Glial tumors have NAA. The higher the Glial tumor grade, the lower the NAA	*Classic Trivia:* NAA peak is super high with Canavans.
Glutamine - "GLX"	2.2-2.4	Neurotransmitter	Increased with Hepatic Encephalopathy	
Creatine - "Cr"	3.0	Energy Metabolism	Decreased in tumor necrosis.	
Choline - "Co"	3.2	Cell Membrane Turnover	More turnover more Choline (thus elevated in high grade tumor, demyelination, inflammation).	
Myoinositol - "mI"	3.5	Cell Volume Regulator and Byproduct of Glucose Metabolism.	- Elevated in low grade gliomas. - Elevated in Alzheimer's (decreased in other dementias) - Elevated in Progressive multifocal leukoencephalopathy (PML)	- Reduced in high grade gliomas - Reduced in Hepatic Encephalopathy

⚖️ THIS vs THAT: Demyelinating vs Dysmyelinating

Demyelinating Disease	Example = MS	Disease that destroys normal myelin
Dysmyelinating Disease	Example = Metachromatic Leukodystrophy	Disease that disrupts the normal formation and turnover of myelin

Leukodystrophies & Friends

On the prior page, I introduced the vocab work "d**y**smyelinating" disease. Leukodystrophies are the classic example of this group of pathologies. Technically speaking Leukodystrophies can occur from deficiencies in lysosomal storage, peroxisomal function, or mitochondrial dysfunction. I'm gonna hit on mitochondrial diseases separately as they tend to be more asymmetric and favor the grey matter. Where as the classic forms target the white matter in a more symmetric and extensive manner.

The distinction between the Leukodystrophy subtypes is totally academic mental masturbation, since they are all untreatable and fatal. Therefore, distinguishing between them is fair game on an intermediate level exam (and specifically listed on the official study guide).

Leukodystrophy = Fucked White Matter in a Kid				
Adreno Leukodystrophy (**ALD**) "X-Linked"	Normal Head Size	Parieto-occipital Predominance "Extends across the Splenium of the Corpus Callosum"	Sex-linked recessive (peroxisomal enzyme deficiency) **Male Predominant** Can Enhance & Restrict	FLAIR
Metachromatic	Normal Head Size	**Frontal Predominance** Periventricular and Deep White Matter - **Tigroid Pattern** (stripes of milder disease).	**Most common Leukodystrophy.** U-fibers are relatively spared	FLAIR
Alexander Disease	Weird Big Head	**Frontal Predominance**	Also hits the cerebellum and middle cerebellar peduncles Can Enhance	FLAIR
Canavan Disease	Weird Big Head	Diffuse Bilateral subcortical U fibers. "Subcortical Predominance"	**Elevated NAA (MRS).**	FLAIR
Krabbe	Small Head	Centrum semiovale and periventricular white matter with parieto-occipital predominance	High density foci on CT (in the thalamus, caudate, and deep white matter). Early sparing of the subcortical U fibers.	FLAIR
Pelizaeus-Merzbacher	Normal Head Size	Typically diffuse "total lack of normal myelination" with extension to the subcortical U fibers. Patchy variant is also described as "**tigroid**" - although that term is more classic for Metachromatic No enhancement. No restricted diffusion.		FLAIR

Leukodystrophies & Friends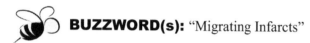

As discussed on the prior page Leukodystrophies can occur from deficiencies in lysosomal storage, peroxisomal function, or mitochondrial dysfunction. The classic forms tend to target the white matter in a more symmetric and extensive manner. This is different than mitochondrial diseases which are more asymmetric and favor the grey matter. Grey Matter needs more oxygen than White Matter (and White Matter needs more oxygen than trial lawyers). Inability to process oxygen (mitochondrial dysfunction) - helps me remember the grey matter > white matter thing.

MELAS – **M**itochondrial **E**ncephalomyopathy, **L**actic **A**cidosis, and **S**troke-like episodes. This is a mitochondrial disorder with lactic acidosis and stroke like episodes.

Tends to have a parietooccipital distribution

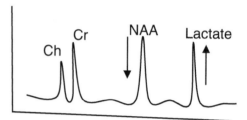

BUZZWORD(s): "Migrating Infarcts"

Typical MRS Pattern for MELAS: Increased Lactate, Decreased NAA.

Leigh Disease - Also called *Subacute Necrotizing Encephalo-Myelopathy* - for the purpose of fucking with you.

White Matter Distribution: Focal areas of subcortical white matter.
Gray Matter Distribution: Basal ganglia and Periaquaductal Gray

Trivia: Head size tends to be normal.

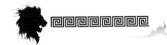 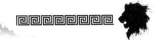

SECTION 7:
BRAIN TUMORS

I want to introduce my idea for multiple choice brain tumor diagnosis. The strategy is as follows; (1) decide if it's single or multiple, (2) look at the age of the patient - *adults and kids have different differentials*, (3) look at the location - *different tumors occur in different spots,* (4) now use the characteristics to separate them. The strategy centers around narrowing the differential based off age and location till you are only dealing with 3-4 common things, then using the imaging characteristics to separate them. It's so much easier to do it that way.

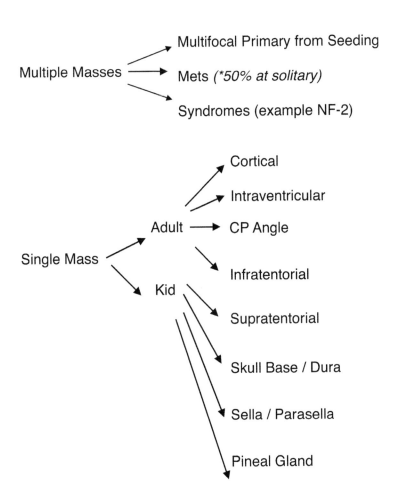

Before we get rolling, the first thing to do is to ask yourself is this a tumor, or is it a mimic? Mimics would be abscess, infarct, or a big MS plaque. This can be tricky. If you see an incomplete ring - you should think giant MS plaque. If they show you diffusion, it is either lymphoma or a stroke (or an abscess) - you'll need to use enhancement to straighten that out (remember lymphoma enhances homogeneously).

Yes... GBM can restrict, but for multiple choice it is way more likely to be lymphoma.

Two more high yield topics before we start crushing the differentials:

"Intra-Axial" vs "Extra-Axial"

The Brant and Helms discussion on brain tumors will have you asking "intra-axial" vs "extra-axial" first. This is not always that simple, but it does lend itself very well to multiple choice test questions (therefore it's high yield).

Basically you need to memorize the "signs of extra-axial location"

- CSF Cleft
- Displaced Subarachnoid Vessels
- Cortical Gray matter between the mass and white matter
- Displaced and expanded Subarachnoid spaces
- Broad Dural Base / Tail
- Bony Reaction

Why Do Things Enhance?

Understanding the WHY is very helpful for problem solving. Let me first answer the question *"Why DON'T things enhance?"* They DON'T enhance because of the blood brain barrier. So, when things DO enhance it's because either:
     (a) They are outside the blood brain barrier (they are extra-axial), or
     (b) They have melted the blood brain barrier.

In other words, extra axial things (classic example is meningioma) will enhance. High grade tumors (and infections) enhance. Low grade tumors just aren't nasty enough to take the blood brain barrier down.

Are there exceptions? HA! There always are. And Yes... they are ALWAYS testable.

Gangliogliomas and Pilocytic Astrocytomas are the exceptions - they are low-grade tumors, but they enhance.

Multiple Masses

In adults or kids, if you see multiple masses you are dealing with mets (or infection). Differentiating between mets and infection is gonna be done with diffusion (infection will restrict). If they want you to decide between those two they must show you the diffusion otherwise only one or the other will be listed as a choice.

Mets — High Yield Trivia:

- Most common CNS met in a kid = neuroblastoma (BONES, DURA, ORBIT - not brain)

- Most common location for mets = Supratentorial at the Grey-White Junction (this area has a lot of blood flow + an abrupt vessel caliber change... so you also see hematogenous infection / septic emboli go there first too).

- Most common morphology is "round" or "spherical"

- Remember that mets do NOT have to be multiple. In fact, 50% of mets are solitary. In an adult, a solitary mass is much more likely to be a met than a primary CNS neoplasm.

- **MRCT** is the mnemonic for bleeding mets (**M**elanoma, **R**enal, **C**arcinoid / **C**horiocarcinoma, **T**hyroid).

- Usually Mets have more surrounding edema than primary neoplasms of similar size.

- *"Next Step Gamesmanship"* - Because the most common intra-axial mass in an adult is a met, if they show you a solitary mass (or multiple masses) and want a next step it's gonna be go hunting for the primary (think lung, breast, colon... the common stuff).

Primary Brain Tumors Can Also Be Multiple:

Tumors that Like to be Multifocal	Tumors that are Multifocal from Seeding
Mets — you should still think this first when you see multiple tumors	Medulloblastoma
Lymphoma	Ependymoma
Multicentric GBM	GBM
Gliomatosis Cerebri	Oligodendroglioma

SYNDROMES - Tumors in Syndromes are more likely to be Multifocal			
NF 1	NF 2 "MSME"	Tuberous Sclerosis	VHL
Optic Gliomas	Multiple Schwannomas	Subependymal Tubers	Hemangioblastomas
Astrocytomas	Meningiomas	IV Giant Cell Astrocytomas	
	Ependymomas		

Cortically Based *(P-DOG):*

Most intra-axial tumors are located in the white matter. So when a tumor spreads to or is primarily located in the gray matter, you get a shorter DDx. High yield piece of trivia regarding the cortical tumor / cortical met is that they often have *very little edema* and so a *small cortical met can be occult without IV contrast.*

P-DOG:
Pleomorphic Xanthoastrocytoma (PXA)
Dysembryoplastic Neuroepithelial Tumor (DNET)
Oligodendroglioma,
Ganglioglioma

PXA (Pleomorphic Xanthroastrocytoma):

Superficial tumor that is ALWAYS supratentorial and usually involves the temporal lobe. They are often in the cyst with a nodule category (50%). There is usually no peritumeral T2 signal. The tumor frequently invades the leptomeninges. Looks just like a Desmoplastic Infantile Ganglioglioma - but is not in an infant.

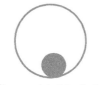
Cyst with Nodule

PXA
PEDS (10-20)
Will Enhance
Dural Tail***
Cyst with Nodule
Temporal Lobe

DNET (Dysembryoplastic Neuroepithelial Tumor):

Kid with drug resistant seizures. The mass will always be in the temporal lobe (on the test – real life 60% temporal). Focal cortical dysplasia is seen in 80% of the cases. It is hypodense on CT, and on MRI there will be little if any surrounding edema. High T2 signal "bubbly lesion."

Bright Rim Sign -
Persistent rim of FLAIR signal
* Looks Similar to T2-FLAIR
  Mismatch of Astrocytomas
  **discussed later*

DNET
PEDS (< 20)
No enhancement
High T2 Signal with Bright FLAIR Rim
"Bubbly"
Temporal Lobe

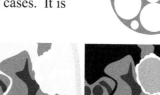
"T2 Bright & Bubbly"   FLAIR Bright Rim

Oligodendroglioma:

Remember this is the guy that **calcifies 90% of the time**. It's most common in the frontal lobe and the buzzword is **"expands the cortex"**. This takes after its most specific feature of cortical infiltration and marked thickening. It's likely you could get asked about this **1p/19q deletion** which I will discuss later when I go into detail about Gliomas (pg 83).

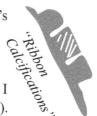
"Ribbon Calcifications"

Oligodendroglioma
ADULT - (40s-50s)
Can Enhance
Calcification Common
"Expands the Cortex"
Frontal Lobe
1p /19q

Ganglioglioma:

This guy can occur at any age, anywhere (usually temporal lobe), and look like anything. However, for the purpose of multiple choice testing the classic scenario would be a 13 year old with seizures, and a temporal lobe mass that is cystic and solid with focal calcifications. There may be overlying bony remodeling.

Mixed Cystic & Solid

Ganglioglioma
Any Age
Can Enhance
NOT Bubbly
Can look like Anything
Temporal Lobe

Intraventricular

Tumors can arise from the ventricular wall, septum pellucidum, or choroid plexus.

Ventricular Wall & Septum Pellucidum	Choroid Plexus	Misc
Ependymoma **(PEDS)**	Choroid Plexus Papilloma **(PEDS in Trigone)** **(ADULT in 4th Vent)**	Mets
Medulloblastoma **(PEDS)**	Choroid Plexus Carcinoma (**PEDS**)	Meningioma
SEGA (Subependymal Giant Cell Astrocytoma) = **PEDS**	Xanthogranuloma ("Found" in **ADULTS**)	Colloid Cyst
Subependymoma **(ADULT)**		
Central Neurocytoma **(YOUNG ADULT)**		

—

Ventricular Wall / Septum Pellucidum Origin:

Ependymoma: Bimodal distribution on this one (large peak around 6 years of age, tiny peak around 30 years of age). I would basically think of this as a **PEDS tumor.**

They come in two flavors:

(a) 4th Ventricle - which is about 70% of the time. There is frequent extension into the foramen of Luschka and Magendie. They are the so-called "plastic tumor" or *"toothpaste" tumor* because they squeeze out of the base of the 4th ventricle.

(b) Parenchymal Supratentorial - which is about 30% of the time. These are usually big (> 4cm at presentation).

Medulloblastoma: Let us just assume we are talking about the "Classic Medulloblastoma" which is a type of PNET. If you want to understand the genetic spectrum of these things, read Osborn's Brain — seriously don't subject yourself to that.

This is a **pediatric tumor** - with most occurring before age 10 (technically there is a second peak at 20-40 but for the purpose of multiple choice tests I'm going to ignore it). These guys are cerebellar arising from vermis / **ROOF** of the 4th ventricle – project into 4th ventricle. They are much more common than their chief differential consideration the Ependymoma (which originates from the FLOOR of the 4th ventricle).

The classic look is a dense mass on CT, heterogeneous on T1 and T2, and enhances homogeneously. They are hypercellular and may restrict. They calcify 20% of the time (less than Ependymoma).

This is a tumor that loves to met via CSF pathways — they like to "drop met." The buzzword is "*zuckerguss*" which apparently is German for sugar icing, as seen on post contrast imaging of the brain and spinal cord (**leptomeningeal carcinomatosis**). As a point of absolute trivia, they are *associated with Basal Cell Nevus Syndrome and Turcots Syndrome.*

 Gorlin Syndrome - If you see a **Medulloblastoma** next look for **dural calcs**. If you see thick dural calcs you might be dealing with this syndrome. They get **basal cell** skin cancer after radiation, and have odontogenic cysts.

 NEXT STEP Trivia: Preoperative imaging of the entire spinal axis should be done in any child with a posterior fossa neoplasm, especially if Medulloblastoma or Ependymoma is suspected. Evidence of tumor spread is a statistically significant predictor of outcome.

Medulloblastoma	Ependymoma
More common	Less Common
Originate from Vermis / ROOF of the 4th Ventricle	Originate from the FLOOR of the 4th ventricle.
Can project into 4th ventricle, do NOT usually extend into basal cisterns	Can extend into basal cisterns like tooth paste pushing though foramina of Luschka and Magendie
Enhance Homogeneously *(more so than Ependymoma anyway)*	Enhance Heterogeneously
Calcify Less (20%)	Calcify More (50%)
Linear "icing-like" enhancement of the brain surface is referred to as "Zuckerguss"	

Subependymal Giant Cell Astrocytoma (SEGA): This is going to be shown in the setting of TS. They will more than likely show you renal AMLs or tell you the kid has seizures / developmental delay.

Because it's syndromic, you see it in kids (average age 11).

It will arise from the lateral wall of the ventricle (near the foramen of Monro), often causing hydrocephalus. It enhances homogeneously.

THIS vs THAT: SEGA vs Subependymal Nodule (SEN) - The SEN will stay stable in size, the SEGA will grow. The SEGA is found in the lateral ventricle near the foramen of Monroe, the SEN can occur anywhere along the ventricle. SENs are way more common. Both SEN and SEGA can calcify.

 Pearl - Enhancing, partially calcified lesion at the foramen of Monro, bigger than 5 mm is a SEGA not a SEN.

— (the next 2 IV tumors are in ADULTS) —

Subependymoma: Found in ADULTS. Well-circumscribed IV mass **most commonly at the foramen of Monro and the 4th ventricle**. They can cause hydrocephalus. They typically don't enhance. They are T2 bright (like most tumors).

Central Neurocytoma:
This is the *most common IV mass in an ADULT aged 20-40*. The buzzword is **"swiss cheese,"** because of the numerous cystic spaces on T2. They **calcify** a lot (almost like oligodendrogliomas).

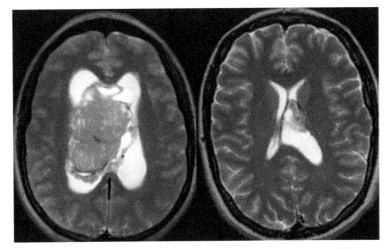

Central Neurocytoma - *Two Examples - Cystic IV Mass*

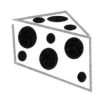

Swiss Cheese + Calcification in the Ventricle

Choroid Plexus Origin:

Choroid Plexus Papilloma / Carcinoma: Can occur in peds (85% under the age of 5) or adults. They make up about 15% of brain tumors in kids under one. Basically you are dealing with an intraventricular mass, which is often making CSF, so it causes hydrocephalus.

 Here is the trick: Brain tumors are usually supratentorial in adults and posterior fossa in kids. This tumor is an exception. Remember exceptions to rules are testable.

 Trivia:

- **In Adults it's in the 4ᵗʰ Ventricle, in Kids it's in the lateral ventricle (usually trigone).**

- Carcinoma type is ONLY SEEN IN KIDS - and are therefore basically ONLY SEEN IN LATERAL VENTRICLE / TRIGONE

- Carcinoma association with Li-Fraumeni syndrome (bad p53)

- Angiography may show enlarged choroidal arteries which shunt blood to the tumor,

- Carcinoma type of this tumor looks very similar (unless it's invading the parenchyma) and is almost exclusively seen in kids.

- The tumor is typically solitary but in rare instances you can have CSF dissemination

Xanthogranuloma –

This is a benign choroid plexus mass. You see it all the time (7%) and don't even notice it.

 The trick is that they restrict on diffusion, so they are trying to trick you into working them up. They are benign… leave them alone.

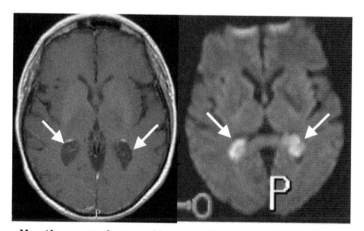

Xanthogranuloma - Note the Restricted Diffusion

Misc:

Mets - The most common location of intraventricular metastasis is the trigone of lateral ventricles (because of the vascular supply of the choroid). The most common primary is controversial - and either lung or renal. If forced to pick I'd go Lung because it's more common overall. I think all things equal renal goes more - but there are less renal cancers. It all depends on how the question is worded.

Colloid Cyst – These are found almost exclusively in the anterior part of the 3rd ventricle behind the foramen of Monro.

They **can cause sudden death via acute onset hydrocephalus**.

Their appearance is somewhat variable and depends on what they are made of. If they have cholesterol they will be T1 bright, T2 dark. If they don't, they can be T2 bright. The trick is a round well circumscribed mass in the anterior 3rd ventricle. If shown on CT, it will be pretty dense.

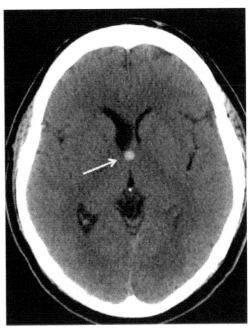

Colloid Cyst -
- Anterior 3rd Ventricle
- Hyperdense on CT

Meningioma – Can occur in an intraventricular location, most commonly (80%) at the **trigone of the lateral ventricles** (slightly more on the left). Details on meningiomas are discussed on the following page.

Cerebellar Pontine Angle (CPA)

Age is actually less of an issue here because the DDx isn't that big. Most of these are adult tumors, but in the setting of NF-2 you could have earlier onset.

Epidemiology: Vestibular Schwannoma is #1 - making up 75% of the CPA masses, #2 is the meningioma making up 10%, and the Epidermoid is #3 making up about 5%. The rest are uncommon.

(75 %) Schwannoma (Vestibular) – These guys account for 75% of CPA masses. When they are bilateral you should immediately think **NF-2** (*one for each side*). Enhances strongly but more heterogeneous than meningomas. May widen the porus acousticus resulting in a "trumpet shaped" IAC. *"Ice Cream Cone IAC."*

Schwannoma	Meningioma
Enhance Less Homogeneously	Enhance Homogeneously
Invade IAC	Don't Usually Invade IAC
IAC can have "trumpeted" appearance	Calcify more often

(10 %) Meningioma – Second more common CPA mass. One of the few brain tumors that is more common in women. They can calcify, and if you are lucky they will have a dural tail (which is pretty close to pathognomonic – with a few rare exceptions). Because they are extradural they will enhance strongly. Radiation of the head is known to cause meningiomas.

 Trivia:

•Most common location of a meningioma is over the cerebral convexity.

 •Meningiomas take up octreotide and Tc-MDP on Nuclear Medicine tests (sneaky).

(5 %) Epidermoid –

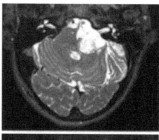

Can be congenital or **acquired** (after trauma – classically after LP in the spine). Unlike dermoids they are usually off midline. They will follow CSF density and intensity on CT and MRI (the exception is this zebra called a *"white epidermoid"* which is T1 bright – just forget I ever mentioned it).

 The key points are

(1) Unlike an arachnoid cyst they are bright on FLAIR (sometimes warm - *they don't completely null)*, and

 (2)They **will restrict diffusion**.

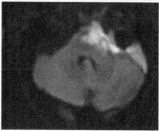

Epidermoid - Follows CSF Signal - Restricts Diffusion

Dermoid Cyst – This is about 4x less common than an epidermoid. It's more common in kids / young adults. Usually midline, and usually are found in the 3rd decade. They contain lipoid material and are usually hypodense on CT and very bright on T1. They are associated with NF2.

 Trivia -

 •These are usually midline

 •Most common location for a dermoid cyst is the suprasellar cistern (posterior fossa is #2)

The Ruptured Dermoid

It is possible for a dermoid cyst to explode -rare in real life, common on multiple choice. Sometimes this is after a trauma, but usually it's spontaneous. The most common clinical scenario is "headache and seizure" - which is pretty much every brain tumor, so that is not helpful. What is helpful is this:

• Buzzword: *"Chemical Meningitis"*

• Aunt Minnie Appearance: <u>Fat droplets</u> (typically shown as low density on CT, or High Signal on T1) <u>floating in the ventricles</u> and/or subarachnoid space.

THIS vs THAT: *Dermoid vs Epidermoid* — The easy way to think of this is that the Epidermoid behaves like CSF, and the Dermoid behaves like fat.

IAC Lipoma - It can occur, and is basically the only reason you get a T1 when you are working up CPA masses. It will fat sat out - because it's a lipoma. There is an association with sensorineural hearing loss, as the vestibulocochlear nerve often courses through it.

Arachnoid Cyst – Common benign lesion that is located within the subarachnoid space and contains CSF. They are increased in frequency in mucopolysaccharidoses (as are perivascular spaces). They are **dark on FLAIR** (like CSF), and **will NOT restrict diffusion**.

How can you tell an epidermoid from an arachnoid cyst?

The epidermoid restricts, the arachnoid cyst does NOT.

Infratentorial - Most are PEDS (Hemangioblastoma is the exception).

Atypical Teratoma / Rhabdoid Tumor ("AT/RT")

– Highly malignant tumors (WHO IV), and rarely occur in patients older than 6 years. The average age is actually 2 years, but they certainly occur in the first year of life.

They can occur in supra and infratentorial locations (most common in the cerebellum). These are usually **large, pissed off looking tumors with necrosis** and heterogeneous enhancement. They believe in nothing Lebowski. They fuck you up. They take the money.

 Buzzword =
"Increased Head Circumference"

THIS vs THAT:
AT/RT vs Medulloblastoma

Both are WHO Grade 4 destroyers (AT/RT is worse) that are often seen in the posterior fossa of a kid.

Technically they are both subtypes of Medulloblastoma - but that's the kind of knowledge that causes you to miss multiple choice questions. For the purpose of multiple choice:

- AT/RT is a 2 year old
- Medulloblastoma is a 6 year old

- AT/RT has calcifications
- Medulloblastoma does not

Medulloblastoma & Ependymoma : *Both are discussed with the IV lesions*

Juvenile Pilocytic Astrocytoma (JPA):

Just think cyst with a nodule in a kid.

They are WHO grade 1, but the nodule will still enhance. This will be located in the posterior fossa (or optic chiasm).

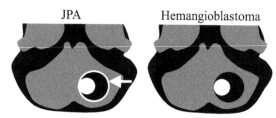
JPA   Hemangioblastoma

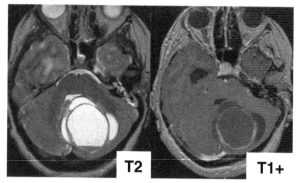
T2   **T1+**

Pilocytic Astrocytoma: Cyst + Nodule in Kid

Gamesmanship — if they don't tell you the age, you can look for enhancement of the cystic wall which JPA can have (~50%) but Hemangioblastomas don't

Hemangioblastoma: First things first – immediately think about this when you see a **cyst with a nodule** in an ADULT. Then think **Von Hippel Lindau**, especially if they are multiple. These things are slow growing, indolent vascular tumors, that can cause hydrocephalus from mass effect. 70% of the time you will see flow voids along the periphery of the cyst. About 90% of the time they are found in the cerebellum. There is an association with <u>polycythemia</u>.

> I Say Posterior Fossa Cyst with a Nodule - PEDS,
>
> you say JPA
>
> I say Posterior Fossa Cyst with a Nodule - ADULT,
>
> you say Hemangioblastoma

Ganglioglioma: Occurs at any age, anywhere, can look like anything - see cortical lesions.

Diffuse Pontine Glioma (DPG): Seen in kids age 3-10. Most common location is the pons, which is usually a high grade fibrillary glioma. It's going to be T2 bright with subtle or no enhancement. 4th ventricle will be flattened. Imaging features are so classic that no biopsy is needed.

Supratentorial - Adults Tumors

Astrocytoma: Most common primary brain tumor in adults. There is a trend towards "genetically classifying" tumors – this actually changes the way they are treated and could be the source of trivia. I'm going to attempt to simply this – because it can get pretty fucking complicated.

In the simplest terms, you have the neurons and you have the glial cells. The glial cells are the "support staff" — there are lots of them and lots of different kinds. Astrocytes and Oligocytes share a common origin (both are support staff – "glial cells") and have a lot of similarities. In other words, they are both "Gliomas" and are going to get lumped together in this discussion.

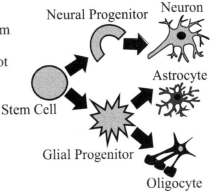

The new way to think about these things is a spectrum of severity based on genetic classification – and the treatment and prognosis follows that.

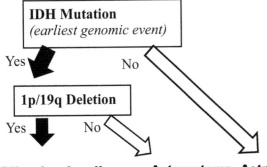

IDH Mutation
(earliest genomic event)

Yes → No →

1p/19q Deletion

Yes → No →

IDH Mutation
(earliest genomic event)

Yes (10%) → No (90 %) →

Oligodendroglioma

Calcification on preoperative CT is associated with codeletion (1p/19q)

Astrocytoma
Low Grade

Astrocytoma
Higher Grade
-Grade 2 – Diffuse
-Grade 3 - Anaplastic

T2 - FLAIR
Mismatch Sign

Astrocytoma
Grade 4 –
Glioblastoma
- Younger Patients
-Better prognosis
-Probably "Secondary GBM" from progression of a previous lower-grade tumor

Astrocytoma
Grade 4 –
Glioblastoma
-Older Patients
-The Worst Prognosis
-Probably "Primary GBM"

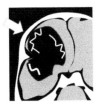

Ribbon pattern of calcification Classic for Oligodendroglioma

Bad Prognosis   **Really Bad Prognosis**   **Abandon All Hope** →

You probably noticed me using this WHO classification (1-4). All brain tumors are bad, but 4 is the worst - this is your GBM. On the following page, I'll get into a few more details on each type but as a general rule low grade tumors don't typically enhance (WHO 2) and higher grades do (mild for grade 3, and intense for grade 4 GBM). The exception to this rule is the pilocytic astrocytoma which often has an enhancing nodule, and the Subependymal Giant Cell Astrocytomas which enhances because of its location (Intraventricular).

GBM is the beast that cannot be stopped. It believes in nothing Lebowski. It grows rapidly, it can necrose (creating the ring of enhancement, with a non-enhancing central necrotic core) , it can cross the midline, and it can restrict diffusion. Remember **Turcot Syndrome** (*that GI polyp thing*), and NF 1 are associated with GBMs.

Astrocytoma *Grade 1*	Astrocytoma *Grade 2 - Diffuse*	Astrocytoma *Grade 3 - Anaplastic*	Astrocytoma *Grade 4- **GBM***
Subependymal Giant Cell Astrocytomas -Intraventricular mass near the foramen of Monro in a *young patient with tuberous sclerosis.* -Can cause obstructive hydrocephalus	White Matter is Preferred **NO** ENHANCEMENT T2 Bright – FLAIR Iso (mismatch sign)	White Matter is Preferred **Mild** ENHANCEMENT T2 Bright – FLAIR Iso (mismatch sign)	White Matter is Preferred - can cross the midline. **RING** ENHANCEMENT (can also be diffuse heterogenous enhancement) T2 & FLAIR Bright
Pilocytic Astrocytoma - Cyst with nodule in the posterior fossa of a kid Remember these tumors break the rule – and enhance despite being low grade.	T2 / FLAIR Mismatch: Seen with WHO 2 (diffuse) and 3 (anaplastic) astrocytoma, not with WHO 1. T2 tumor has high signal with surrounding vasogenic edema. On FLAIR the tumor signal become isointense.		Central locations (like the thalamus) are worse than normal. NF type 1, <u>Turcot syndrome</u> , Li Fraumeni syndrome

Gliomatosis Cerebri: A diffuse glioma with extensive infiltration. It involves at least 3 lobes and is often bilateral. The finding is usually mild blurring of the gray-white differentiation on CT, with extensive T2 hyperintensity and little mass effect on MR. It's low grade, so it **doesn't typically enhance**.

Mets: The most common supratentorial mass. Just like mets favor the lower lobes in the lungs, the cerebrum is favored over the cerebellum (it is a blood flow thing). They are usually multiple, but can be solitary — some sources say 50% of the time, so don't be fooled a solitary lesion can totally be a met. Some other trivia worth knowing — <u>melanoma can be T1 bright even if it doesn't bleed</u>. CT-MR is a good way to remember the ones that like to bleed (<u>C</u>horiocarcinoma / <u>C</u>arcinoid, <u>T</u>hyroid, <u>M</u>elanoma, <u>R</u>enal).

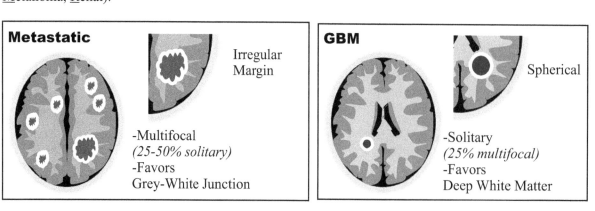

Metastatic — Irregular Margin
-Multifocal *(25-50% solitary)*
-Favors Grey-White Junction

GBM — Spherical
-Solitary *(25% multifocal)*
-Favors Deep White Matter

Supratentorial - Adults Tumors - Continued

Primary CNS Lymphoma: Seen in end stage AIDS patients, and those post-transplant. EB virus plays a role. Most common type is **Non-Hodgkin B cell**.

*Classic picture would be an intensely enhancing homogeneous solid mass in the periventricular region, with **restricted diffusion**.* However, it can literally look like and do anything.

 Classic Multiple choice test question is that it is **Thallium Positive on SPECT** (toxo is not).

 I say restricting brain tumor, you say Lymphoma (although GBM can do this also)

THIS vs THAT: Periventricular / Ependymal Enhancement Patterns

Thin Smooth and Linear

Ependymitis - (Classic Example = CMV)

Thick and Irregular

Lymphoma *"Rim Phoma"*

Supratentorial - Peds Tumors

DNET & PXA (Pleomorphic Xanthroastrocytoma):
Discussed under the cortical tumors .

Desmoplastic Infantile Ganglioglioma / Astrocytoma "DIG":

These guys are **large cystic tumors** that like to involve the superficial cerebral cortex and leptomeninges. Unlike the Atypical Teratoma / Rhabdoid, these have an ok prognosis (WHO 1). They **ALWAYS arise in the supratentorial location,** usually involve more than one lobe (frontal and parietal most commonly), and usually <u>present before the first birthday.</u>

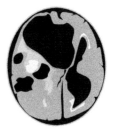

Big Cystic Tumor with Hydro

 -**Buzzword** is "rapidly increasing head circumference."

Skull Base:

Chordoma – This is a locally aggressive tumor that originates from the notochord. *WTF is the "notochord" ?* It's an embryology thing that is related to spine development.

The thing you need to know is that the notochord is a midline structure. Therefore all Chordomas are midline - either in the clivus, vertebral bodies (especially C2), or Sacrum. You can NOT get them in the hips, ribs, legs, arms, or any other structure that is not totally midline along the axis of the axial skeleton.

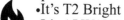

- •It is most common in the sacrum (#2 is the clivus)
- •When it involves the spine, it's most common at C2 - but typically extends across a disc space to involve the adjacent vertebral body.
- •It's T2 Bright
- •It's ALWAYS Midline. — it is never in a leg, arm, etc... ONLY MIDLINE structures.

Chondrosarcoma – This is the main differential of the chordoma in the clivus. The thing to know is that it is **nearly always lateral to midline** *(chordoma is midline)*. These are also T2 bright, but will have the classic "arcs and rings" matrix of a chondrosarcoma. Obviously you'll need a CT to describe that matrix.

Dura:

Meningioma – As described above, it is common and enhances homogeneously. The most common location is over the cerebral convexity and it has been <u>known to cause hyperostosis</u>.

Hemangiopericytoma – This is a soft tissue sarcoma that can **mimic an aggressive meningioma** because they both enhance homogeneously. They also can mimic a dural tail, with a narrow base of dural attachment. They **won't calcify or cause hyperostosis , but will invade the skull.**

Mets – The most common met to the dura is from breast cancer. 80% will be at the gray-white junction. They will have more edema than a primary tumor of similar size.

Sella / Parasella - Adults

Pituitary Adenoma – The most common tumor of the sella. They are seen 97% of the time in adults. If they are greater than 1 cm they are "macroadenomas." When functional, most are prolactin secreting (especially in women). Symptoms are easy to pick up in women (menstrual irregularity, galactorrhea). Men tend to present later because their symptoms are more vague (decreased libido). On MR, 80% are T1 dark and T2 bright. They take up contrast more slowly than normal brain parenchyma. Next step = Dynamic contrast enhanced MR.

Things to know (about Pituitary adenomas):

- Microadenoma under 10 mm,
- Macroadenoma over 10 mm.
- Microadenomas typically form in the adenohypophysis (anterior 2/3).
- Prolactinoma is the most common functional type.
- Typically they enhance less than normal pituitary.

Pituitary Apoplexy – Hemorrhage or Infarction of the pituitary, usually into an enlarged gland (either from pregnancy or a macroadenoma). Here are the multiple choice trivia association: taking **bromocriptine** (or other prolactin drugs), "**Sheehan Syndrome**" in postpartum woman, Cerebral Angiography. They will be **T1 bright** (remember adenoma is usually T1 dark). Supposedly this is an emergent finding because the lack of hormones can cause hypotension.

Rathke Cleft Cyst – Usually an incidental finding. Rarely symptomatic. The "cleft" is between the anterior and posterior pituitary. They are variable on T1 and T2, but are usually very bright on T2. They do NOT enhance.

Epidermoid - Discussed on page 80. Remember these guys restrict diffusion.

I say "Midline Suprasellar Mass that Restricts Diffusion", You say Epidermoid.

Craniopharyngioma – They come in two flavors: (a) Papillary - 10% and (b) Adamantinomatous - 90%. The Papillary type is the adult type (Papi for Pappi). They are solid and do not have calcifications. They recur less frequently than the Adamantinomatous form (because they are encapsulated). They strongly enhance. The relationship to the optic chiasm is key for surgery. These things occur along the infundibulum. Pediatric type is discussed below (under on the next page with the peds tumors).

Sella / Parasella - Peds

Craniopharyngioma – As stated above, they come in two flavors: (a) Papillary and (b) Adamantinomatous. The kid type is the Adamantinomatous form. These guys are **calcified** (papillary is not). These guys recur more (Papillary does less – because it has a capsule).
Buzzword is "machinery oil."

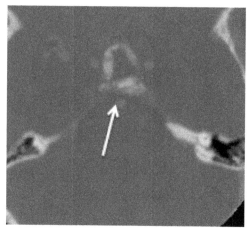

Craniopharyngioma
- *Shown on bone window*
- *Calcifications in the Sella*

- T1 Bright
- T2 Bright
- CT / GRE = Calcifications
- Enhance Strongly (in the solid parts)

Hypothalamic Hamartoma – A classic Aunt Minnie. This is a hamartoma of the tuber cinereum (part of the hypothalamus located between the mammillary bodies and the optic chiasm). The location is the key.

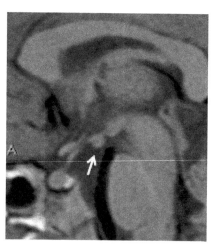

Hamartoma of the Tuber Cinereum

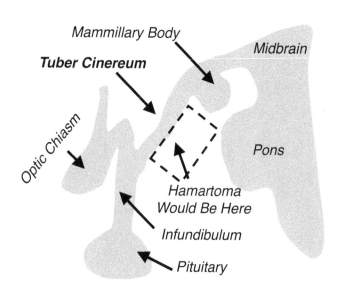

- T1 Iso
- T2 Iso
- Do NOT enhance.

 The Classic History is **Gelastic Seizures**
(although *precocious puberty is actually more common*).

Pineal Region -

There are 3 main characters here, all of which can present with "vertical gaze palsy" (dorsal Parinaud syndrome).

Germinoma: The **most common of the 3**, and seen almost exclusively in boys (Germinomas in the suprasellar region are usually in girls). Precocious puberty may occur from secretion of hCG. Characteristic findings are a **mass containing fat and calcification** with variable contrast enhancement. It is heterogeneous on T1 and T2 (because of its mixed components).

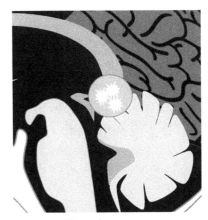

Germinoma:
"Engulfed" Calcification Pattern

Pineoblastoma: Does occur in childhood. Unlike the pineocytoma, these guys are **highly invasive**. Some people like to think of these as PNETs in the pineal gland. They are **associated with retinoblastoma ("trilateral").** They are heterogeneous and enhance vividly.

Pineocytoma: Rare in childhood. Well-circumscribed, and **non-invasive**. Tend to be more solid, and the solid components do typically enhance.

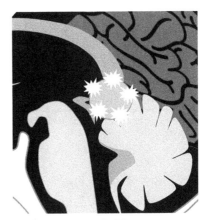

Pineoblastoma & Pineocytoma:
"Expanded" Calcification Pattern

Pineal Cyst - An incidental findings that is meaningless… although frequently obsessed over. They can have thin enhancement. Calcifications occur in 25%.

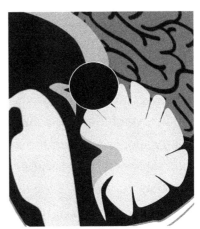

Pineal Cyst:
Classically— looks like a cyst

Special Topics - A Few Extra Tips on Characterization:

"Restriction"

If they show a supratentorial case with restriction it's likely to be one of two things (1) **Abscess** or (2) **Lymphoma**. Technically any hypercellular tumor can restrict (**GBM & Medulloblastoma**), but lymphoma is the one they classically show restricting.

If it's a CP angle case, then it's an **Epidermoid**.

Lastly, a dirty move could be to show **Herpes** encephalitis restricting in the temporal horns.

"Midline Crossing"

If they show it crossing the midline, it's most likely going to be a **GBM or Lymphoma**. Alternative sneaky things they could show doing this would be **radiation necrosis**, a big **MS** plaque in the corpus callosum, or Meningioma of the falx simulating a midline cross.

"Calcification"

If they show it in the brain it is probably an **Oligodendroglioma**. The trick is that Oligodendrogliomas calcify 90% of the time by CT (and 100% by histopathology), whereas astrocytomas only calcify 20% of the time. But astrocytoma is very common and oligodendroglioma is not. So in other words, in real life it's probably still an astrocytoma.

"T1 Bright"

Most tumors are T1 dark (or intermediate). Exceptions might include a tumor that has bled (Pituitary apoplexy or hemorrhagic mets). Hemorrhagic mets are classically seen on **MR** and **CT** (**M**elanoma, **R**enal, **C**arcinoid / **C**horiocarcinoma, **T**hyroid). Tumors with fat will also be T1 bright (Lipoma, Dermoid). Melanin is T1 bright (Melanoma). Lastly think about cholesterol in a colloid cyst.

T1 Bright:

Fat: Dermoid, Lipoma

Melanin: Melanoma

Blood: Bleeding Met or Tumor

Cholesterol: Colloid Cyst

Special Topics - Syndromes

NF-1	Optic Nerve Gliomas
NF-2	MSME: Multiple Schwannomas, Meningiomas, Ependymomas
VHL	Hemangioblastoma (brain and retina)
TS	Subependymal Giant Cell Astrocytoma, Cortical Tubers
Nevoid Basal Cell Syndrome (Gorlin)	Medulloblastoma
Turcot	GBM, Medulloblastoma, Intestinal Polyposis
Cowdens- "COLD"	Lhermitte-Duclos (Dysplastic Cerebellar Gangliocytoma)

MSME

If you see tumors EVERYWHERE then you are dealing with NF-2. Ironically there are no neurofibromas in neurofibromatosis type 2 (obviously that would make a great distractor).

Just remember **MSME**
- **M**ultiple **S**chwannomas,
- **M**eningiomas,
- **E**pendymomas

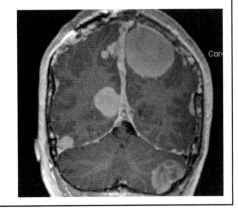

Lhermitte-Duclos *(Dysplastic Cerebellar Gangliocytoma)*

This thing is very uncommon, but when you see it you need to have the following thoughts:

- Hey! That is Lhermitte Dulcos….
- I guess she has Cowdens syndrome….
- I guess she has breast CA

Next Step? - Mammogram

The appearance is classic, with a "tiger stripe" mass, typically contained in one cerebellar hemisphere (occasionally crosses the vermis). It's not a "cancer", but actually a hamartoma - which makes sense since Cowdens is a hamartoma syndrome.

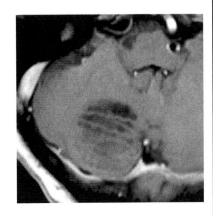

Brain Tumors - MRS Pearls

As cell walls get broken down NAA (a maker for neuronal viability) will go down, Creatine (marker for cellular metabolism) will go down, and Choline (a maker for cell membrane turnover) will go up. This is why the ratios of NAA/Cho, Cho/Cr and NAA/Cr get throw around.

Other relevant marker changes:

• **Lactate** may go up. You see this in the scenario of a high grade tumor outgrowing its blood supply and changing over to anaerobic pathways.

• **Lipids** may go up. You see this in the scenario of a necrotic tumor. Lipids are associated with necrosis.

• **Alanine** - is associated with meningiomas.

• **NAA** - This is a glioma maker. Non gliomas tend to have little or no NAA.

Tumor Grade:

Higher Grade Tumors will have more cellular destruction, inflammation, and more ischemia / necrosis.

Higher Grade Will Have:

Less NAA
Less Creatine
More Lactate
More Choline
More Lipids

Relative to a lower grade tumor.

Recurrent Tumor vs Radiation Necrosis

Recurrent Tumor: Rising choline infers that cell walls are being turned over (something is growing).

Mo Choline, Mo Problems

Radiation Necrosis: When you think necrosis you should think elevated lipids (found in necrotic tissue) and elevated lactate. You could also reason that NAA, Creatinine, and Choline (makers of cell integrity, metabolism, and turnover) would also be low - if the tissue in that region was fried like chicken (or bananas - if you enjoy denying your true nature as the apex predator).

GBM vs Met:

Both can look gnarly on conventional MR (big enhancing tumor).

The GBM is classically underestimated on brain MRI (if you are just looking at the solid enhancing tumor). The surround T2 edema often contains infiltrative mirco-tumor. By using a multiple voxel analysis (looking at the tumor, and also surrounding tissue) MRS supposedly adds value (allegedly).

For the purpose of multiple choice, <u>elevated Choline in the T2 signal surrounding the tumor = infiltrating glioma</u> (rather than a met)

Voxel Selection: It is important to choose an area of interest with enhancing tumor (avoid cystic parts of the tumor, calcifications, blood, or frank necrosis).

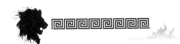 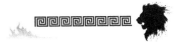

Neonatal Infections:

We are talking about TORCH infections. The first critical thing is that they only really matter in the first two trimesters (doesn't cause as much harm in the third trimester). Calcifications and microcephaly are basically present in all of them.

	Trivia	Classic Look	Highest Yield Trivia
CMV	**Most Common TORCH** (3x more common than Toxo – which is the second most common).	It prefers to target the germinal matrix resulting in periventricular tissue necrosis. The result is the most likely test question = **Periventricular calcifications**. Of the TORCHs **CMV has the highest association with polymicrogyria.**	Most Common TORCH Periventricular Calcifications Polymicrogyria
Toxoplasmosis	This is the second most common TORCH.	It's seen in the children of women who clean up cat shit. The calcification pattern is more random, and targets the basal ganglia (like most other TORCH infections). The frequency is increased in the 3rd trimester (but only causes a problem in the first two). Associated with **Hydrocephalus**.	Hydrocephalus, Basal Ganglia Calcifications
Rubella	Less common because of vaccines	Calcifications are less common than in other TORCHs. Focal high T2 signal might be seen in white matter (related to vasculopathy and ischemic injury).	Vasculopathy / Ischemia. High T2 signal Fewer Calcifications
HSV	It's HSV-2 in 90% of cases.	Unlike adults, the virus does not primarily target the limbic system but instead prefers the endothelial cells resulting in **thrombus and hemorrhagic infarction** with resulting **encephalomalacia** and **atrophy.**	Hemorrhagic Infarct, with resulting Bad Encephalomalacia (Hydranencephaly)
HIV	Not a TORCH but does occur during pregnancy, at delivery, or via breast feeding.	You may have faint basal ganglia enhancement seen on CT and MRI preceding the appearance of basal ganglia calcification. Brain atrophy pattern favors the Frontal Lobes	**Brain Atrophy, predominantly in the Frontal Lobes**

Infections of the Immunosuppressed (people with AIDS)

The most common opportunistic infection in patients with AIDS is toxo. The most common fungal infection (in people with AIDS) is Cryptococcus. Two other infections worth talking about are JC Virus, and CMV.

Gamesmanship:
- Nipple Rings = AIDS
- From South Africa = AIDS

HIV Encephalitis:

The encephalitis that people with AIDS get. This is actually pretty common and affects about 50% of AIDS patients.

We are talking about a situation with a CD4 < 200.

Symmetric increased T2 / FLAIR signal in the deep white matter.

T1 will be normal.

The lesions will not enhance.

These tend to **spare the subcortical U-fibers** *(PML will involve them)*.

There may be associated brain atrophy.

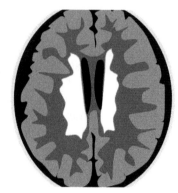

HIV Encephalitis
-Symmetric, and Spare Cortical U Fibers

Progressive Multifocal Leukoencephalopathy (PML):

Caused by the JC virus.

We are talking about a situation with a CD4 < 50.

CT will show single or multiple scattered Hypodensities, with corresponding **T1 hypointensity** (remember HIV was T1 normal),

Will involve **subcortical U-fibers**

T2/FLAIR hyperintensities out of proportion to mass effect - buzzword

PML
-Asymmetric, and Involves Cortical U Fibers

CMV: Think about brain **atrophy**, periventricular hypodensities (that are T2/FLAIR bright), and thin **ependymal enhancement**.

Ependymal cells are the cells that line the ventricles and central portion of the spinal cord.

Cryptococcus: The most common fungal infection in AIDS. The most common presentation is meningitis that involves the base of the brain (leptomeningeal enhancement). The most likely way this will be shown on a multiple choice exam is **dilated perivascular spaces filled with mucoid gelatinous crap (these will not enhance)**. The second most likely way this will be shown is lesions in the basal ganglia "cryptoccomas" – these are T1 dark, T2 bright, and may ring enhance.

Infections of the Immunosuppressed (people with AIDS) - part 2

Toxo: Most common opportunistic infection in AIDS. Classically we are talking about T1 dark, T2 bright, ring enhancing (when larger than 1 cm) lesions. These guys will NOT show restricted diffusion. Just think **"ring enhancing lesion, with LOTS of edema."**

High Yield Trivia = Toxo is Thallium Cold, and Lymphoma is Thallium hot.

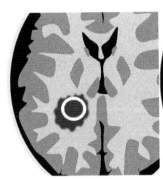 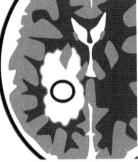 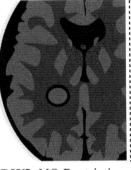

WTF ?!
I thought abscesses restrict diffusion?

Typical they do.

However, atypical infections like Toxo or fungal don't always follow this rule.

T1+C Ring Enhancing   **T2** Lots of Edema   **DWI:** NO Restriction

THIS vs **THAT:**	
Toxo	**Lymphoma**
Ring Enhancing	Ring Enhancing
Hemorrhage more common after treatment	Hemorrhage less common after treatment
Thallium Cold	**Thallium HOT**
PET Cold *(acts like necrosis)*	PET Hot *(acts like a tumor)*
MR Perfusion: Decreased CBV	MR Perfusion: Increased (or Decreased) CBV

Infections of the Immunosuppressed (people with AIDS) - Summary

AIDS Encephalitis	PML	CMV	Toxo	Cryptococcus
Symmetric T2 Bright	Asymmetric T2 Bright	Periventricular T2 Bright	Ring Enhancement + Lots of Edema	Dilated Perivascular Spaces
	T1 Dark	<u>Thin</u> Ependymal Enhancement	No Restricted Diffusion	Basilar Meningitis
Spare U Fibers	Involve U Fibers		Thallium Cold	

Characteristic Infections:

TB Meningitis:

Has a predilection for the basal cisterns (**enhancement of the basilar meninges with minimal nodularity**).

May have dystrophic calcifications.

Complications include vasculitis which may result in infarct (more common in children). Obstructive hydrocephalus is common.

Enhancement of the Basilar Meninges + Hydrocephalus = TB

*Sarcoid can have a nearly identical appearance.
If it looks like TB - but that isn't a choice, it's probably Sarcoid.

HSV - "Herpes" or "The Dirty Herp"

HSV 1 in adults and HSV 2 in neonates. I mention that because

(1) It seems like testable trivia and

(2) They actually have different imaging appearances (as previously mentioned, type 1 prefers the limbic system).

Earliest Sign = Restricted Diffusion – related to vasogenic edema.

This could be tested by asking *"What sequence is more sensitive?"*, with the answer being that **diffusion is more sensitive than T2**.

Blooming on gradient means it's bleeding (common in adults, rare in neonate form).

For the purpose of a multiple choice test think swollen T2 bright (unilateral or bilateral) **medial temporal lobe**.

THIS vs THAT:

HSV **spares the basal ganglia** (distinguishes it from MCA stroke).

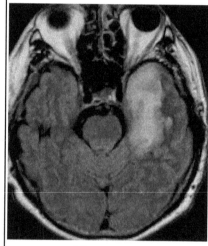

Herpes -
Edema in the Temporal Lobe

Limbic Encephalitis:

Not an infection, but a commonly tested mimic.

It is a **paraneoplastic syndrome (usually small cell lung cancer)**, that looks very **similar to HSV**.

This could be asked by showing a classic HSV image, but then saying the HSV titer is negative. The second order question would be to ask for lung cancer screening.

West Nile:

Several viruses characteristically involve the basal ganglia (Japanese Encephalitis, Murray Valley Fever, West Nile…), the only one realistically testable is West Nile.

Classic Look: **T2 bright basal ganglia and thalamus, with corresponding restricted diffusion.** Hemorrhage is sometimes seen.

CJD: Creutzfeldt-Jakob Disease

The imaging features are variable and can be unilateral, bilateral, symmetric, or asymmetric.

Three most likely testable appearances diagramed below.

Random Factoids:

- Characteristic look on EEG the *"periodic sharp wave"* (whatever the fuck that is).

- "14-3-3" protein assay is a CSF test neurologists order.

There are 3 types:

- Sporadic (80-90%),
- Variant "Mad Cow" (rare)
- Familial (10%).

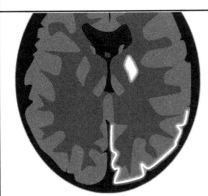

DWI Cortical Gyriform Restricted Diffusion–

Supposedly <u>diffusion is the most sensitive sign</u>, & the cortex is the most common early site of manifestation.

Basal Ganglia may also be involved.

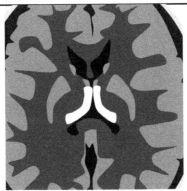

Hockey Stick Sign:
- Bilateral FLAIR bright dorsal medial thalamus
- Described in the variant subtype.

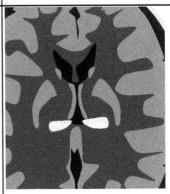

Pulvinar Sign:
- Bilateral FLAIR bright pulvinar thalamic nuclei (posterior thalamus).
- Classic in the variant subtype.

Another way to show this (which would be more work for the test writer - and is therefore less likely) would be a series of MRs or CTs showing <u>rapidly progressive atrophy.</u>

Neurocysticercosis

Caused by eating pig shit (or undercooked pork). The bug is tinea solium (pork tapeworm).

Trivia: <u>Involvement of the basal cisterns carries the worst outcome.</u>

Most common locations (in descending order):

1- Subarachnoid over the cerebral hemispheres,

2- Basal cisterns,

3- Brain parenchyma,

4- Ventricles

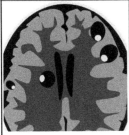

Stage 1: Vesicular
Cyst + Scolex
No Enhancement

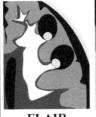

FLAIR   **T1+C**

Stage 2: Colloidal
CT: Hyperdense Cyst
MR: Edema + Enhancement

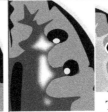

FLAIR   **T1+C**

Stage 3: Granular
CT: Early Calcification
MR: Smaller Cysts,
Less Edema,
Less Enhancement

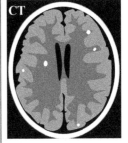

CT

Stage 4: Calcified / Involution
CT: Calcification
MR: Blooming on SWI (T2* etc..)

Meningitis and Cerebral Abscess

You can think of meningitis in 4 main categories: bacterial (acute pyogenic), viral (lymphocytic), chronic (TB or Fungal), and non-infectious (sarcoid).

Vocab

Leptomeningeal: Pial +Arachnoid
Pachymeningeal: Dural

Essentially, we are talking about thick leptomeningeal enhancement, in the appropriate clinical setting.

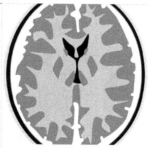

This pattern can be seen with Bacterial Meningitis or Carcinomatous Meningitis

Leptomeningeal (Pia-Arachnoid) Enhancement: Fills the subarachnoid spaces & <u>extends into the</u> sulci & cisterns.

Complications include:

Venous thrombosis,
Vasospasm (leading to the stroke),
Empyema,
Ventriculitis,
Hydrocephalus,
Abscess

Fungal and Carcinomatous meningitis tend to be "more lumpy" and "thicker"

A very testable piece of trivia is that infants will often get sterile reactive subdurals (much less common in adults).

Abscess Facts (trivia)
- DWI - Restricts
- MRS – Lactate High
- FDG PET – Increased Metabolic

Pachymeningeal (Dural) Enhancement

Key Feature: <u>Enhancement does NOT extend into the sulci</u>

Seen this with lots of stuff: Intracranial Hypotension, Dural attachment of a Meningioma , Sarcoid, TB, Wegener's , Fugal Infections.

Both Breast and Prostate Cancer can deposit a solitary dural met.

Secondary CNS Lymphoma is often extra-axial and can be dural based or fill the subarachnoid space (*"Rim Phoma"*)

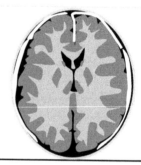

Empyema

Can be subdural or epidural (just like blood).

Follows the same rules as far as crossing dural attachments (epidurals don't) and crossing the falx (subdurals don't).

Subdurals are more common and have more complications relative to epidurals.

The vast majority of subdurals are the sequela of frontal sinusitis. The same is true of epidurals with some sources claiming 2/3 of epidurals are secondary to sinusitis.

Classic Look: **T1 bright** and **restrict diffusion**.

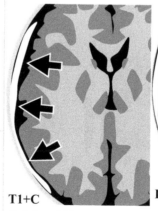
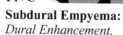
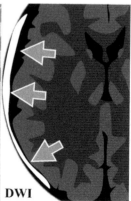

T1+C   DWI

Subdural Empyema:
Dural Enhancement,   *Restricts Diffusion*

Abscess: A cerebral abscess is a cavity that contains pus, debris, and necrotic tissue. These can develop secondary to to bacterial, fungal, or parasitic infection - most commonly via hematogenous spread. For the purpose of multiple choice, remember to think about right-to-left shunts and pulmonary AVMs. Direct spread (example = sinus) is possible, but just less common because of the dura.

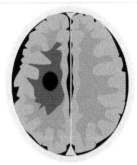 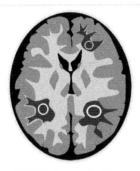 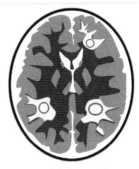 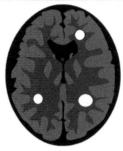

| CT: Focal area of low density with surrounding low density vasogenic edema. | T1+C: Smooth Ring Enhancement with Multiple Lesions - Suggests Abscesses | T2: Multiple Lesions with Vasogenic Edema — this is nonspecific (could be mets) | DWI: Typical Abscess (bacteria) will restrict. Remember Atypical (Toxo etc..) doesn't always restrict |

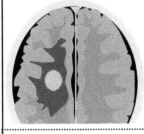 CT: Hypercellular Tumor (classic example would be Lymphoma) will be hyper dense instead on low density like an abscess

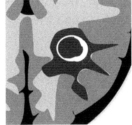 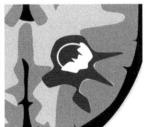

Multiple Rings Mets vs Abscess

The smooth margin suggests Abscess, but doesn't exclude mets. The difference is that tumor usually starts out as a solid enhancing mass then becomes ring enhancing with necrosis. Also, Abscesses tend to be smaller (usually less than 10mm).

Smooth Ring = Abscess | Irregular Ring = Tumor

Abscess Rings tend to be thicker on the "Oxygen Side" or "Grey Matter Side" of the Brain - and thinner towards the ventricle.

"Bumpy" or "Shaggy" inner lip of the ring is supposed to suggest necrosis

Both Tumor & Abscess will have Vasogenic Edema

Cerebritis is the early form of intra-axial infection, which can lead to **Abscess** if not treated. The typical look is the vasogenic edema without the well defined central enhancing lesion. There may be spotty restricted diffusion.

Ventriculitis: Usually the result of a shunt placement or intrathecal chemo - as discussed on page 51. The ventricle will enhance and you can sometimes see ventricular fluid-fluid levels

If septa start to develop you can end up with obstructive patterns of hydrocephalus.

The intraventricular extension of abscess is a very serious / ominous "pre-terminal event".

MRI Gamesmanship - Enhancement Patterns

In general, to solve MR puzzles you will need to be able to work through some MR sequences. The trick is to have a list of things that are T1 bright, T2 bright, Restrict diffusion, and Enhance. Plus you should know the basic enhancement patterns (homogenous, heterogenous, ring, and incomplete ring).

STROKE vs TUMOR vs ABSCESS vs MS Plaque

T2: For the most part, T2 is not super helpful for lesion characterization
- as stroke, tumors, abscess, MS, all have edema.

DWI: This is helpful only if they follow the classic rules. Out of those 4 (stroke, tumors, abscess, MS) the classical diffusion restrictors are: Abscess, and Stroke. Certain hypercellular tumors (classically lymphoma) can restrict, and demyelinating lesions with acute features can restrict.

Enhancement: In this situation this is probably the most helpful.
Out of those 4 (Tumor, Abscess, MS, and Stroke) each should have a different pattern.

- *Tumor* usually heterogeneous or homogenous if high grade (or none if low grade). Technically ring enhancement can also be seen with Gliomas, and Mets (though I expect this is less likely to be shown on multiple choice).

- *Abscess* will classically have RING pattern.

- *MS* will classically have an INCOMPLETE RING pattern.

- *Stroke* will have cortical ribbon (GYRIFORM) type enhancement in the sub-acute time period (around 1 week).

> ### How Many Rings ?
>
> The number of rings can be a helpful strategy. <u>A single ring is more likely to be tumor</u> (around half of mets and 3/4 of gliomas are solitary).
>
> Abscess and MS Lesions are almost always (like 75-85%) multiple.

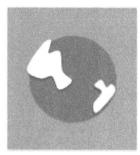  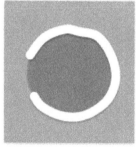 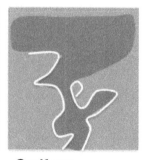

Heterogeneous
-Most likely Tumor (higher grade)

Ring
-Can be lots of stuff: <u>Abscess</u> and Tumor are both prime suspects

Incomplete Ring
-Classic for <u>demyelinating lesion</u>

Gyriform
-Classic for <u>subacute stroke</u> *(can also be seen with PRES or encephalopathy / encephalitis)*

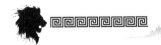 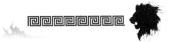
Parenchymal Contusion: The rough part of the skull base can scrape the brain as it slides around in a high speed MVA. Typical locations include the anterior temporal lobes and inferior frontal lobes. The concept of coup (site of direct injury) and contre-coup (opposite side of brain along vector of force). Contusion can look like blood with associated edema in the expected regions.

Diffuse Axonal Injury/Shear Injury: There are multiple theories on why this happens (different density of white and gray matter etc…) they don't matter for practical purposes or for multiple choice.

Things Worth Knowing:

- Initial Head CT is often normal

- Favorite sites of DAI are the posterior corpus callosum, and GM-WM junction in the frontal and temporal lobes

- Multiple small T2 bright foci on MRI

DAI Grading

Grade 1 = Grey-White Interface

Grade 2 = Corpus Callosum

Grade 3 = Brainstem

Subarachnoid Hemorrhage: Trauma is the most common cause. FLAIR is the most sensitive sequence. This is discussed in more later in the chapter.

THIS vs THAT: Subdural vs Epidural

Epidural	Subdural
Classic History: Trauma Patient – with a skull fracture	*Classic History:* Elderly alcoholic with a shriveled up atrophic brain spent the evening with a bottle of "Rotgut - Hobo Tranquilizer" brand whiskey, then fell over stretching & tearing his cortical bridging veins. A week later he seems to be acting progressively more confused.
"Bi-convex" or Lenticular	"Bi-concave"
Can cross the midline	Does not cross the midline, may extend into interhemispheric fissure
Can NOT cross a suture	Can cross a suture
Usually arterial	Usually venous
Can rapidly expand and kill you	More mass effect than expected for size

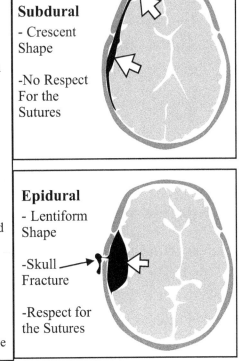

Subdural
- Crescent Shape

-No Respect For the Sutures

Epidural
- Lentiform Shape

-Skull Fracture

-Respect for the Sutures

How Old is that Blood?

CT: This is an extremely high yield topic. Maybe the most high yield topic in all of neuro, with regard to multiple choice. The question can be asked with CT or MRI (MRI more likely). If they do ask the question with CT it's most likely to be the subacute subdural that is isointense to brain, with loss of sulci along the margins. They could also show the "swirl sign" – see below.

Blood on CT	
Hyperacute Acute (< 1 hour)	Hypodense
Acute (1 hour – 3 days)	Hyperdense
Subacute (4 days – 3 weeks)	Progressively less dense, eventually becoming isodense to brain. **Peripheral rim enhancement may occur with contrast**.
Chronic (> 3 weeks)	Hypodense

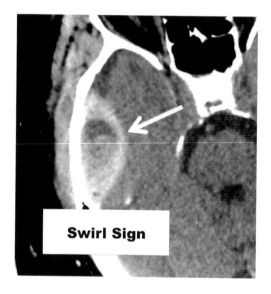

Swirl Sign

Swirl Sign – This is an ominous sign of active bleeding. The central low attenuation blood represents hyper-acute non-clotted blood, with surrounding acute clotted blood.

Blood Age Via MR:

MRI is more difficult to remember. Some people use the mnemonic "IB, ID, BD, BB, DD" or "**It Be Iddy Biddy, BaBy, Doo-Doo**" which I find very irritating. I prefer mnemonics that employ known words (just my opinion). Another one with actual words is "**G**eorge **W**ashington **B**ridge" For T1 (Gray, White, Black), and Oreo Cookie for T2 (Black, White, Black).

Blood Age Via MR (continued): Instead of memorizing baby babbling noises, I use this graph showing a clockwise movement. This thing may seem tricky and too much to bear, at first, but it does actually work and once you draw it twice, you'll have it memorized. You'll also notice a few things: (1) you won't feel like a dipshit for making baby noises, (2) you'll have a renewed sense of self-esteem, and (3) you are likely to notice marked improvement in your golf-swing.

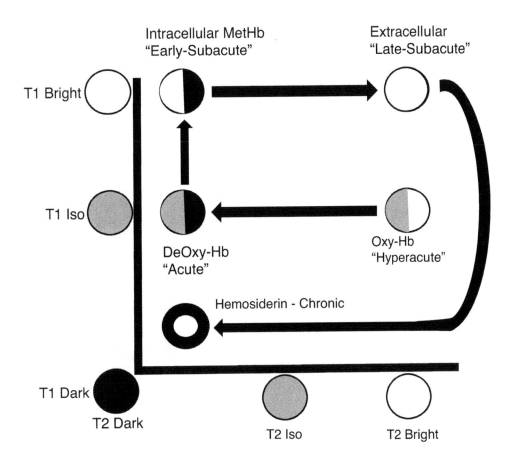

Another strategy (which is somewhat unconventional) is to actually try and understand the MRI changes (I strongly discourage this). If you insist on trying to understand this I have a 40 min lecture on TitanRadiology.com explaining it (this lecture is also free on my YouTube Channel — google "Prometheus Lionhart Blood Age").

Hyperacute	< 24 hours	Oxyhemoglobin, Intracellular	T1- Iso, T2 Bright
Acute	1-3 days	Deoxyhemoglobin, Intracellular	T1 – Iso, T2 Dark
Early Subacute	> 3 days	Methemoglobin, Intracellular	T1 Bright, T2 Dark
Late Subacute	>7 days	Methemoglobin, Extracellular	T1 Bright, T2 Bright
Chronic	> 14 days	Ferritin and Hemosiderin, Extracellular	T1/ T2 Dark Peripherally, Center may be T2 bright

Hemorrhage (Non-Traumatic)

Subarachnoid Hemorrhage:

Yes, the most common cause is trauma. A common point of trivia is that the **most sensitive sequence on MRI for acute SAH is FLAIR** (because it won't suppress out - making it hyperintense). Be aware that **supplemental oxygen** (usually 50-100%) **can give you a fake out that looks like SAH on FLAIR**.

When the blood is real, in the absence of trauma, there are a few other things to think about.

Aneurysm – Discussed later in the chapter.

Benign Non-Aneurysm Perimesencephalic hemorrhage: This is a well described entity (although not well understood). This is NOT associated with aneurysm (usually – 95%), and may be associated with a venous bleed. *You have to prove that - you need a negative CTA. The location of the blood – around the midbrain and pons without extension into the lateral Sylvian cisterns or interhemispheric fissures is classic. **Just think anterior to the brainstem**. Re-bleeding and ischemia are rare- and they do extremely well.

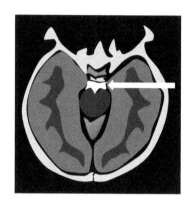

Superficial Siderosis: This is a side effect of repeated episodes of SAH. I like to think about this as *"staining the surface of the brain with hemosiderin."* The classic look is curvilinear **low signal on gradient coating the surface of the brain**. The classic history is **sensorineural hearing loss and ataxia**.

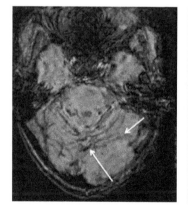 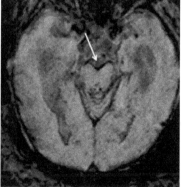

Superficial Siderosis - Hemosiderin Staining

Pseudo-Subarachnoid Hemorrhage

This is a described mimic of SAH that is seen in the setting of diffuse cerebral edema (most commonly anoxic brain injury). Near drowning, or suicide attempt by hanging would be classic clinical vignettes.

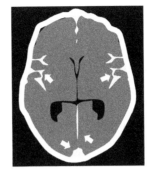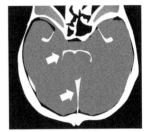

What you are seeing is actually two things at once. (1) You are seeing diffuse edema which lowers the attenuation of the brain (makes it darker). (2) You are seeing compression and collapse of the sub arachnoid spaces which gives them a hyper dense appearance. The combination of these factors gives the suggestions of hyper density in the cerebral sulci, fissures, and cisterns which can mimic SAH (hence the name).

THIS vs **THAT:** Pseudo SAH vs Real SAH: If they give you history that should help (anoxic brain injury vs headache / trauma). The absence of any intraventricular bleeding can suggest pseudo SAH. Lastly density of the Pseudo SAH will be less than 40. Acute blood tends to be around 60-70 HU.

Intraparenchymal Hemorrhage:

- **Hypertensive Hemorrhage:** Common locations are the basal ganglia, pons, and cerebellum. For the purpose of multiple choice tests, the **basal ganglia is the most common location (specifically the putamen).** You typically have intraventricular extension of blood.

- **Amyloid Angiopathy:** History of an old dialysis patient (or some other history to think Amyloid). *The classic look is multiple lobes at different ages with scattered microbleeds on gradient.*

- **Septic Emboli:** These are seen in certain clinical scenarios (**IV drug user**, organ transplant, cyanotic heart disease, AIDS patients, people with lung AVMs). **The classic look is numerous small foci of restricted diffusion. Septic emboli to the brain result in abscess and mycotic aneurysms (most commonly in the distal MCAs),** The location favors the gray-white interface and the basal ganglia. There will be surrounding edema around the tiny abscesses. The classic scenario should be parenchymal bleed in a patient with infection.

- **Other Random Causes:** These would include AVMs, vasculitis, brain tumors (primary and mets) - these are discussed in greater detail in various sections of the text.

Intraventricular Hemorrhage:

- Not as exciting. Just think about trauma, tumor, hypertension, AVMs, and aneurysms – all the usual players.

Epidural / Subdural Hemorrhage:

- Obviously these are usually post-traumatic.

- **Dural AVFs and High Flow AVMs** can bleed causing subdurals / subarachnoid hemorrhage. These are discussed further later in the chapter.

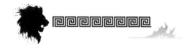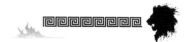
Stroke

Stroke is a high yield topic. You can broadly categorize stroke into ischemic (80%) and hemorrhagic (20%). It's critical to remember that stroke is a clinical diagnosis and that imaging findings compliment the diagnosis (and help exclude clinical mimic of stroke - tumor etc..).

Vascular Territories: Below is a diagram showing the various vascular territories. The junction between these zones is sometimes referred to as a "*watershed*". These areas are prone to ischemic injury, especially in the setting of hypotension or low oxygen states (near drowning or Roger Gracie's mounted cross choke or a Marcello Garcia high elbow guillotine).

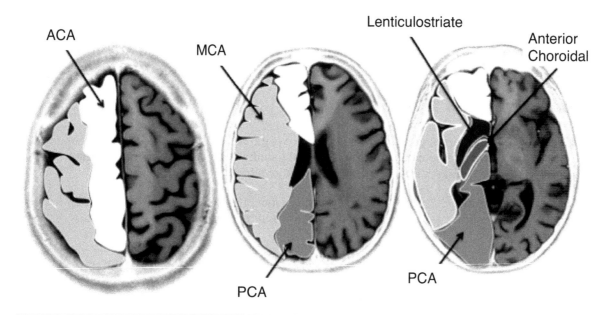

Watershed Ischemia favors the border zones of different vascular territories (just like the bowel).

The classic clinical scenario for watershed infarcts would be severe hypotension (shock / CPR / Etc..) , severe carotid stenosis, or a 2009 IBFFJ worlds match up with Roger Gracie.

 Gamesmanship: Watershed Infarcts in a Kid = Moyamoya (Idiopathic supraclinoid ICA vasculo-occlusive disease)

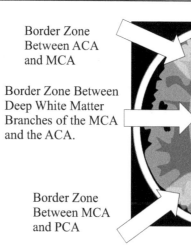

Border Zone Between ACA and MCA

Border Zone Between Deep White Matter Branches of the MCA and the ACA.

Border Zone Between MCA and PCA

Imaging Signs on CT:

Subacute Infarct:
Unique that it <u>Enhances but creates NO Mass Effect</u>

Dense MCA Sign	Intraluminal thrombus is dense, usually in the M1 and/or M2 segments
Insular Ribbon Sign	Loss of normal high density insular cortex from cytotoxic edema
Loss of GM-WM differentiation	Basal Ganglia / Internal Capsular Region and Subcortical regions
Mass Effect	Peaks at 3-5 days
Enhancement	Rule of 3s: Starts in 3 days, peaks in 3 weeks, gone by 3 months.

Fogging:

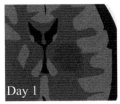 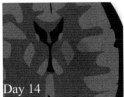 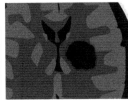

Day 1   Day 14

This is a phase in the evolution of stroke when the infarcted brain looks like normal tissue. This is seen around 2-3 weeks post infarct, as the edema improves.

"Fogging" is classically described with non-contrast CT, but T2 MRI sequences have a similar effect (typically occurring around day 10). In the real world, you could give IV contrast to demarcate the area of infarct or just understand that fogging occurs.

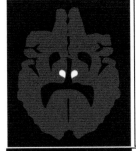

Artery of Percheron Stroke:

Classic V Shaped bilateral infarct of the paramedian thalami.

This can only occur in the setting of the Artery of Percheron vascular variant . This variant is characterized by a solitary trunk originating from one of the two PCAs to feed the rostral midbrain and both thalami (normally there are several bilateral paramedic arteries originating from the PCAs).

Recurrent Artery of Heubner Stroke

Classic Caudate Infarct

The Artery of H is a deep branch off the proximal ACA

This thing can get "bagged" during the clipping of ACOM artery aneurysm.

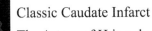

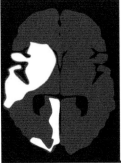 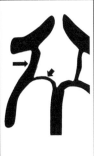

Cardioembolic Stroke:

This has the classic pattern of multiple foci of restricted diffusion scattered bilaterally along multiple vascular territories.

The clinical history is usually A-Fib or endocarditis.

Fetal PCOM Stroke Pattern

This pattern demonstrates infarcts in both the anterior and posterior circulation of the same hemisphere.

This pattern is possible as the variant anatomy with the PCA feeds primarily from the ICA.

Restricted Diffusion:

Acute infarcts usually are bright from about 30 mins after the stroke to about 2 weeks.

Restricted diffusion without bright signal on FLAIR should make you think hyperacute (< 6 hours).

Not Everything That Restricts is a Stroke
Bacterial Abscess, CJD (cortical), Herpes, Epidermoids, Hypercellular Brain Tumors (Classic is lymphoma), Acute MS lesions, Oxyhemoglobin, and Post Ictal States. Also artifacts (susceptibility and T2 shine through).

Enhancement: The rule of 3's is still useful. Starts day 3, peaks ~ 3 weeks, gone by 3 months.

	0-6 hours	6-24 hours	24 hours -1 week
Diffusion	Bright	Bright	Bright
FLAIR	**NOT BRIGHT**	Bright	Bright
T1	Iso	Dark	Dark, with Bright Cortical Necrosis
T2	Iso	Bright	Bright

Hemorrhagic Transformation:

This occurs in about 50% of infarcts, with the typical time period between 6 hours and 4 days. If you got TPA it's usually within 24 hours of treatment.

People break these into (1) tiny specs in the gray matter called "petechial" which is the majority (90%) and (2) full on hematoma – about 10%.

Who gets it? People on anticoagulation, people who get TPA, people with embolic strokes (especially large ones), people with venous infarcts.

Predictors of Hemorrhagic Transformation in Patients Getting TPA
• Multiple Strokes, • Proximal MCA occlusion, • **Greater than 1/3 of the MCA territory,** • Greater than 6 hours since onset "delayed recanalization", • Absent collateral flow

Venous Infarct:

Not all infarcts are arterial, you can also stroke secondary to venous occlusion (usually the sequelae of dural venous sinus thrombosis or deep cerebral vein thrombosis). In general, venous infarcts are at higher risk for hemorrhagic transformation. In little babies think dehydration, in older children think about mastoiditis, in adults think about coagulopathies (protein C & S def) and oral contraceptives. The most common site of thrombosis is the superior sagittal sinus, with associated infarct occurring 75% of the time.

Venous thrombosis can present as a dense sinus (on non-contrast CT) or "empty delta" (on contrast enhanced CT). Venous infarcts tend to have *heterogeneous restricted diffusion*. Venous thrombosis can result in vasogenic edema that eventually progresses to stroke and cytotoxic edema.

- Arterial stroke = Cytotoxic Edema

- Venous Stroke = Vasogenic Edema + Cytotoxic Edema

Stigmata of chronic venous thrombosis include the development of a dural AVF, and/or increased CSF pressure from impaired drainage.

ASPECTS (Alberta Stroke Program Early CT Score)

This was developed to give "providers" a more specific guideline for giving TPA - as an alternative to the previous 1/3 vascular territory rule. The idea being that the greater the vascular territory involved, the worse the clinical outcome (post TPA bleed etc..).

The way this works is that you start out with 10 points, and lose points based on findings of acute cytotoxic ischemia to various locations (example: minus 1 for caudate, or lentiform nucleus, or insular ribbon, etc.. etc.. so on and so forth).

Testable Pearls:

• This is for MCA ONLY (not other vascular territories)

• This is for ACUTE ischemia (don't subtract points for chronic lacunar infarcts etc..)

• A score of 8 or greater has a better chance of a good outcome (score of 7 or less may contraindicate TPA — depending on the institutional policy.

CT Perfusion - Crash Course

After an arterial occlusion perfusion pressure is going to be rapidly reduced. Millions of neurons will suddenly cry out in terror then suddenly silenced, unless they are lucky to have arteriolar dilation with capillary recruitment to bring in as much blood to that area of brain as possible. This process is called physiologic auto-*regulation* and should result in an increase in capillary blood pool. The key point is that you need live neurons (penumbra) to cry out for help. If they cry out and are suddenly silenced (infarct core) you won't see any auto regulation attempts. This physiology makes up the basis of perfusion for stroke.

Parameters:

• Cerebral Blood Flow (CBF): Represents instantaneous capillary flow in tissue.
• Cerebral Blood Volume (CBV): Describes the blood volume of the cerebral capillaries and venules per cerebral tissue volume.
• Mean Transit Time (MTT) = **CBV divided by CBF** ; it is the average length of time a certain volume of blood is present in the capillary circulation.
• Time to Peak (TTP): This is the opposite of CBF. Less flow = Longer Time to reach maximum concentration of contrast.

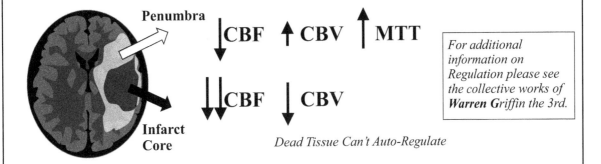

For additional information on Regulation please see the collective works of **Warren Griffin the 3rd.**

Dead Tissue Can't Auto-Regulate

The primary role of perfusion is to distinguish between salvagable brain (penumbra), and dead brain. The penumbra may benefit from therapy. The dead brain will not- *"He's Dead Jim"* - Dr. McCoy

Aneurysm

Who gets them? People who smoke, people with polycystic kidney disease, connective tissue disorders (Marfans, Ehlers-Danlos), aortic coarctation, NF, FMD, and AVMs.

Where do they occur? They occur at branch points (why do persistent trigeminals get more aneurysms ? – because they have more branch points). They favor the anterior circulation (90%) – with the **anterior communicating artery being the most common site**. As a piece of random trivia, the basilar is the most common posterior circulation location (PICA origin is the second most common).

When do they rupture? Rupture risk is increased with size, a posterior location, history of prior SAH, smoking history, and female gender.

Which one did it? A common dilemma is SAH in the setting of multiple aneurysms. The things that can help you are location of the SAH/Clot, location of the vasospasm, size, and which one is the most irregular *Focal out-pouching - "Murphy's tit"*)

Aneurysm Types:

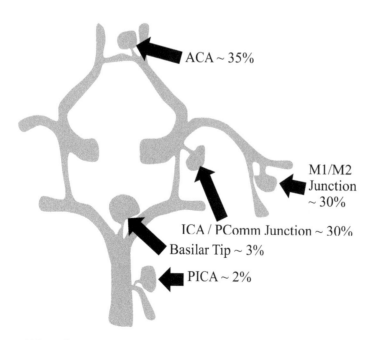

ACA ~ 35%

M1/M2 Junction ~ 30%

ICA / PComm Junction ~ 30%
Basilar Tip ~ 3%

PICA ~ 2%

Note that around 90% arise from the Anterior Circulation

Dolichoectasia of the Basilar Artery

This refers to a widened elongated twisty appearance of the basilar artery. This is probably the result of chronic hypertension (abnormal vessel remodeling).

The height of the bifurcation and the more lateral the position of the vessel (relative to the clivus) the more severe - so says the Smoker criteria.

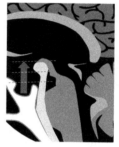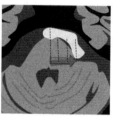

Complications include: nothing (most have no symptoms), dissection, compression of cranial nerves (hemi-facial spasm), stroke (brainstem), and hydrocephalus.

Saccular (Berry):

The most common type and the most common cause of non-traumatic SAH. They are commonly seen at bifurcations.

The underlying pathology may be a congenital deficiency of the internal elastic lamina and tunica media (at branch points).

Remember that most are idiopathic (with the associations listed above). They are multiple 15-20% of the time.

Aneurysm Types Continued:

Fusiform Aneurysm – Associated with PAN, Connective Tissue Disorders, or Syphilis. These more commonly affect the posterior circulation. May mimic a CPA mass.

Pseudoaneurysm – Think about this with an irregular (often saccular) arterial out-pouching at a strange / atypical location. You may see focal hematoma next to the vessel on non-contrast.

Traumatic – Often distal secondary to penetrating trauma or adjacent fracture.

Mycotic – Often distal (most commonly in the MCA), with the associated history of endocarditis, meningitis, or thrombophlebitis.

Blister Aneurysm – This is a sneaky little dude (the angio is often negative). It's broad-based at a non-branch point (supraclinoid ICA is the most common site).

Infundibular Widening – Not a true aneurysm, but instead a funnel-shaped enlargement at the origin of the Posterior Communicating Artery at the junction with the ICA. *Thing to know is "not greater than 3 mm."*

AVM Associated Pedicle Aneurysm:

Aneurysm associated with an AVM.

The trivia to know is that it's **found on the artery feeding the AVM** (15% of the time).

These may be higher risk to bleed than the AVM itself (because they are high flow).

Aneurysm Rupture Trivia:

- Aneurysm > 10mm have a 1% risk of rupture per year.

- Although controversial, 7 mm is often thrown around as a treatment threshold for anterior circulation aneurysms

- In general, posterior circulation aneurysms have a higher rate of rupture per mm in size.

Aneurysm Subtypes Summary

Saccular (Berry)	Branch Points – in the Anterior Circulation
Fusiform	Posterior Circulation
Pedicle Aneurysm	Artery feeding the AVM
Mycotic	Distal MCAs
Blister Aneurysm	Broad Based Non-Branch Point (Supraclinoid ICA)

Maximum Bleeding – Aneurysm Location

ACOM	Interhemispheric Fissure
PCOM	Ipsilateral Basal Cistern
MCA Trifurcation	Sylvian Fissure
Basilar Tip	Interpeduncular Cistern, or Intraventricular
PICA	Posterior Fossa or Intraventricular

Vascular Malformations

High Flow AVM	• Most Common Most Common Type of High Flow • Congenital malformation • Supratentorial location (Usually) • Most common complication = bleeding (3% annual) • Risk increased with: Smaller AVMs (they are under higher pressure), Small Draining Veins (can't reduce pressure), Perinidal Aneurysm, and Basal Ganglia location • Symptoms: Headache (#1), Seizure (#2)	Arterial Component Nidus Draining veins Adjacent brain may be gliotic (T2 bright) and atrophic.
Dural AVF	• Flow Rate is Variable (can be high or low flow) • SPINAL AVFs are actually the most common type of AVFs - a helpful hint is the classic clinical history of "gradual onset LE weakness" • Risk of Bleeding - increased with direct cortical venous drainage. • These aren't congenital (like AVMs) but instead are acquired — classically from dural sinus thrombosis • Symptoms: Tinnitus — especially if the sigmoid sinus is involved.	• No Nidus • Can be occult on MRI/MRA - need catheter angio if suspicion high
DVA	• Variation in normal venous drainage • Resection is a bad idea = venous infarct • **Associated with cavernous malformations.** • They almost never bleed in isolation. If you see evidence of prior bleeding (blooming on gradient) there is probably an associated cavernoma.	• "Caput medusa" or "large tree with multiple small branches" - collection of vessels converging towards an enlarged vein (seen on venous phase only). • Can have a halo of T2 bright gliosis.
Cavernous Malformation *(cavernoma, or cavernous angioma)*	• Low Flow - WITHOUT intervening normal tissue • Can be induced from radiotherapy • Can ooze some blood, but typically don't have full-on catastrophic bleeds. Presence of a "fluid-fluid" level suggests recent intralesional hemorrhage • Single or multiple (more common in Hispanics). • Classic gamesmanship is to show you a nearby DVA	• "Popcorn-like" with "Peripheral Rim of Hemosiderin." • Best seen on gradient
Capillary Telangiectasia	• Low Flow - WITH intervening normal tissue • Can also be radiation induced • Usually don't bleed (thought of as an incidental finding) • Classic Look = Single lesion in the Pons	• Brush-like" or "Stippled pattern" of enhancement • Best seen on gradient (slow flow and deoxyhemoglobin)
Mixed	• Wastebasket term, most often used for DVA with AV shunting or DVAs with telangiectasias	

Calcification Rapid Review / Summary

Pineal Gland - Common in adults, Rare in kids. If you see calcification in a kid under 7, it could suggest underlying neoplasm.
—Germinoma = "Engulfed" Pattern "1"
—Pineoblastoma & Pineocytoma: "Expanded" Pattern "2"

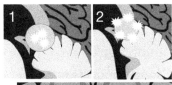

Habenular - Curvilinear structure (solid white arrow) located a few millimeters anterior to the pineal body (open arrow). About 1 in 5 normal adults will have calcification here. The trivia is an increased association with schizophrenia.

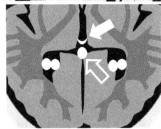

Choroid plexus - Common in adults. Remember there is no choroid plexus in the frontal/occipital horn of the lateral ventricles or the cerebral aqueduct.

Dural Calcifications - Common in adults. If the calcs are bulky and there are a bunch of tooth cysts (Odontogenic keratocysts) think Gorlin Syndrome.

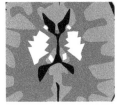

Fahr

Basal Ganglia - Very common with age, favors the globus pallidus. If extensive & symmetrical think Fahr disease.

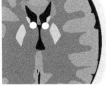 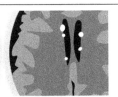

Tuberous Sclerosis - Calcifications of the subependymal nodules are pathognomonic typically found at the caudothalamic groove and atrium. You can see calcified subcortical tubers - more typical in older patients.

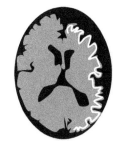

Sturge-Weber - Tram track / double-lined gyriform pattern parallel to the cerebral folds.

Etiology = subcortical ischemia secondary to pial angiomatosis.

Congenital **CMV** - Periventricular calcifications. Can also have brain atrophy

Congenital **Toxo** - Basal Ganglia Calcifications + Hydrocephalus,

Neurocysticercosis - Etiology: Eating Mexican pork sandwiches -end-stage will have scattered quiescent calcified cyst remnants.

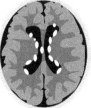 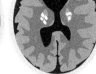

CMV   Toxo   Neurocysticercosis

Cavernoma— scattered dots or stippled "popcorn" calcification	Brain Tumors can calcify. The ones most people talk about are Old Elephants Age Gracefully
	O: Oligodendroglioma - variable, but "ribbon" pattern is most commoon E: Ependymoma (Medulloblastomas can also calcify - just less often) A: Astrocytoma G: Glioblastoma - mural calcified nodule
AVM — calcifications in the tortuous veins or the nidus	Even though more Oligodendrogliomas calcify, Astrocytoma is still the most common calcified tumor (because there are alot more of them).
	Craniopharyngioma, Meningioma, Choroid plexus tumors are all known to calcify as well. Osteosarcoma mets famously calcify.

Vasospasm

Vessels do not like to be bathed in blood (SAH), it makes them freak out (spasm). The **classic timing for this is 4-14 days after SAH (NOT immediately)**. It usually looks like smooth, long segments of stenosis. It typically involves multiple vascular territories. It can lead to stroke.

Who gets it? It's usually in patients with SAH and the more volume of SAH the greater the risk. In 1980 some neurosurgeon came up with this thing called the Fisher Score, which grades vasospasm risk. The gist of it is greater than 1 mm in thickness or intraventricular / parenchymal extension is at higher risk.

Are there Non-SAH causes of vasospasm? Yep. Meningitis, PRES, and Migraine Headache.

Critical Take Home Point - Vasospasm is a delayed side effect of SAH. It does NOT occur immediately after a bleed. You see it 4-14 days after SAH.

Vascular Dissection

Vascular dissection can occur from a variety of etiologies (usually penetrating trauma, or a trip to the chiropractor).

Penetrating trauma tends to favor the carotids, and blunt trauma tends to favor the vertebrals.

This would be way too easy to show on CT as a flap, so if it's shown it's much more likely to be the T1 bright "crescent sign", or intramural hematoma.

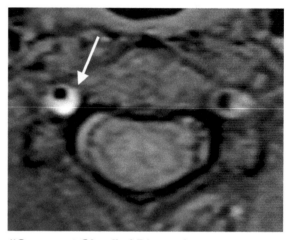

"Crescent Sign" of Dissection
- it's the T1 bright intramural blood.

Vasculitis

You can have a variety of causes of CNS vasculitis. One way to think about it is by clumping it into (a) Primary CNS vasculitis, (b) Secondary CNS vasculitis from infection, or sarcoid, (c) systemic vasculitis with CNS involvement, and (d) CNS vasculitis from a systemic disease.

Primary CNS Vasculitis	Primary Angiitis of the CNS (PACNS)
Secondary CNS vasculitis from infection, or sarcoid	**Meningitis** (bacterial, TB, Fungal), Septic, Embolus, Sarcoid,
Systemic vasculitis with CNS involvement	**PAN**, Temporal Arteritis, Wegeners, Takayasu's,
CNS vasculitis from a Systemic Disease	**Cocaine Use**, RA, SLE, Lyme's

They all pretty much look the same with multiple segmental areas of vessel narrowing, with alternating dilation ("beaded appearance"). You can have focal areas of vascular occlusion.

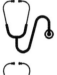 **Trivia:**

PAN is the Most Common systemic vasculitis to involve the CNS (although it is a late finding).

SLE is the Most Common Collagen Vascular Disease

Misc Vascular Conditions

Moyamoya – This poorly understood entity (originally described in Japan – hence the name), is characterized by progressive non-atherosclerotic stenosis of the supraclinoid ICA, eventually leading to occlusion. The progressive stenosis results in an enlargement of the basal perforating arteries.

 **Trivia:**

- Buzzword = *"Puff of Smoke"* – for angiographic appearance
- Watershed Distribution
- In a child think sickle cell
- Other notable associations include: NF, prior radiation, Downs syndrome
- Bi-Modal Age Distribution (early childhood and middle age)
- Children Stroke, Adults Bleed

Crossed Cerebellar Diaschisis (CCD):

Depressed blood flow and metabolism affecting the cerebellar hemisphere after a contralateral supratentorial insult (infarct, tumor resection, radiation).

Creates an Aunt Minnie Appearance:

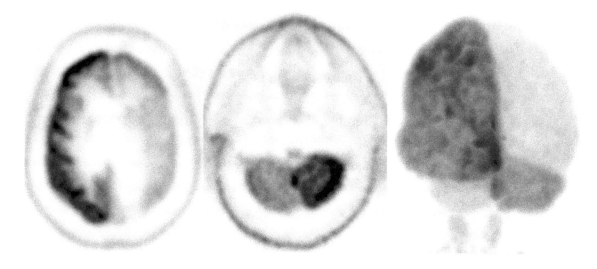

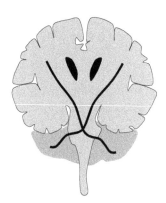

Mechanism / Gamesmanship: When I was a medical student, I had to memorize a bunch of tiny little tracks and pathways all over the brain, cerebellum, and spine. It (like many things in medical school) made me super angry because it was such a colossal waste of time. More PhD bullshit, lumped right in with those step 1 *"what chromosome is that on?"* questions.

Redemption for the PhDs has arrived. Apparently, one of these pathways, the *"corticopontine-cerebellar pathway,"* is actually important. Sorta....

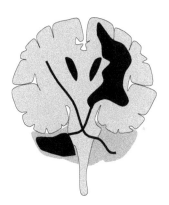

Allegedly, this pathway connects one cerebral hemisphere to the opposite cerebellar hemisphere. If the pathway gets disrupted (by tumor, radiation, etc...), then metabolism shuts down in the opposite cerebellum even though there is nothing structurally wrong with it. That is why you get this criss-crossed hypo-metabolic appearance on FDG-PET.

The trick is to show you the FDG-PET picture, and try and get you to say there is a pathology in the cerebellum. There isn't! The cerebellum is normal - the problem is in the opposite cerebrum where the pathway starts.

NASCET Criteria: The North American Symptomatic Carotid Endarterectomy Trial (NASCET) criteria, are used for carotid stenosis.

The rule is: measure the degree of stenosis using the maximum internal carotid artery stenosis ("A") compared to a parallel (non-curved) segment of the distal cervical internal carotid artery ("B").

You then use the formula:

[1- A/B] X 100% = % stenosis

Carotid endarterectomy (CEA) is often performed for symptomatic patients with > 50% stenosis.

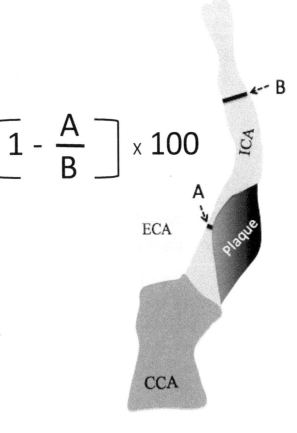

$$\left[1 - \frac{A}{B} \right] \times 100$$

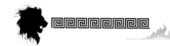 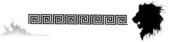
The LeFort Fracture Pattern System: In the dark ages, Rene LeFort beat the shit out of cadavers with clubs and threw them off buildings — it was "science". He then described three facial fracture patterns that interns in ENT and people who write multiple test questions think are important. It can be overly complicated but the most common way a test question is written about these is either by asking the buzzword or the essential component (or showing them).

 Buzzwords:

LeFort 1: "The Palate Separated from the Maxilla" or **"Floating Palate"**

LeFort 2: "The Maxilla Separated from the Face" or **"Pyramidal"**

LeFort 3: "The Face Separated from the Cranium"

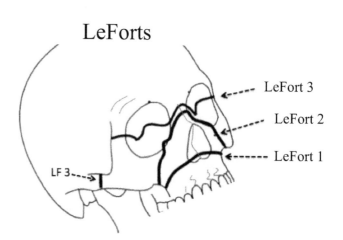

Essential Elements: All three fracture types share the pterygoid process fracture. If the pterygoid process is not involved, you don't have a LeFort. Each has a unique feature (which lends itself easily to multiple choice).

* LeFort 1: Lateral Nasal Aperture
* LeFort 2: Inferior Orbital Rim and Orbital Floor
* LeFort 3: Zygomatic Arch and Lateral Orbital Rim/Wall

Mucocele: If you have a fracture that disrupts the frontal sinus outflow tract (usually nasal-orbital-ethmoid types) you can develop adhesions, which obstruct the sinus and result in mucocele development. The **buzzword is "airless, expanded sinus."** They are usually T1 bright, with a thin rim of enhancement (tumors more often have solid enhancement). The frontal sinus is the most common location – occurring secondary to trauma (as described above). More on this later....

CSF Leak: Fractures of the facial bones, sinus walls, and anterior skull base can all lead to CSF leak. The most common fracture site to result in a CSF leak is the anterior skull base. *"Recurrent bacterial meningitis"* is a known association with CSF leak.

Temporal Bone Fractures:

The traditional way to classify these is longitudinal and transverse, and this is almost certainly how the questions will be written. In the real world that system is old and worthless, as most fractures are complex with components of both. The real predictive finding of value is violation of the otic capsule - as described in more modern papers.

Longitudinal	Transverse
Long Axis of T-Bone	Short Axis of T-Bone
More Common	Less Common
More Ossicular Dislocation	More Vascular Injury (Carotid / Jugular)
Less Facial Nerve Damage (around 20%)	More Facial Nerve Damage (>30%)
More Conductive Hearing Loss	More Sensorineural Hearing Loss

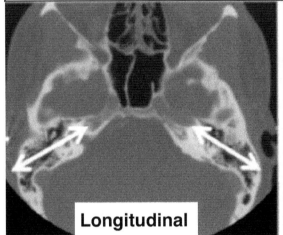

Longitudinal

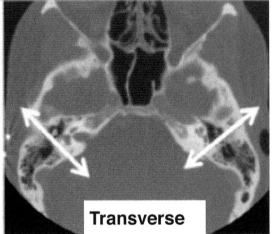

Transverse

Things to Know About Facial Fractures:

• Nasal Bone is the most common fracture

• Zygomaticomaxillary Complex Fracture (Tripod) is the most common fracture pattern, and involves the zygoma, inferior orbit, and lateral orbit.

• Le-Fort Fractures are both a stupid and a high yield topic in facial trauma – for multiple choice. Floating Palate = 1, Pyramidal = 2, Separated Face = 3

• Transverse vs Longitudinal Temporal Bone Fractures – this classification system is stupid and outdated since most are mixed and otic capsule violation is a way better predictive factor... but this is still extremely high yield

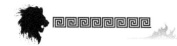 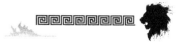

It would be very easy to get completely carried away with this anatomy and spend the next 20 pages talking about all the little bumps and variants. I'm gonna resist that urge and instead try and give you some basic framework. Then as we go through the various pathologies I'll try and give "normal" anatomy comparisons and point out some landmarks that are relevant for pathology. Additionally, I'm gonna do a full anatomy T-Bone talk for RadiologyRonin this year - so if your really want to understand this deeper, that might be helpful.

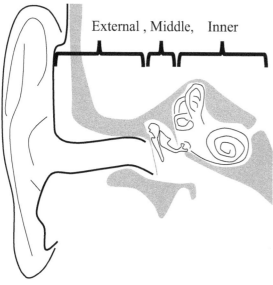

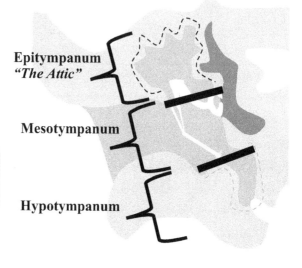

At the most basic level you can think about 3 general locations: External, Middle, and Inner.

The External ear is everything superficial to the ear drum (tympanic membrane).

The Inner ear is everything deep to the medial wall of the tympanic cavity.

The Middle ear is everything in-between.

A closer look at the middle ear gives us 3 more general locations

The Epitympanum, also called "the attic" is basically everything above the tip of the scutum (see below).

The Hypotympanum is everything below the tympanic membrane. This is where the Eustachian tube arises.

The Mesotympanum is everything in-between (or everything directly behind the ear drum).

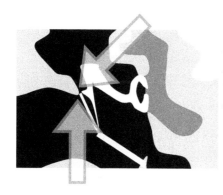

The **scutum** (arrows) is a "shield" like osseous spur formed via the lateral wall of the tympanic cavity. This anatomic land mark is often brought up with discussion of the erosion pattern of Cholesteatomas.

Cholesteatoma – The simple way to think about this is "a bunch of exfoliated skin debris growing in the wrong place." It creates a big inflammation ball which wrecks the temporal bone and the ossicles.

There are two parts to the ear drum, a flimsy whimpy part "Pars Flaccida", and a tougher part "Pars Tensa." The flimsy flaccida is at the top, and the tensa is at the bottom.

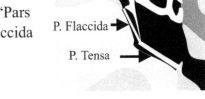

P. Flaccida →
P. Tensa →

If you "acquire" a hole with some inflammation / infection involving the Pars Flaccida you can end up with this ball of epithelial crap growing and causing inflammation in the wrong place.

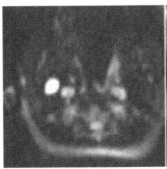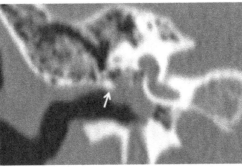

- Typical location of this soft tissue blob with erosion of scutum (arrow)

- They restrict diffusion

There are two subtypes based on the location.

Pars Flaccida Type	Pars Tensa Type:
<ul><li>Acquired Types are more common – typically involving the pars flaccida. They grow into **Prussak's Space**</li><li>The **Scutum is eroded early** (maybe first)- considered a very specific sign of acquired cholesteatoma</li><li>The Malleus head is displaced medially</li><li>**The long process of the incus is the most common segment of the ossicular chain to be eroded.**</li><li>Fistula to the semi-circular canal most commonly involves the lateral segment</li></ul>	•The inner ear structures are involved earlier and more often •This is less common than the Flaccida Type

Prussak's Space and Scutum Erosion:

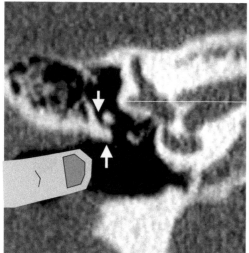

This is a coronal view of the T-Bone. To orient you I drew I cartoon finger in the ear. That finger is running right up to the ear drum (tympanic membrane). The membrane is usually too thin to see, but it's right around there. Remember the flimsy Flacida is at the top and the thicker Tensa is at the bottom.

There are two white arrows here.

The top arrow is pointing to a space between an ossicle (incus) and the lateral temporal bone. This is called **"Prussak's space"** and is the most common location of a Pars Flacida Cholesteatoma. Remember the incus was the most common ossicle eroded.

The bottom arrow is pointing to a bony shield shaped bone - "the **scutum**" which will be the first bone eroded by a pars flaccida.

Labyrinthine Fistula (perilymphatic fistula):

This is a potential complication of cholesteatoma (or other things - iatrogenic, trauma, etc…). What we are talking about here is a bony defect creating an abnormal communication between the normally fluid filled inner ear and normally air filled tympanic cavity. In the case of cholesteatoma, **the lateral semicircular canal** (arrows) **is most often involved.**

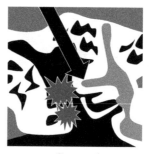 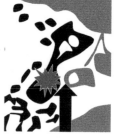

Coronal   Axial

The classic clinical history is "sudden <u>fluctuating</u> sensorineural hearing loss and vertigo."

On CT, you want to see the soft tissue density of the cholesteatoma eating through the otic capsule into the semicircular canal. The presence of air in the semicircular canal **(pneumolabyrinth)** is definitive evidence of a fistula (although it's not often seen in the real world).

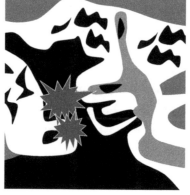 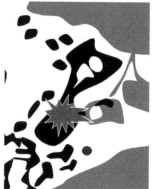

Otitis Media (OM) – This is a common childhood disease with effusion and infection of the middle ear. It's more common in children and patients with Down Syndrome because of a more horizontal configuration of the Eustachian tube. It's defined as chronic if you have fluid persisting for more than six weeks.

It <u>can look a lot like a cholesteatoma (soft tissue density in the middle ear)</u>.

THIS vs THAT:

	Chronic Otitis Media	Cholesteatoma
Mastoids	Poorly pneumatized	Poorly pneumatized
Middle Ear Opacification	Can completely opacity	Can completely opacity
For the Purpose of Multiple Choice - this could be a hint	Thickened mucosa	Non-Dependent Mass
Erosions (scutum and ossicular chain)	Rare (< 10%)	Common (75%)
Displacement of the ossicular chain	NEVER	It can happen

Complications of OM

Coalescent Mastoiditis	Erosion of the mastoid septae with or without intramastoid abscess
Facial Nerve Palsy	Secondary to inflammation of the tympanic segment (more on this later in the chapter).
Dural Sinus Thrombosis	Adjacent inflammation may cause thrombophlebitis or thrombosis of the sinus. This in itself can lead to complications: *Venous Infarct:* This can occur secondary to dural sinus thrombosis *Otitic Hydrocephalus:* Lateral sinus thrombosis can alter resorption of CSF and lead to hydrocephalus.
Meningitis, and Labyrinthitis	It can happen

Labyrinthitis Ossificans -

- Gamesmanship - *"history of childhood meningitis."*
- You see it in kids (ages 2-18 months).
- Classic Appearance on CT – *Ossification of the membranous labyrinth.*
- They present with sensorineural hearing loss.
- **Calcification in the cochlea is often considered a contraindication for cochlear implant.**

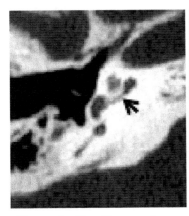 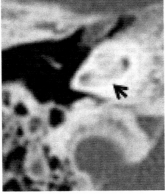

Normal - For Comparison   Labyrinthitis Ossificans

> *WTF is a "membranous labyrinth" ?*
>
> The world "Labyrinth" most commonly refers to the timeless 1986 science fiction adventure staring David Bowie as Jareth the Mother Fucking Goblin King.
>
> Another less popular use of the word "Labyrinth" is the anatomical blanket term encompassing the Vestibule, Cochlea, and Semicircular Canals.
>
> Under the umbrella of the "Labyrinth" you can have the *bony* portion (the series of canals tunneled out of the t-bone), and the *membraneous* portion (which is basically the soft tissue lining inside the bony part).
>
> You can then further divide the "membranous" portion into the cochlear & vestibular labyrinths.

Labyrinthitis – This is an inflammation of the membranous labyrinth, probably most commonly the result of a viral respiratory track infection. Acute otomastoiditis can also spread directly to the inner ear (this is usually unilateral). Bacterial meningitis can cause bilateral labyrinthitis.

Classic Look: The cochlea and semicircular canals will be shown enhancing on T1 post contrast imaging.

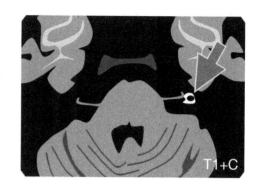

The Facial Nerve (CN 7)

Most people will describe 6 segments to the facial nerve.

- Intracranial ("Cisternal") segment
- Meatal ("Canalicular") segment - the part inside the Internal Auditory Canal "IAC").
- **Labyrinthine segment** (LS) - from the IAC to geniculate ganglion (GG).
- **Tympanic segment** (TS) - GG to pyramidal eminence
- **Mastoid segment** (MS) - from pyramidal eminence to stylomastoid foramen "SMF"
- Extratemporal segment - Distal to the SMF

Enhancement

The facial nerve is unique in that portions of it can enhance normally. The trick is which parts are normal and which parts are NOT.

Normal Enhancement: Tympanic & Mastoid Segments including the Geniculate Ganglia. The Labyrinthine segment can also sometimes.

No normal enhancement = Cisternal, Canalicular, or Extratemporal

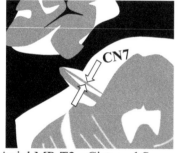

Axial MR T2 - Cisternal Segment -CN8 is posterior also entering the IAC

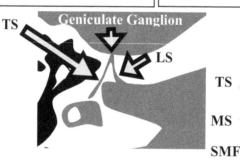

Axial CT- Level of IAC -the bend at the GG = "anterior genu" -

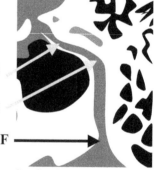

Sagittal CT-

What causes abnormal enhancement?
Big one is Bell's Palsy. Lymes, Ramsay Hunt, and Cancer can do it too.

When do you think Cancer ?
Nodular Enhancement.

When do you damage the facial nerve?
T-Bone fracture (transverse > longitudinal).

Bells Palsy & Ramsey Hunt

Bells: Etiology is probably viral. Usually a clinical diagnosis. Abnormal enhancement in the Canalicular Segment (in the IAC) is probably the most classic finding.

RH: Caused by reactivation varicella zoster virus. Classic rash around ear. CN 5 is usually also involved.

Otosclerosis (Fenestral and Retrofenestral):

A better term would actually be "otospongiosis," as the bone becomes more lytic (instead of sclerotic). When I say conductive hearing loss in an adult female, you say this.

Fenestral – This is **bony resorption anterior to the oval widow** at the fissula ante fenestram. If not addressed, the footplate will fuse to the oval window.

Retro-fenestral – This is a **more severe** form, which has progressed to have **demineralization around the cochlea**. This form usually has a sensorineural component, and is **bilateral and symmetric nearly 100% of the time**.

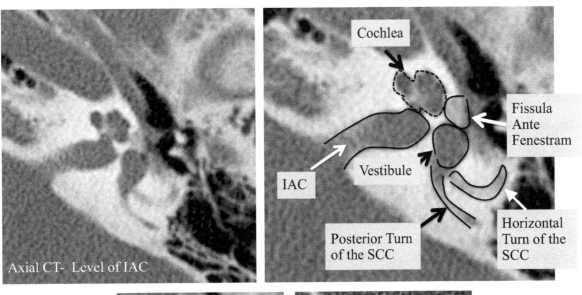

Bony resorption anterior to the oval widow at the fissula ante fenestram

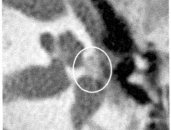

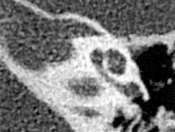

Normal Comparison

Treatment Options:

Early on (if the focus is small) dietary supplementation with Fluoride may be useful. Although this is controversial - may or may not work… and may or may not be part of a new world order David Icke Reptilian conspiracy to lower IQs (Alex Jones has the documents).

Later on they might try a stapedectomy (partial removal of the stapes with implantation of a prosthetic device) or a Cochlear implant.

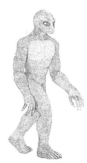

Slithery space born illuminati villains advocate for Fluoride treatment.

Superior Semicircular Canal Dehiscence

This is an Aunt Minnie. It's supposedly from long standing elevated ICP. The most likely way this will be asked is either (1) what is it? with a picture or (2) **"Noise Induced Vertigo"** or "Tullio's Phenomenon."

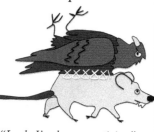
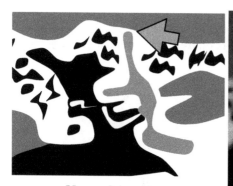

Normal Anatomy
Note the intact Bony Roof (Arrow)

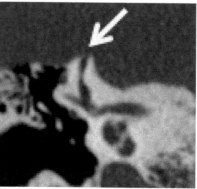

Superior Semicircular Canal Dehiscence Note the Absence of a Bony Covering

Large Vestibular Aqueduct Syndrome

The vestibular aqueduct is a bony canal that connects the vestibule (inner ear) with the endolymphatic sac. The enlargement of the aqueduct (> 1.5 mm) has an Aunt Minnie appearance. The classic history is **progressive sensorineural hearing loss.** Supposedly the underlying etiology is a failure of the endolymphatic sac to resorb endolymph, leading to endolymphatic hydrops and dilation.

Trivia:
- This is the most common cause of congenital sensorineural hearing loss
- The finding is often (usually) bilateral.
- There is an association with cochlear deformity - near 100%
(absence of the bony modiolus in more than 90%)
- Progressive Sensorineural Hearing Loss (they are NOT born deaf)

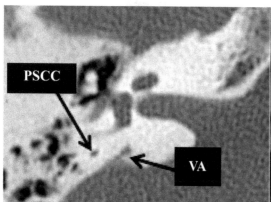

The normal Vestibular Aqueduct (VA) is NEVER larger than the adjacent Posterior Semicircular Canal (PSCC)

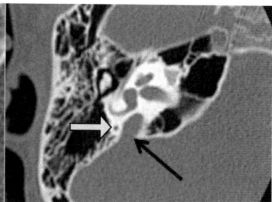

Enlarged Vestibular Aqueduct
(larger than PSCC - grey arrow)

Congenital malformations of the inner ear can be thought about along a spectrum of severity. As the construction of the hearing machinery is complicated business, you can imagine that the earlier things go wrong in this multi-stage anatomical development the more severe the anomaly.

Along those lines, we can discuss two disorders on opposite ends of that severity spectrum with the **Michel's Aplasia** being the earliest and most severe, and the **Classic Mondini's Malformation** (incomplete partition II) being the latest and least severe.

Mondini Malformation - Type of cochlear hypoplasia where the basal turn is normal, but the middle and apical turns fuse into a cystic apex. This is usually written as "only 1.5 turns" - instead of the normal 2.5. There is an association with an enlarged vestibule, and enlarged vestibular aqueduct. They have sensorineural hearing loss, although high frequency sounds are typically preserved (as the basal turn is normal).

Michel's Aplasia - This is also referred to as complete labyrinthine aplasia or "CLA." As above, this represents the most severe of the congenital abnormalities of the inner ear - with absence of the cochlea, vestibule, and vestibular aqueduct. No surprise these kids are completely deaf.

Associations: Anencephaly, Thalidomide Exposure

Gamesmanship: Some people think this looks like labyrinthitis ossificans. Look for the absent vestibular aqueduct to help differentiate.

THIS vs THAT: Mondini vs Michel		
	Mondini	**Michel**
Timing	Late (7th Week)	Early (3rd Week)
Severity	Some Preserved High Frequency Hearing	Total Deafness
Cochlea:	Cystic Apex (basilar turn is normal)	**Absent**
Vestibule	Sometimes Enlarged (can be normal)	**Absent**
Vestibular Aqueduct	Large	**Absent**
Frequency	Common (relative to other malformations)	Rare As Fuck

Endolymphatic Sac Tumor

Rare tumor of the endolymphatic sac and duct. Although most are sporadic, when you see this tumor you should immediately think **Von-Hippel-Lindau**.

Classic Look: They almost always have **internal amorphous calcifications on CT**. There are T2 bright, with **intense enhancement**. They are **very vascular** often with **flow voids**, and **tumor blush** on angiography.

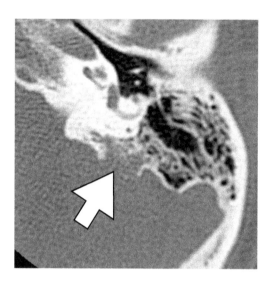
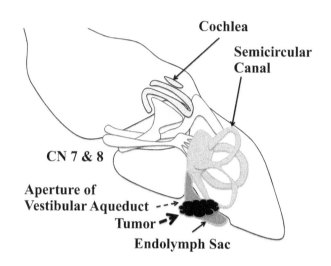

Paraganglioma

On occasion, paraganglioma of the jugular fossa (glomus jugulare or jugulotympanic tumors) can invade the occipital bone and adjacent petrous apex.

Trivia:

• **40% of the time it's hereditary, and they are multiple**.
• The **most common presenting symptom is hoarseness** from vagal nerve compression.
• They are very vascular masses and enhance avidly with a **"salt and pepper"** **appearance on post contrast MRI, with flow voids**.
• They are FDG avid.

More on these later in the chapter

Petrous Apex - Anatomic Variations:

Variation can occur in the amount of pneumatization, marrow fat, bony continuity, and vascular anatomy.

Asymmetric Marrow: - Typically the petrous apex contains significant fat, closely following the scalp and orbital fat (T1 and T2 bright). When it's asymmetric you can have two problems (1) falsely thinking you've got an infiltrative process when you don't, and (2) overlooking a T1 bright thing (cholesterol granuloma) thinking it's fat. The key is to use STIR or some other fat saturating sequence.

Cephaloceles: - A cephalocoele describes a herniation of CNS content through a defect in the cranium. In the petrous apex they are a slightly different animal. They don't contain any brain tissue, and simply represent cystic expansion and herniation of the posterolateral portion of Meckel's cave into the superomedial aspect of the petrous apex. Describing it as a **herniation of Meckel's Cave would be more accurate**. These are usually unilateral and are classically described as *"smoothly marginated lobulated cystic expansion of the petrous apex."*

Aberrant internal carotid. The classic history is **pulsatile tinnitus** (although other things can cause that). This term is used to describe the situation where the C1 (cervical) segment of the ICA has involuted/underdeveloped, and middle ear collaterals develop (enlarged caroticotympanic artery) to pick up the slack. The hypertrophied vessel runs through the tympanic cavity and <u>joins the horizontal carotid canal.</u> The ENT exam will show a vascular mass pulsing behind the ear drum (don't expect them to make it that easy for you).

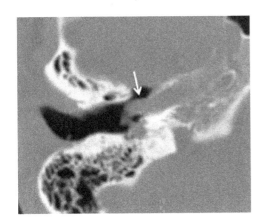

The oldest trick in the book is to try and fool you into calling it a paraganglioma.

<u>Look for the connection to the horizontal carotid canal</u> - that is the most classic way to show this.

DO NOT BIOPSY !

Apical Petrositis

Infection of the petrous apex is a rare complication of infectious otomastoiditis. It can have some bad complications if it progresses including osteomyelitis of the skull base, vasospasm of the ICA (if it involves the carotid canal), subdural empyema, venous sinus thrombosis, temporal lobe stroke, and full on meningitis.

In children, it can present as a primary process. In adults it's usually in the setting of chronic otomastoiditis or recent mastoid surgery.

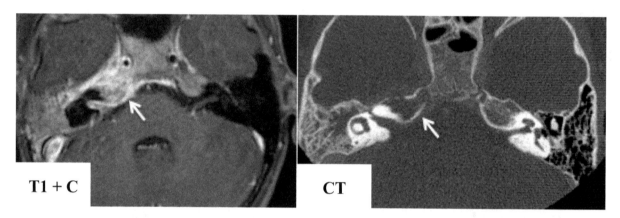

T1 + C   CT

Gradenigo Syndrome

This is a complication of apical petrositis, when Dorello's canal (CN 6) is involved. They will show you (or tell you) that the patient has a **lateral rectus palsy**.

> **Dorello's Canal**
>
> The most medial point of the pertrous ridge - between the pontine cistern and cavernous sinus

Classic Triad:
- Otomastoiditis,
- Face pain (trigeminal neuropathy), and
- Lateral Rectus Palsy

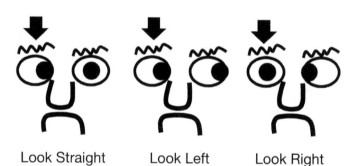

Look Straight   Look Left   Look Right

Petrous Apex - Inflammatory Lesions

Cholesterol Granuloma

The **most common primary petrous apex lesion**. Mechanism is likely obstruction of the air cell, with repeated cycles of hemorrhage and inflammation leading to expansion and bone remodeling. The most common symptom is hearing loss.

On CT the margins will be sharply defined. On MRI it's gonna be **T1 and T2 bright,** with a T2 dark hemosiderin rim, and faint peripheral enhancement.

Key Point:
Cholesterol Granuloma = T1 and T2 Bright.

The slow growing ones can be watched. The fast growing ones need surgery.

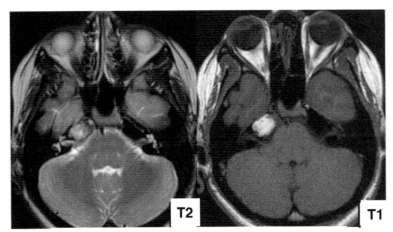

Cholesterol Granuloma = *T1 and T2 Bright*

Cholesteatoma

This is basically an epidermoid (ectopic epithelial tissue). Unlike the ones in the middle ear, these are congenital (not acquired) in the petrous apex. They are typically slow growing, and produce bony changes similar to cholesterol granuloma.

The difference is their MRI findings; T1 dark, T2 bright, and restricted diffusion.

Key Point: **Cholesteatoma = T1 Dark, T2 Bright, Restricted Diffusion**

THIS vs **THAT:**	
Cholesterol Granuloma	**Cholesteatoma**
T1 Bright	T1 Dark
T2 Bright	T2 Bright
Doesn't Restrict	**Does Restrict**
Smooth Expansile Bony Change	Smooth Expansile Bony Change

External Ear

Regular and Necrotizing Otitis Externa:

Otitis Externa - the so called "swimmers ear" is an infection (usually bacterial) of the external auditory canal. The more testable version **Necrotizing Otitis Externa** (also called *"Malignant"* Otitis Externa - for the purpose of fucking with you) is a more aggressive version seen almost exclusively in diabetics.

You are going to see swollen EAC soft tissues, probably with a bunch of small abscesses, and adjacent bony destruction.

They always (95%) have diabetes and the causative agent is always (98%) Pseudomonas.

External Auditory Canal Exostosis ("Swimmers Ear") - This is an overgrowth of tissue in the ear canal, classically seen in Surfers who get repeated bouts of ear infections. It's usually bilateral, and when chronic will look like bone. Unlike Necrotizing Otitis, these patients are immunocompetent and non-diabetes (although they are dirty hippie surfers).

External Auditory Canal Osteoma - This is a benign bone tumor, maybe best thought of as an overgrowth of normal bone. They are usually incidental and unilateral (*remember exostosis was bilateral*) occurring near the junction of cartilage and bone in the ear canal.

External Auditory Canal Atresia:

This is a developmental anomaly where the external auditory canal (secondary crayon storage compartment) doesn't form. As you might imagine, this results in a hearing deficit (conductive subtype). There may or may not be a mashed up ossicular chain.

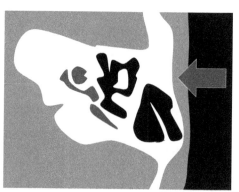

Normally, there is a place to stick a crayon right around here (arrow).

Trivia: ENT will want to know: (1) if the tissue covering the normally open ear hole (atretic plate) is soft tissue or bone, and (2) if there is an aberrant course of the facial nerve.

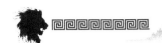
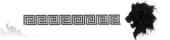
Pagets – This is discussed in great depth in the MSK chapter. Having said that, I want to remind you of the Paget skull changes. You can have osteolysis as a well-defined large radiolucent region favoring the frontal and occipital bones. Both the inner and outer table are involved. The buzzword is **osteolysis circumscripta**.

Paget's Skull related complications:
* Deafness is the most common complication
* Cranial Nerve Paresis
* Basilar Invagination -> Hydrocephalus -> Brainstem Compression
* Secondary (high grade) osteosarcoma.

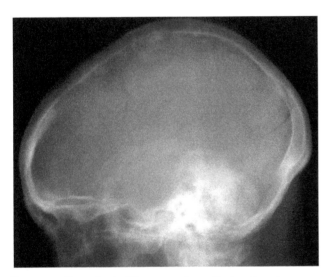

Pagets - *Osteolysis Circumscripta (lytic phase)*   *Thickened Expanded Skull (Sclerotic Phase)*

Chordoma *(midline)* & **Chondrosarcoma** *(off midline) discussed in MSK chapter.*

Fibrous Dysplasia - The <u>ground-glass</u> lesion. If you are getting ready to call it Pagets, stop and look at the age. Pagets is typically an older person (8% at 80), whereas fibrous dysplasia is usually in someone less than 30.

* Classically, fibrous dysplasia of the skull spares the otic capsule
* McCune Albright Syndrome - Multifocal fibrous dysplasia, cafe-au-lait spots, and precocious puberty.
* The outer table is favored (Pagets tends to favor in the inner table)

Sinus Disease Strategy Intro: You will see CT and MRI used in the evaluation of sinus disease. It is useful to have some basic ideas as to why one modality might be preferred over the other (for gamesmanship and distractor elimination). CT is typically used for orbital and sinus infections. In particular it is useful to see if the spread of infection involves the anterior 2/3 of the orbit. If you wanted to know if the patient has cavernous sinus involvement, or involvement of the posterior 1/3 (orbital apex) MRI will be superior.

CT also has the ability to differentiate common benign disease (inspissated secretion and allergic fungal sinusitis) from the more rare sinus tumors. The trick being that a hyperdense opacified sinus is nearly always benign (tumor will not be dense). In addition to that CT is useful for characterization of anatomical variation (justification of endoscopic nasal surgery for recurrent sinusitis).

- Hyper Dense Sinus -
• Blood   • Dense (inspissated) Secretions   • Fungus

MRI is going to be more valuable for tumor progression / extension (perineural spread, marrow involvement etc..).

Fungal Sinusitis

This comes in two flavors; the good one (allergic) and the bad one (invasive). The chart below will contrast the testable differences:

Allergic Fungal Sinusitis	Acute Invasive Fugal Sinusitis
Opacification of multiple sinuses, ususually bilateral favoring the ethmoid and maxillary sinuses.	Opacification of multiple sinuses. Stranding / Extension into the fat around the sinuses in the key finding.
Normal Immune System (Asthma is common)	Immunocompromised - Neutropenic = Aspergillus - Diabetic in DKA = Zygomycetes / Mucor
CT: **Hyperdense** centrally or with layers. Can erode and remodel sinus walls if chronic.	CT: Opacified Sinus with is NOT hyperdense. Fat stranding in the orbit, masticator fat, pre-antral fat, or PPF suggests invasion. This does NOT require bone destruction.
MRI: T1-T2 Dark - because of the high protein content / heavy metals. Can mimic an aerated sinus. Inflamed (T2 bright) mucosa which will enhance. The glob of fungus snot will not enhance (thats how you know it is not a tumor).	MRI: Also can be T1/T2 Dark. However, the mucosa may not enhance (suggesting it is necrotic). The **extension of disease out of the sinus** will be bright on STIR and enhance.

Chronic Inflammatory Sinonasal Disease

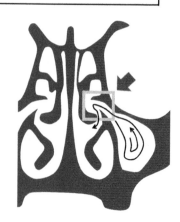

This is typically thought of as an inflammation of the paranasal sinuses that lasts at least 12 weeks. The causes are complex and people write long boring papers about the various cytokines and T-Cell mediation pathways are involved but from the Radiologist's point of view the issue is primarily anatomical patency of sinus Ostia (box with arrow).

Chronic Inflammatory Sinonasal Disease Continued...

There are several described patterns of recurring sinonasal disease.

Infundibular Pattern.

The most common pattern.

In this pattern, disease is limited to the maxillary sinus and occurs from the obstruction at the ipsilateral ostium / infundibulum (star).

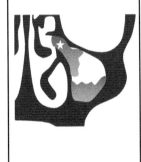

Ostiomeatal Unit Pattern

Second most common pattern. I'm not going to get into depth on the various subtypes -

just think about this as more centered at the middle meatus (star) with disease involving the ipsilateral maxillary, frontal and ethmoid sinuses.

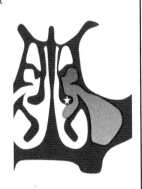

The contributors to this pattern involve all the usually suspects (hypertrophied turbinates, anatomic variants - concha bullosa, middle turbinates which curl the wrong way "paradoxical", and septal deviation).

Sinonasal Polyposis Pattern.

The pattern is characterized by a combination of soft tissue nasal polyps (found throughout the nasal cavity) and variable degrees of sinus opacification. About half the time fluid levels will also be present.

A key feature is the bony remodeling and erosion. In particular the "widening of the infundibula" is the classic description. This erosion and remodeling is important to distinguish between the "expansion" of the sinus - which is more classic for a mucocele.

Testable associations include CF and Aspirin Sensitivity.

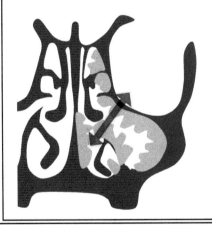

Mucocele

This is how I think about these things. You have an obstructed sinus. Maybe you had trauma which fucked the drainage pathway or you've got CF and the secretions just clog things up. Mucus continues to accumulate in the sinus, but it can't clear (because it's obstructed). Over time the sinus become totally filled and then starts to expand circumferentially. Hence the buzzword "expanded airless sinus." The frontal sinus is the most common location. It won't enhance centrally (it is not a tumor), but the periphery may enhance from the adjacent inflamed mucosa.

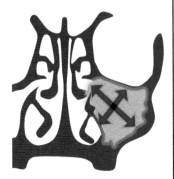

Antrochoanal Polyp

Seen in young adults (30s-40s), classically presenting with nasal congestion / obstruction symptoms. Arises within the maxillary sinuses and passes through and enlarges the sinus ostium (or accessory ostium).

 Buzzword is **"widening of the maxillary ostium."**

Classically, there is no associated bony destruction but instead smooth enlargement of the sinus. The polyp will extend into the nasopharynx. This thing is basically a monster inflammatory polyp with a thin stalk arising from the maxillary sinus.

Juvenile Nasal Angiofibroma (JNA)

Often you can get this one right just from the history - **Male teenager with nose bleeds** (obstruction is actually a more common symptom in real life, but not so much on multiple choice).

- Location = Centered on the sphenopalatine foramen
- Bone Remodeling (not bone destruction)
- Extremely <u>vascular</u> (super enhancing) with intratumoral <u>Flow Voids</u> on MR
- Pre-surgical embolization is common (via internal maxillary & ascending pharyngeal artery)

Inverted Papilloma:

This uncommon tumor has distinctive imaging features (which therefore make it testable). The **classic location is the lateral wall of the nasal cavity – most frequently related to the middle turbinate.** Impaired maxillary drainage is expected.

- A <u>focal hyperostosis</u> tends to occur at the tumor origin.
- Another high yield pearl is that <u>10% harbor a squamous cell CA.</u>
- MRI **"cerebriform pattern"** – which sorta looks like brain on T1 and T2.

Esthesioneuroblastoma:

This is a neuroblastoma of olfactory cells so it's gonna start at the cribiform plate. It classically has a dumbbell appearance with growth up into the skull and growth down into the sinuses, with a waist at the plate. There are often cysts in the mass. There is a bi-modal age distribution.

- Dumbbell shape with wasting at the cribiform plate is classic
- Intracranial posterior cyst is a "diagnostic" look
- Octreotide scan will be positive – since it is of neural crest origin

Squamous Cell / SNUC:

Squamous cell is the **most common head and neck cancer.** The maxillary antrum is the most common location. It's highly cellular, and therefore low on T2. Relative to other sinus masses it enhances less. *SNUC* (the undifferentiated squamer), is the monster steroided-up version of a regular squamous cell. They are massive and seen more in the ethmoids.

Epistaxis (Nose Bleeds)

This is usually idiopathic, although it can be iatrogenic (picking it too much - *or not enough*). They could get sneaky and work this into a case of HHT (hereditary hemorrhagic telangiectasia). The most common location is the anterior septal area (Kiesselbach plexus) - these tend to be easy to compress manually. The posterior ones are less common (5%) but tend to be the ones that "bleed like stink" (need angio). Most cases are given a trial of nasal packing. When that fails, the N-IR team is activated.

 The main supply to the posterior nose is the sphenopalatine artery (terminal internal maxillary artery) and tends to be the first line target. Watch out for the variant anastomosis between the ECA and ophthalmic artery (you don't want to embolize the eye).

Nasal Septal Perforation

Typically involves the anterior septal cartilaginous area.

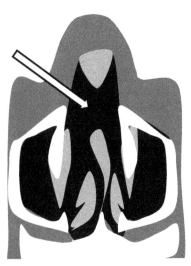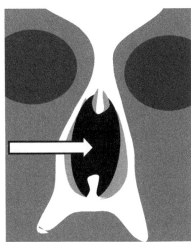

There are a bunch of things that can do this. These are the ones I'd think about:

- **Surgery** - Old school Septoplasty techniques - essentially resecting the thing (Killian submucous resection)
- **Cocaine** use (> 3 months)
- **Too much nose picking** (or perhaps not picking it enough)
- Granulomatosis with polyangiitis (**Wegener granulomatosis**) — Triad of renal masses, sinus mucosal thickening and nasal septal erosion, disease, and cavitary lung nodules / fibrosis. cANCA positive.
- **Syphilis** - affects the bony septum (most everything else effect the cartilaginous regions).

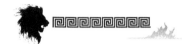 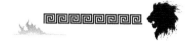

Sialolithiasis - Stones in the salivary ducts. The testable trivia includes: (1) **Most commonly in the submandibular gland duct (wharton's)**, (2) can lead to an infected gland "sialoadenitis", and (3) chronic obstruction can lead to gland fatty atrophy.

Submandibular = Wharton
Parotid = Stenson
Sublingual = Rivinus

Odontogenic Infection – These can be dental or periodontal in origin. If I were writing a question about this topic I would ask three things. The first would be that infection is **more common from an extracted tooth** than an abscess involving an intact tooth.

The second would be that the **attachment of the mylohyoid muscle to the mylohyoid ridge dictates the spread of infection to the sublingual and submandibular spaces**. Above the mylohyoid line (anterior mandibular teeth) goes to the sublingual space, and below the mylohyoid line (second and third molars) goes to the submandibular space.

The third thing I would ask would be that an **odontogenic abscess is the most common masticator space "mass" in an adult.**

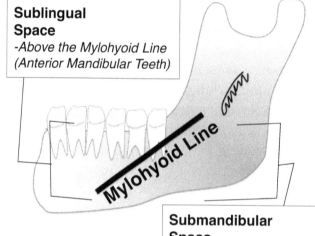

Sublingual Space
-Above the Mylohyoid Line (Anterior Mandibular Teeth)

Submandibular Space
-Below the Mylohyoid Line (2nd and 3rd Molars)

Ludwig's Angina:

This is a super aggressive cellulitis in the floor of the mouth. If they show it, there will be gas everywhere.

Trivia: most cases start with an odontogenic infection.

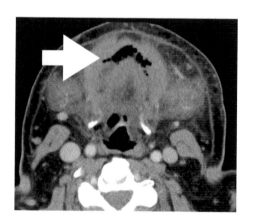

Torus Palatinus:	**Osteonecrosis of the Mandible:**	**Ranula:**
This is a normal variant that looks scary. Because it looks scary some multiple choice writer may try and trick you into calling it cancer. **It's just a bony exostosis** that comes off the hard palate in the midline. *Classic History*: "Grandma's dentures won't stay in."	The trivia is most likely gonna be etiology. Just remember it is related to prior radiation, licking a radium paint brush, or **bisphosphonate treatment.**	This is a mucous retention cyst. They are typically **lateral**. There are two testable pieces of trivia to know: (1) They **arise from the sublingual gland / space**, and (2) Use the word **"plunging"** once it's **under the mylohyoid muscle.**
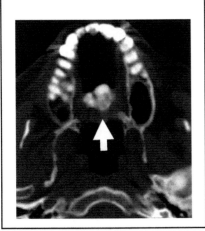	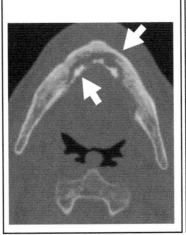	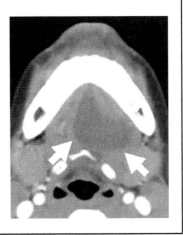

Thyroglossal Duct Cyst – This can occur anywhere between the foramen cecum (the base of the tongue) and the thyroid gland. They are usually found in the midline. It looks like a thin-walled cyst. Further discussion in the endocrine & peds chapters.

Floor of Mouth Dermoid / Epidermoid - There isn't a lot of trivia about these other than the buzzword and what they classically look like. The **buzzword is "sack of marbles"** - fluid sack with globules of fat. They are typically **midline**. Further discussion in the peds chapter.

Cancer - Squamous cell is going to be the most common cancer of the mouth (and head and neck). In an older person think drinker and smoker.

In a younger person think **HPV**. HPV related SCCs tend to be present with large necrotic level 2a nodes (don't call it a branchial cleft cyst!).

Classic Scenario = Young adult with new level II neck mass = HPV related SCC.

Lesions of the Jaw

There are a BUNCH of these and they all look pretty similar. Lesions in the jaw are broadly grouped into either odontogenic (from a tooth) or non-odontogenic (not from a tooth). The non-odontogenic stuff you see in the mandible is the same kind of stuff you see in other bones (ABCs, Simple Bone Cysts, Osteomyelitis, Myeloma / Plasmacytoma etc…). I think if a test writer is going to show a jaw lesion - they probably are going to go for odontogenic type. Obviously your answer choices will help you decide what they are going for. The other tip is that odontogenic lesions are usually associated with a tooth.

I'm going to pick 5 that I think are most likely to be asked and focus on how I would tell them apart.

Periapical Cyst (Radicular Cyst) - This is the most common type of odontogenic cyst. They are typically the result of inflammation from dental caries (less commonly trauma). The inflammatory process results in a cystic degeneration around the periodontal ligament.

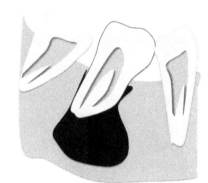

- Located at the <u>apex of a non-vital tooth</u>
- Round with a Well Corticated Border
- Usually < 2 cm

Dentigerous Cyst (Follicular Cyst) - This is a cyst that forms around the crown of an un-erupted tooth. It's best thought of as a developmental cyst (peri-apicals are acquired). These things like to displace and resorb adjacent teeth - usually in an apical direction. This is the kind of cyst that will displace a tooth into the condylar regions of the mandible or into the floor of the orbit.

- Located at the <u>crown of an un-erupted tooth</u>
- Tend to displace the tooth

Keratogenic Odontogenic Tumor

(Odontogenic Keratocyst) - Unlike the prior two lesions (which were basically fluid collections) this is an actual tumor. They tend to occur at the mandibular ramus or body. Although they can be uni-locular the classic look is multi-locular (*"daughter cysts"*) and that's how I would expect them to look on the test.

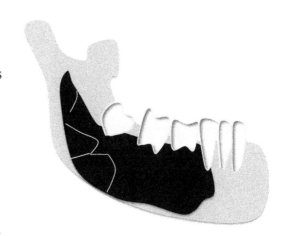

- Body / Ramus Mandible
- They typically grow along the length of the bone
- Without significant cortical expansion
- May have daughter cysts
- When multiple think _Gorlin Syndrome_

Ameloblastoma (Adamantinoma of the jaw) - This is another tumor (locally aggressive).
The appearance is variable but for the purpose of multiple choice I would expect the most classic look - multi-cystic with solid components and expansion of the mandible.

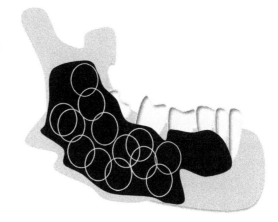

Out of the four I've discussed, this will be the most aggressive-looking one. If they show you a really aggressive-looking lesion, especially if it has multiple "soap bubbles" - you should consider this.

- Hallmark = Extensive Tooth Root Absorption
- Mandibular Expansion
- Solid component (shown on MR or CT) favors the Dx of Ameloblastoma
- About 5% arise from Dentigerous Cysts

Odontoma - This is the easy one to pick out because it's most likely to be shown in it's mature solid form (they start out lucent). It's actually the most common odontogenic tumor of the mandible. It's basically a "tooth hamartoma."

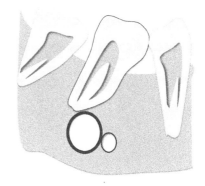

- <u>Radiodense</u> with a lucent rim

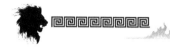
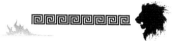

- Can be LARGE with "fluffy" calcifications

The suprahyoid neck is usually taught by using a "spaces" method. This is actually the best way to learn it. What space is it? What is in that space? What pathology can occur as the result of what normal structures are there? Example: lymph nodes are there – thus you can get lymphoma or a met.

Parotid Space:

The parotid space is basically the parotid gland, and portions of the facial nerve. You can't see the facial nerve, but you can see the retromandibular vein (which runs just medial to the facial nerve).

Another thing to know is that the parotid is the only salivary gland to have lymph nodes, so pathology involving the gland itself, and anything lymphatic related, is fair game.

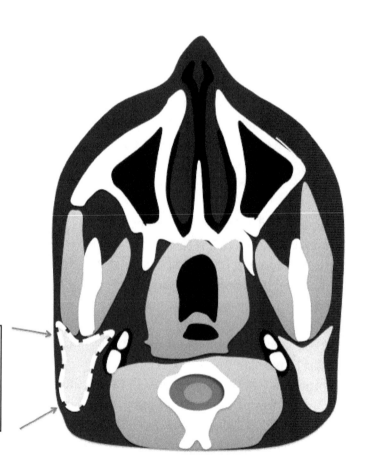

Parotid Space Contains:
- The Parotid Gland
- Cranial Nerve 7 (Facial)
- Retro-mandibular Vein

Pathology:

Pleomorphic Adenoma (benign mixed tumor) -
This is the most common major *(and minor)* salivary gland
tumor. It occurs most commonly in the parotid, but can also
occur in the submandibular or sublingual glands. 90% of
these tumors occur in the superficial lobe. They are
commonly T2 bright, with a rim of low signal. **They have a
small malignant potential** and are treated surgically.

```
Major Salivary Glands:
• Parotid
• Submandibular
• Sublingual

Minor Salivary Glands
• Literally 100s of un-
  named minor glands
```

- *Superficial vs Deep:* Involvement of the superficial (lateral to the facial nerve) or deep
  (medial to the facial nerve) lobe is critical to the surgical approach. A line is drawn
  connecting the lateral surface of the posterior belly of the digastric muscle and the
  lateral surface of the mandibular ascending ramus to separate superficial from deep.

- Apparently, if you resect these like a clown you can spill them, and they will have a
  massive, ugly recurrence.

Warthins: This is the second most common benign tumor. This one ONLY occurs in the
parotid gland. This one is **usually cystic, in a male, bilateral (15%), and in a smoker**. As a
point of total trivia, this tumor **takes up pertechnetate** (it's basically the only tumor in the
parotid to do it , *ignoring the ultra rare parotid oncocytoma*).

Mucoepidermoid Carcinoma – This is the **most common malignant tumor of minor
salivary glands**. The general rule is – the smaller the gland, the more common the malignant
tumors; the bigger the gland, the more common the benign tumors. There is a variable
appearance based on the histologic grade. There is an association with radiation.

Adenoid Cystic Carcinoma – This is another malignant salivary gland tumor, which
favors minor glands but can be seen in the parotid. The number one thing to know is
perineural spread. This tumor likes perineural spread.

When I say adenoid cystic, you say perineural spread.

Pearl: I used to think that perineurial tumor spread would widen a neural foramen
(foramen ovale for example). It's still might… but it's been my experience that a nerve
sheath tumor (schwannoma) is much more likely to do that. Let's just say for the
purpose of multiple choice that neural foramina widening is a schwannoma - unless
there is overwhelming evidence to the contrary.

Lymphoma

Because the parotid has lymph nodes (it's the only salivary gland that does), you can get lymphoma in the parotid (primary or secondary). If you see it and it's bilateral, you should think Sjogrens. Sjogrens patients have a big risk (like 1000x) of parotid lymphoma. Like lymphoma is elsewhere in the body, the appearance is variable. You might see bilateral homogeneous masses. For the purposes of the exam, **just knowing you can get it in the parotid (primary or secondary) and the relationship with Sjogrens is probably all you need**.

Sjogrens

Autoimmune lymphocyte-induced destruction of the gland. "Dry Eyes and Dry Mouth." Typically seen in women in their 60s. **Increased risk** (like 1000x) risk of non-Hodgkins MALT type **lymphoma**. There is a **honeycombed appearance of the gland**.

Benign Lymphoepithelial Disease:

You have **bilateral mixed solid and cystic lesions** with <u>diffusely enlarged</u> parotid glands. This is **seen in HIV**. The condition is painless (unlike parotitis – which can enlarge the glands).

Acute Parotitis:

Obstruction of flow of secretions is the most common cause. They will likely show you a stone (or stones) in Stensen's duct, which will be dilated. The stones are calcium phosphate. Post infectious parotitis is usually bacterial. Mumps would be the most common viral cause. As a point of trivia, sialography is contraindicated in the acute setting.

Parapharyngeal Space

Also referred to as the *"pre-styloid"* parapharyngeal space - for the purpose of fucking with you.

The primary utility of the space is when it is displaced (discussed below).

Mets and infections can spread directly in a vertical direction through this space (squamous cell cancer from tonsils, tongue, and larynx).

A cystic mass in this location could be an atypical 2nd Branchial Cleft Cyst (but is more likely a necrotic lymph node).

The parapharyngeal space is bordered on four sides by different spaces. If you have a mass dead in the middle, it can be challenging to tell where it's coming from. Using the displacement of fat, you can help problem solve. Much more important than that, this lends itself very well to multiple choice.

Parotid **M**ass **P**ushes **M**edially (PMPM)

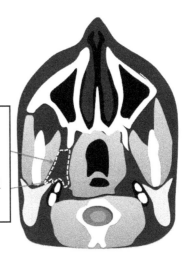

The parapharyngeal space is primarily a ball of fat with a few branches of the trigeminal nerves, and the pterygoid veins.

Parapharyngeal Fat (PPF) Displacement

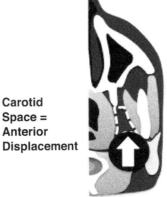

Carotid Space = Anterior Displacement

Parotid Space = Medial Displacement

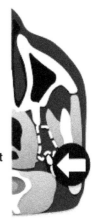

Masticator Space = Posterior Medial Displacement

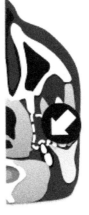

Superficial Mucosal Space = Lateral Displacement

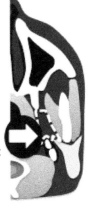

Carotid Space:

The carotid space is also sometimes called the *"post styloid" or "retro-styloid"* parapharyngeal space — for the purpose of fucking with you.

There are **3 Classic Carotid Space Tumors:**
(1) Paraganglioma
(2) Schwannoma
(3) Neurofibroma

Although it is worth noting that this space is commonly involved in secondary spread of aggressive multi-spatial disease - such as infectious path (necrotizing otitis external) or malignant spread (nasopharyngeal , squamous cell etc..).

Metastatic squamous cell is what you should think for nodal disease in this region.

Carotid Space Contains:
- Carotid artery
- Jugular vein
- Portions of CN 9, CN 10, CN 11
- Internal jugular chain lymph nodes

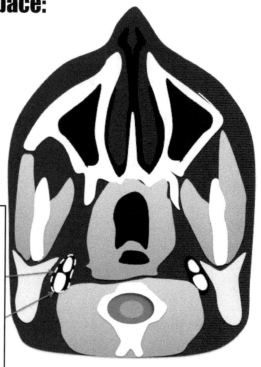

Lesions Displace the Parapharyngeal Fat ANTERIOR

Paragangliomas: There are three different ones worth knowing about – based on location. The imaging features are the same. They are **hypervascular (intense tumor blush)**, with a **"Salt and Pepper" appearance on MRI** from the flow voids. They can be multiple and bilateral in familial conditions (10% bilateral, 10% malignant, etc.). **[111]In-octreotide accumulates in these tumors** (receptors for somatostatin).

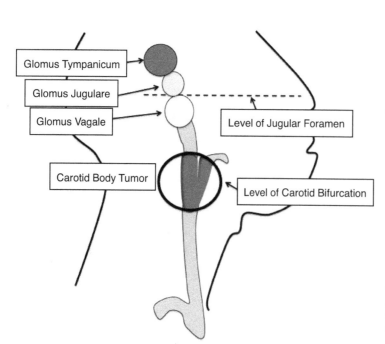

Glomus Tympanicum
Glomus Jugulare
Glomus Vagale
Carotid Body Tumor
Level of Jugular Foramen
Level of Carotid Bifurcation

Carotid Body Tumor = Carotid Bifurcation (*Splaying ICA and ECA*)

Glomus Jugulare = Skull Base (*often with destruction of jugular foramen*)

Middle Ear Floor Destroyed = Glomus Jugulare.

Glomus Vagale = Above Carotid Bifurcation, but below the Jugular Foramen

Glomus Tympanicum = Confined to the middle ear. Buzzword is *"overlying the cochlear promontory."*

Middle Ear Floor Intact = Glomus Tympanum

Schwannoma

Most commonly in this location we are talking about vagal nerve (CN 10), but if the lesion is pretty high up near the skull base it could also be involving CN 9, 11, or even 12. The typical MR appearance is an oval mass, heterogenous (cystic and sold parts) with heterogenous bright signal on T2.

These things enhance a ton (at least the solid parts anyway). They enhance so much you might even think they were vascular. Ironically, schwannomas are considered hypo vascular lesions and the only reason they enhance is because of extravascular leakage (and poor venous drainage).

Neurofibroma

These are less common than the schwannoma. About 10% of the time they are related to NF-1 (in which case you should expect them to be bilateral and multiple). In contrast to schwannomas they tend to be more homogenous, and demonstrate the classic target sign on T2 with decreased central signal.

Neurofibroma	Schwannoma	Paraganglioma
Mildly Heterogenous Enhancement	Although they enhance intensely they are not vascular on Angio	Hypervascular (tumor blush on angio)
T2: Target Sign (bright rim, dark middle)	T2: Moderate to High Signal - Heterogenous	T2: Light Bulb Bright with Salt and Pepper (flow voids)
NF-1 Association	NF-2 Association	^{111}In-Octreotide avid

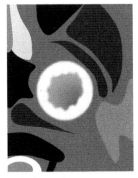 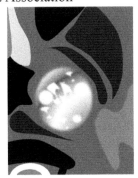 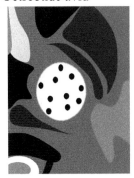

Neck Infection Syndromes

Lemierre's Syndrome - This is a thrombophlebitis of the jugular veins with septic emboli in the lung. It's found in the setting of oropharyngeal infection (pharyngitis, tonsillitis, peritonsillar abscess) or recent ENT surgery. Buzzword bacteria = "Fusobacterium Necrophorum"

Grisel's Syndrome - Torticollis with atlanto-axial joint inflammation seen in H&N surgery or retropharyngeal abscess

Masticator Space:

As the name implies this space contains the **muscles of mastication** (masticator, temporalis, medial and lateral pterygoids).

Additionally, you have the angle and **ramus of the mandible**, plus the **inferior alveolar nerve** *(branch of V3).*

A trick to be aware of is that the space extends superiorly along the side of the skull via the temporalis muscle. So, aggressive neoplasm or infection may ride right up there.

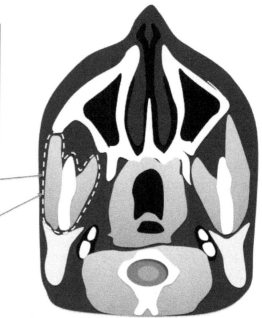

Lesions Displace the Parapharyngeal Fat
POSTERIOR and MEDIAL

Odontogenic Infection –

In an adult, this is the most common cause of a masticator space mass. If you see a mass here, the next move should be to look at the mandible on bone windows. Just in general, you should be on the look out for spread via the pterygopalatine fossa to the orbital apex and cavernous sinus. The relationship with the mylohyoid makes for good trivia - as discussed above.

Sarcomas –

In kids, you can run into nasty angry masses like Rhabdomyosarcomas. You can also get sarcomas from the bone of the mandible (chondrosarcoma favors the TMJ).

Cavernous Hemangiomas –

These can also occur, and are given away by the presence of phleboliths. Venous or lymphatic malformations may involve multiple compartments / spaces.

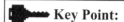 **Key Point:**
Congenital Stuff and Aggressive Infection/ Cancer tends to be Trans-Spatial.

Perineural Spread – You can have perineural spread from a head and neck primary along V3.

When I say *"perineural spread"* you should think two things:
(1) **Adenoid Cystic** Carcinoma of the minor salivary gland
(2) Melanoma

Nerve Sheath Tumors – Since you have a nerve, you can have a schwannoma or neurofibroma of V3. Remember the schwannoma is more likely to cause the foramina expansion vs perineural tumor spread.

Retropharyngeal Space / Danger Space

The retropharyngeal space has some complex anatomy. Simplified, this is a midline space, deep to the oral & nasal pharynx. The retropharyngeal space has an anterior "true" space which extends caudal to around C6-C7, and a more posterior "danger space" - which is dangerous because it listens to rap music and plays first person shooter video games - plus it extends into the mediastinum - so you could potentially dump pus, or cancer, right into the mediastinum.

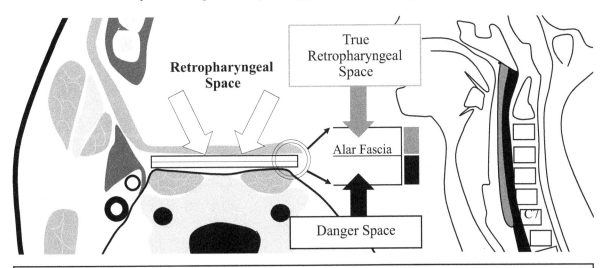

Infectious behind this deep cervical fascia (the **Prevertebral Space**) are different than the ones discussed below in that they are not spread from the neck but instead the spine/disc (osteomyelitis).

Infection

Infection – Involvement of the retropharyngeal space most often occurs from spread from the tonsillar tissue. You are going to have centrally low density tissue and stranding in the space. You should evaluate for spread of infection into the mediastinum.

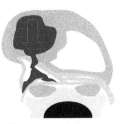

Cartoon Axial Showing Infection Spreading from a Tonsillar Abscess to the Danger Zone

Don't Forget:

Delays are often critical for differentiate phlegmon and drainable abscess

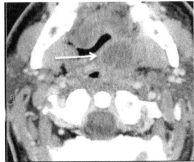

Peritonsillar Abscess

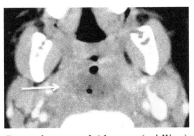

Retropharyngeal Abscess (midline)

Necrotic Nodes

Necrotic Nodes (nodes of Rouviere) - These things are located in the lateral retropharyngeal region. In kids you can see suppurative infection in these, but around age 4 they start to regress - so adults are actually much less to get infection in this region. Now, you can still get mets (squamous cell, papillary thyroid, etc..). Lymphoma can involve these nodes as well - but won't be necrotic until treated.

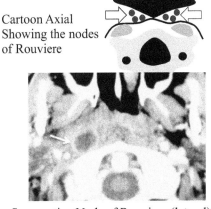

Cartoon Axial Showing the nodes of Rouviere

Suppurative Node of Rouviere (lateral)

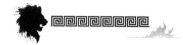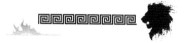
When you are talking about head and neck cancer, you are talking about squamous cell cancer. Now, this is a big complex topic and requires a fellowship to truly understand / get good at. Obviously, the purpose of this book is to prepare you for multiple choice test questions not teach you practical radiology. If you want to actually learn about head and neck cancer in a practical sense you can try and find a copy of Harnsberger's original legendary handbook (which has been out of print for 20 years), but who has time for that ? Now, for the trivia....

Lymph Node Anatomy:

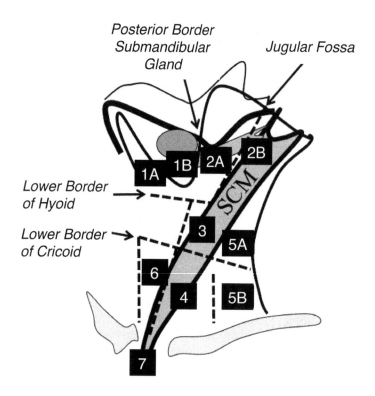

Testable Trivia:

Anterior Belly of Digastric separates 1A from 1B

Stylohyoid muscle *(posterior submandibular gland)* separates 1B from 2A

Jugular Vein *(Spinal Accessory Nerve)* separates 2A from 2B *see below

Vertical borders:
2-3 = Lower Hyoid
3-4 = Lower Cricoid

 2A: Anterior, Medial, Lateral or Abutting the Posterior Internal Jugular

 2B: Posterior to the Internal Jugular, with a clear fat plane between node and IJ

Cancers

Floor of the Mouth SCC:

I touched on this once already. Just remember smoker/drinker in an old person. HPV in a young person. Necrotic level 2 nodes can be a presentation (not a branchial cleft cyst).

Nasopharyngeal SCC:

This is more common in Asians and has a bi-modal distribution:
- group 1 (15-30) typically Chinese
- group 2 (> 40).

Involvement of the parapharyngeal space results in worse prognosis (compared to nasal cavity or oropharynx invasion).

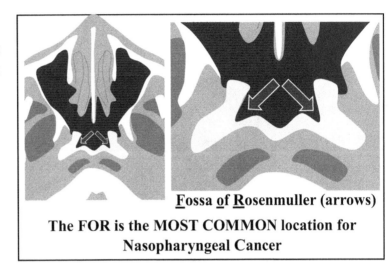

Fossa of Rosenmuller (arrows)

The FOR is the MOST COMMON location for Nasopharyngeal Cancer

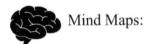 Mind Maps:

See a Unilateral Mastoid Effusion

OR

See a Pathologic Retropharyngeal Node

→ Look at the FOR →

"Earliest Sign" of nasopharyngeal SCC is the effacement of the fat within the FOR.

See a Pathologic Retropharyngeal or Supraclavicular Node

Nodal mets are present in 90% of nasopharyngeal tumors, with the retropharyngeal nodes usually the first involved.

Look at the Clivus

About 30% of the patients with nasopharyngeal tumors have skull base erosion.
(MRI > CT for skull base invasion)

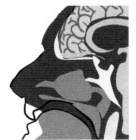

Normal Comparison (T1 Bright Marrow Signal)

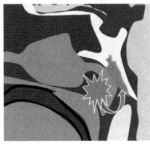

Invasion (loss of Normal T1 Marrow Signal)

Neck Anatomy Blitz

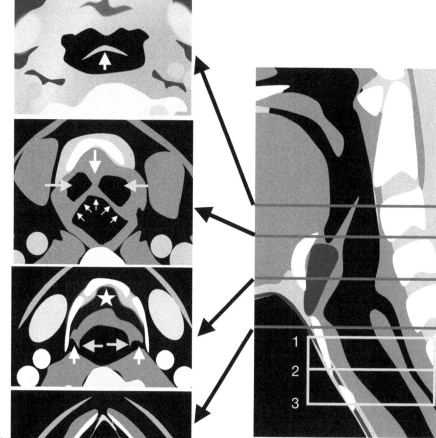

Supraglottic Region: Arrow on the Tip of the Epiglottis

Supraglottic Region: Valleculae (grey arrows), Hypoepiglottic Ligament (white arrow), Epiglottis (multiple tiny white arrows)

Supraglottic Region: Pre-Epiglottic Fat (star), Aryepiglottic folds (grey arrows), piriform sinuses (white arrows)

Supraglottic Region: Para-Epiglottic Spaces (open arrows), Aryepiglottic folds (grey arrows), piriform sinuses (white arrows)

The Para-Epiglottic communicates with the Pre-Epiglottic Space / Fat superiorly.

The Pre-Epiglottic fat is rich in lymphatics, makes tumor invasion of these regions important for tumor staging.

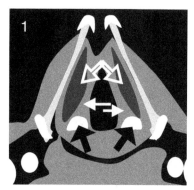

Supraglottic Region: Level of the False Cords (white arrows), with para-glottic spaces (open arrows), and arytenoid cartilages (black arrows)

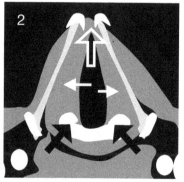

Glottic Region: Level of the True Cords (white arrows), with the cricoarytenoid joint (black arrows), and Anterior Commissure (open arrow)

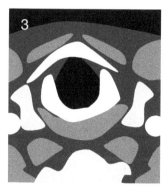

Sub- Glottic Region: Level of the Cricoid Ring

152

Larynx

Laryngocele:

When the laryngeal "saccule" dilates with air you call it a laryngocele. If it is filled with fluid you still might call it a larygocele (but if *saccular cyst* is a choice - consider that). If it is filled with fluid and air you still might call it a larygocele (but it *laryngopyocele* is a choice — and you have any hint of infection - consider that).

What the fuck is a "saccule"? The "saccule" is the appendix of the laryngeal ventricle (a blind ending sac that extends anterior and upwards). It's usually closed or minimally filled with fluid (you don't typically see it in normal adults).

Why does it dilate? Usually because it's obstructed (ball-valve mechanics at the neck of the saccule), and the testable point is that <u>15% of the time that obstruction is a tumor</u>. You can also see them in forceful blowers (trumpet players, glass blowers) — well maybe, this depends on what you read. Simply read the mind of the question writer to know if they are on team trumpet player laryngocele.

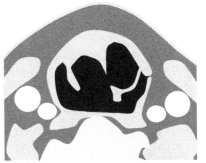

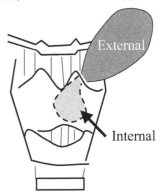

There are internal and external version of this (based on containment of violation of the thyrohyoid membrane).

Vocal Cord Paralysis:

The **involved side will have an expanded ventricle** (it's the opposite side with a cancer). If you see it on the left, a good "next step" question would be to look at the chest (for recurrent laryngeal nerve involvement at the AP window).

 Buzzword = "**Hoarseness**" - If you see "Hoarseness" in the question header, you need to think recurrent laryngeal nerve compression in the AP Window - either from a mass/node or aortic path. *Hoarseness is also a classic Laryngeal CA buzzword (so look there too).*

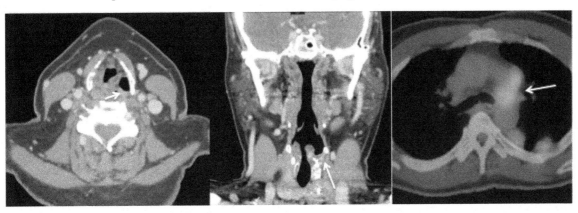

Vocal Cord Paralysis - Ipsilateral Expanded Ventricle   AP Window PET Avid Node

Laryngeal Cancer
(Nearly Always ~ 85% Squamous Cell)

Risk Factors: Smoking, Alcohol, Radiation, Laryngeal Keratosis, HPV, GERD, & Blasphemy against the correct religion (false religions are safe to talk shit about).

The role of the Radiologist is not to make the primary cancer diagnosis here, but to assist in staging. Laryngeal cancers are subdivided into (a) supraglottic, (b) glottic, and (c) subglottic types. "Transglottic" would refer to an aggressive cancer that crosses the laryngeal ventricle.

Supra-Glottic

-More Aggressive
-Early Lymph Node Mets
-They don't get hoarseness

You always need to find (guess at) the inferior margin of a supraglottic mass.

Partial laryngectomy usually can only be done if the tumor is restricted to the supraglottis and does not involve the arytenoids or laryngeal ventricle.

Supra-Glottic: Epiglottic Centered

-Anterior
-Likes to Invade the Pre-Epigolttic Space /Fat (which is rich in lymphatics

Supra-Glottic: False Cord / Fold Centered

-Posterior Lateral
-Likes to Invade the Para-Glottic Space /Fat (which communicates superiorly with the Pre-Epiglottic Space

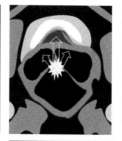

Epiglottic mass spreading anterior across the hypo epiglottic ligament into the preepiglottic space and into the paired vallecula.

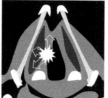

False Cord mass spreading into the para-glottic space

Paraglottic space involvement makes the tumor T3 and "transglottic."
*Best seen in coronals.

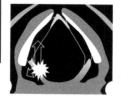

Aryepiglottic fold mass spreading into the paraglottic space & piriform sinus

Glottic

-Most Common
-Best Outcome
-Grow Slowly
-Metastatic Disease is Late

Usually involve the anterior cord and spread into the anterior commissure (typically defined as soft tissue thickening of > 2mm)

Classic Clinical History: "Progressive and Continuous Hoarseness."

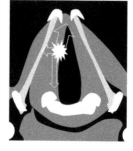

Glottic mass spreading forward towards the anterior commissure

Fixation of the cords indicates at least a T3 tumor - this is best assessed with a scope but can be suspected with disease in the cricoarytenoid joint.

Sub-Glottic

-Least Common
-Often small compared to nodal burden
-Bilateral nodal disease & mediastinal extension

The typical look is soft tissue thickening between the airway and the cricoid ring.

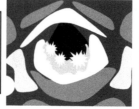

The only reliable sign of cricoid invasion is tumor on both sides of the cartilage *(irregular sclerotic cartilage can be normal)*.

Invasion of the cricoid cartilage is a contraindication to all types of laryngeal conservation surgery *(cricoid cartilage is necessary for postoperative stability of the vocal cords)*.

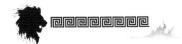 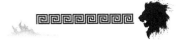
Tumors and Tumor Like Conditions:

Retinoblastoma - This is the most common primary malignancy of the globe. **If you see calcification in the globe of a child - this is the answer.**

The step 1 question is RB suppressor gene (chromosome 13 — "unlucky 13"). That's the same chromosome osteosarcoma patients have issues with and why these guys are at increased risk of facial osteosarcoma after radiation.

The globe should be normal in size (or bigger), where Coats' is usually smaller. It's **usually seen before age 3** (rare after age 6). The trivia is gonna be where else it occurs. They can be bilateral (both eyes - 30%), *trilateral* (both eyes and the pineal gland), and *quadrilateral* (both eyes, pineal, and suprasellar).

Coats' Disease - The cause of this is retinal telangiectasia which results in leaky blood and subretinal exudate. It can lead to retinal detachment. It's seen in young boys and typically unilateral. The key detail is that it is NOT CALCIFIED (retinoblastoma is).

CT - Dense
T1 - Hyper
T2 - Hyper

Coats disease has a smaller globe. Retinoblastoma has a normal sized globe.

Persistent Hyperplastic Primary Vitreous (PHPV) -

This is a failure of the embryonic ocular blood supply to regress. It can lead to retinal detachment. The classic look is a **small eye (microphthalmia) with increased density of the vitreous**. No calcification.

Retinal Detachment - This can occur secondary to PHPV or Coats. It can also be caused by trauma, sickle cell, or just old age. The imaging finding is a "V" or "Y" shaped appearance due to lifted up retinal leaves and subretinal fluid.

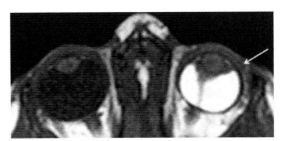
Retinal Detachment in the setting of PHPV

Globe Size Comparison
- A Strategy for Eliminating Distractors

- *Retinoblastoma* - Normal Size
- *Toxocariasis* - Normal Size

- *PHPV* - Small Size *(Normal Birth Age)*
- *Retinopathy of Prematurity* - Bilateral Small
- Coats' - Smaller Size

Melanoma - This is the **most common intra-occular lesion in an adult.** If you see an enhancing soft tissue mass in the back of an adult's eye this is the answer.

Here are 4 ways you could ask a question about this:
(1) show a picture - what is it?,
(2) ask what the most common intra-occular lesion in an adult is?
(3) ask the buzzword *"collar button shaped" ?* - which is related to Bruch's membrane,
(4) strong predilection for liver mets - next step Liver MR.

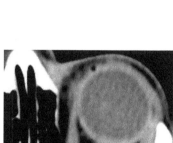

Optic Nerve Glioma: These almost always (90%) occur under the age of 20. You see expansion / enlargement of the entire nerve. If they are bilateral you think about **NF-1**. They are most often WHO grade 1 *Pilocytic Astrocytomas*. If they are sporadic they can be GBMs and absolutely destroy you.

Optic Nerve Sheath Meningioma: The buzzword is *"tram-track" calcifications.* Another buzzword is "doughnut" appearance, with **circumferential enhancement around the optic nerve.**

"Tram-Track" = Meningioma

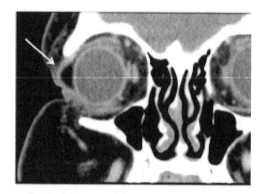

Dermoid: This is the most common benign congenital orbital mass.

It's usually **superior and lateral,** arising from the frontozygomatic suture, and presenting in the first 10 years of life. It's gonna have fat in it (like any good dermoid). The location is classic.

Orbital Dermoid - Classic Location

Rhabdomyosarcoma - *Most common extra-occular orbital malignancy in children* (dermoid is most common benign orbital mass in child). Favors the superior-medial orbit and classically has bone destruction. Just think **"bulky orbital mass in a 7 year old."**

When they do occur - 40% of the time it's in the head and neck - and then most commonly it's in the orbit. It's still rare as hell.

Lymphoma - There is an association with **Chlamydia Psittaci** (the bird fever thing) and MALT lymphoma of the orbit. It usually involves the upper outer orbit - closely associated with the lacrimal gland. It will enhance homogeneously and restricts diffusion - just like in the brain.

Metastatic Neuroblastoma - This has a very classic appearance of **"Raccoon Eyes"** on physical exam.

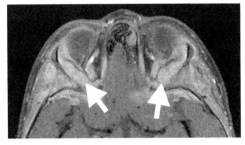

The *classic location is periorbital tumor infiltration with associated proptosis.* Don't forget a basilar skull fracture can also cause Raccoon Eyes... so clinical correlation is advised. Neuroblastoma mets tend to be more

Another thing worth mentioning is the bony involvement of the greater wing of the sphenoid. Neuroblastoma is gonna be bilateral. Ewings favors this location also - but will be unilateral.

Metastatic Scirrhous (fibrosing) Breast Cancer -

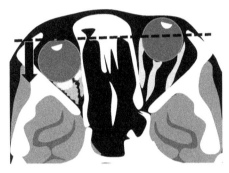

This is classic gamesmanship here. The important point to know is that unlike primary orbital tumors that are going to cause proptosis, classically the **breast cancer met causes a desmoplastic reaction and enophthalmos** *(posterior displacement of the globe).*

Trivia: Mets are actually more common to the eye relative to the orbit (like 8x more common).

Infiltrative retrobulbar mass + enophthalmos = scirrhous carcinoma of the breast

---

IgG4 - Orbit

Orbital Pseudotumor:

This is one of those IgG4 idiopathic inflammatory conditions that involves the extraoccular muscles. It looks like an expanded muscle. The things to remember are that this thing is **painful**, unilateral, it **most commonly involves the lateral rectus** and it **does NOT spare the myotendinous insertions**. Remember that Graves does not cause pain, and does spare the myotendinous insertions. It gets better with steroids. It's classically T2 dark.

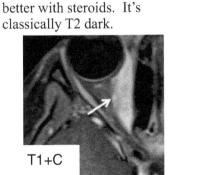

T1+C

Tolosa Hunt Syndrome:

This is histologically the same thing as orbital pseudotumor but instead involves the cavernous sinus.

It is painful (just like pseudotumor), and presents with multiple cranial nerve palsies. It responds to steroids (just like pseudotumor).

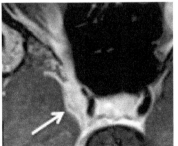
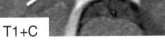

T1+C

Lymphocytic Hypophysitis:

This is the same deal as orbital pseudotumor and Tolosa Hunt, except it's the pituitary gland. Just think enlarged pituitary stalk in a postpartum / 3rd trimester woman. It looks like a pituitary adenoma, but it classically has a <u>T2 dark rim</u>.

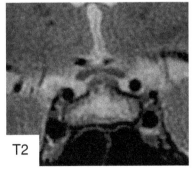

T2

Thyroid Orbitopathy: This is seen in 1/4th of the Graves cases and is the most common cause of exophthalmos. The antibodies that activate TSH receptors also activate orbital fibroblasts and adipocytes.

Things to know:
- Risk of compressive optic neuropathy
- Enlargement of ONLY MUSCLE BELLY (spares tendon) - different than *pseudo tumor*
- NOT Painful - different than *pseudo tumor*
- Order of Involvement:
  IR > MR > SR > LR > SO/IO

Inferior, **M**iddle, **S**uperior, **L**ateral, **O**blique

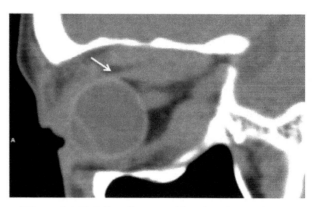

Thyroid Orbit - *Spares Tendon Insertion*

Orbital Vascular Malformations

Lymphangioma	Varix	Carotid-Cavernous Fistula
These are actually a mix of venous and lymphatic malformations. They are ill-defined and lack a capsule. The usual distribution is infiltrative (**multi-spatial**), involving, pre-septal, post-septal, extraconal, and intraconal locations.	These occur secondary to weakness in the post-capillary venous wall (gives you massive dilation of the valveless orbital veins).	These come in two flavors: (1) Direct - which is secondary to trauma, and (2) Indirect - which just occurs randomly in post menopausal women.
Fluid-Fluid levels are the most classic finding , with regard to multiple choice.	Most likely question is going to pertain to the fact that **they distend with provocative maneuvers** (valsalva, hanging head, etc...).	The direct kind is a communication between the intracavernous ICA and cavernous sinus. The indirect kind is usually a dural shunt between meningeal branches of the ECA and the Cavernous Sinus.
<u>Do NOT distend with provocative maneuvers (valsalva).</u>	Another piece of trivia is that they are the *most common cause of spontaneous orbital hemorrhage.* They can thrombose and present with pain.	*Buzzword: Pulsatile Exophthalmos *although this can also be a buzzword for NF-1 in the setting of sphenoid wing dysplasia.*

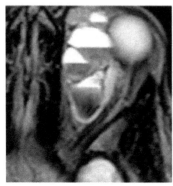

Fluid-Fluid Levels

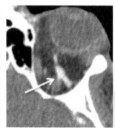

Prominent left cavernous sinus

Prominent left superior ophthalmic vein with proptosis

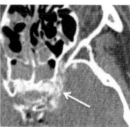

Orbital Infection

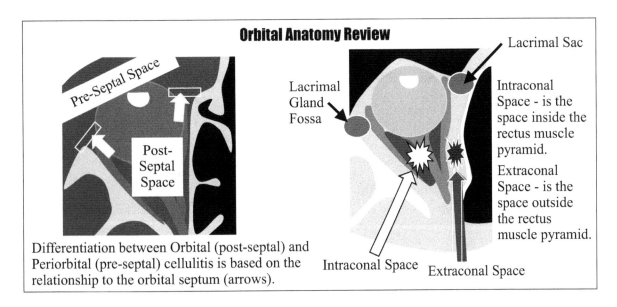

Orbital Anatomy Review

Pre-Septal Space

Post-Septal Space

Lacrimal Gland Fossa

Lacrimal Sac

Intraconal Space - is the space inside the rectus muscle pyramid.

Extraconal Space - is the space outside the rectus muscle pyramid.

Intraconal Space   Extraconal Space

Differentiation between Orbital (post-septal) and Periorbital (pre-septal) cellulitis is based on the relationship to the orbital septum (arrows).

Pre-Septal/ Post-Septal Cellulitis -

As above, location of orbital infections are described by their relationship to the orbital septum. The testable trivia is probably (1) that the orbital septum originates from the periosteum of the orbit and inserts in the palpebral tissue along the tarsal plate, (2) that pre-septal infections usually start in adjacent structures (likely teeth and the face), (3) post-septal infections are usually from paranasal sinusitis, and (4) pre-septal infections are treated medically, post septal is surgical.

Trivia: Periorbital abscess can cause thrombosis of the ophthalmic veins or cavernous sinus (in extreme examples infection — usually aspergillosis — can even cause a cavernous-carotid fistula).

Dacryocystitis -

This is inflammation and dilation of the lacrimal <u>sac</u>. It has an Aunt Minnie look, with a well circumscribed, round rim enhancing lesion centered in the lacrimal fossa. The etiology is typically obstruction followed by bacterial infection (staph and strep).

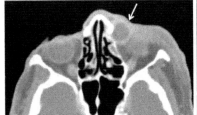
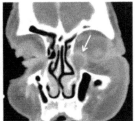

Usually this is diagnosed clinically unless there is an associated peri-orbital cellulitis in which can CT is needed to exclude post septal infection (treated surgically) from simple dacryocystitis (treated non-surgically).

Orbital Subperiosteal Abscess:

If you get inflammation under the periosteum it can progress to abscess formation.

This is usually associated with ethmoid sinusitis. This also has a very classic look.

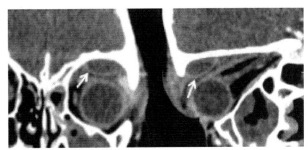

Misc Orbital Conditions

Optic Neuritis:

There will be **enhancement of the optic nerve**, *without enlargement* of the nerve/ sheath complex. Usually (70%) unilateral, and painful.

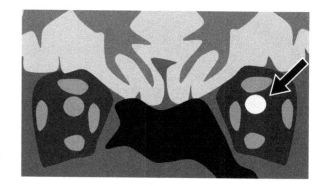

You will often see intracranial or spinal cord demyelination – in the setting of Devics (neuromyelitis optica). 50% of patient's with acute optic neuritis will develop MS.

 If the optic nerve is enlarged, think glioma… then think NF-1.

Papilledema:

This is really an eye exam thing.

Having said that you can sometimes see dilation/ swelling of the optic nerve sheath.

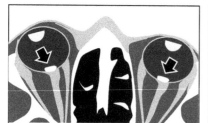

Drusen - Mineralization at the optic disc. Supposedly there is an association with age-related maculopathy

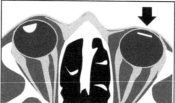

Intraocular Lens Implant -
The standard treatment for cataracts. A replaced lens has a thin linear appearance.

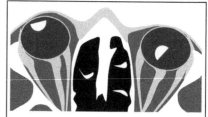

Ectopia Lentis (lens dislocation) - Causes include Trauma, Marfans, and Homocystinuria.

Coloboma:

This is a focal discontinuity of the globe (failure of the choroid fissure to close). They are usually posterior. If you see a unilateral one - think sporadic.

If you see bilateral ones - think CHARGE (coloboma, heart, GU, ears).

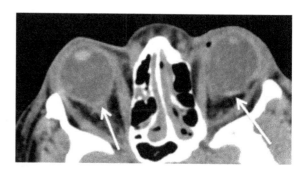

Bilateral Coloboma - CHARGE Syndrome

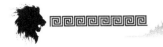 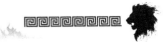

Anatomy Trivia

Cord Blood Supply: There is an anterior blood supply and a posterior blood supply to the cord. These guys get taken out with different clinical syndromes.

Anterior spinal artery - arises bilaterally as two small branches at the level of the termination of the vertebral arteries. These two arteries join around the level of the foramen magnum.

Artery of Adamkiewicz – This is the most notable reinforcer of the anterior spinal artery. In 75% of people it **comes off the left side of the aorta between T8 and T11.** It supplies the lower 2/3 of the cord. This thing can get covered with the placement of an endovascular stent graft for aneurysm or dissection repair leading to spine infarct.

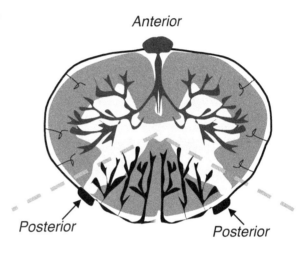

Posterior Spinal Artery – Paired arteries which arise either from the vertebral arteries or the posterior inferior cerebellar artery. Unlike the anterior spinal artery this one is somewhat discontinuous and reinforced by multiple segmental or radiculopial branches.

Conus Medullaris: This is the terminal end of the spinal cord. It usually terminates at around L1. Below the inferior endplate of the L2 / L3 body should make you think tethered cord (especially if shown in a multiple choice setting).

Epidural Fat: The epidural fat is not evenly distributed. The epidural space in the cervical cord is predominantly filled with venous plexus (as opposed to fat). In the lumbar spine there is fat both anterior and posterior to the cord. *"Epidural Lipomatosis"* = is a hypertrophy of this fat that only occurs with patients on steroids ("on corticosteroids" would be a huge clue).

Stenosis: Spinal stenosis can be congenital (associated with short pedicles) or be acquired. The Torg-Pavlov ratio can be used to call it (cervical canal diameter to vertebral body width < 0.85).
Symptomatic stenosis is more common in the cervical spine (versus the thoracic spine or lumbar spine). You can get some congenital stenosis in the lumbar spine from short pedicles, but it's generally not symptomatic until middle age.

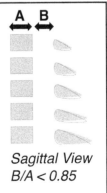

Sagittal View
B/A < 0.85

Degenerative Changes

What is this degenerative change you speak of ? The best way to understand this is through two mechanisms; **Spondylosis Deformans** and **Intervertebral Osteochondrosis.**

Spondylosis Deformans

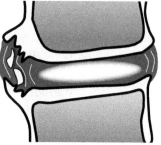

This is probably part of "normal aging"

"Degenerative Change" or spine osteoarthritis. This is more rim / margin centered. Process is characterized by osteophyte formation.

Intervertebral Osteochondrosis

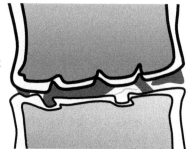

Pathologic (but not necessarily symptomatic)

"Deteriorated Disc" - This process is more centered in the disc space favoring the nucleus pulposus & vertebral body endplates.

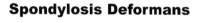 **THIS** vs **THAT**: Osteophytes vs Syndesmophytes

Osteophytes:

- More horizontal / oblique with a "claw" like appearance.
- Formed also the vertebral margin.
- Seen in "DJD" / Spondylosis

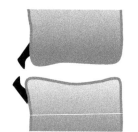

Syndesmophytes:

- More vertical symmetric, and thinner
- Represent ossification of the annulus fibrosis.
- Seen in Ankylosing Spondylitis.

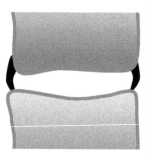

Endplate Changes: Commonly referred to as "**Modic Changes**."

There is a progression in the MRI signal characteristics that makes sense if you think about it. You start out with degenerative changes causing irritation / inflammation so there is edema (T2 bright). This progresses to chronic inflammation which leads to some fatty change – just like in the bowel of an IBD patient – causing T1 bright signal. Finally, the whole thing gets burned out and fibrotic and it's T1 and T2 dark. As a prominent factoid, Type 1 changes look a lot like Osteomyelitis (clinical correlation is recommended).

Type 1 "Edema"	T1 Dark, T2 Bright
Type 2 "Fat"	T1 Bright, T2 Bright
Type 3 "Scar"	T1 Dark, T2 Dark

Type 1
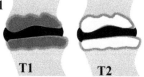
T1   T2

Type 2
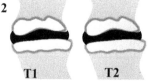
T1   T2

Type 3
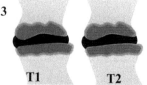
T1   T2

Annular Fissure:

As the disc ages, it tends to dry out making it more friable and easily torn. "Tears" in the annulus (which are present in pretty much every degenerated disc) aren't called "tears" but instead "fissures". People who write the papers on this stuff make a big fucking deal about that - with the idea being that "tear" implies pathology. Fissuring can be asymptomatic and part of the aging process.

Even though fissures are present in basically every degenerated disc you don't always see them on MRI. What you do see (some of the time) is a fluid signal gap in the annulus - which has been given the official vocabulary word "**High Intensity Zone**," and anything with official vocabulary nomenclature should be respected as possible multiple choice fodder.

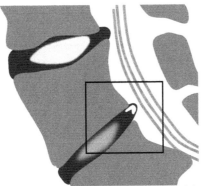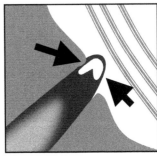

"High Intensity Zone" -MR with Fluid Signal in the Annulus

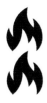
- Annular fissures may be a source of pain
(radial pain fibers - trigger "discogenic pain") but are also seen as incidentals.
- Fissures are found in all degenerative discs but are not all fissures are visualized as HIZs.
- Discography is more sensitive to fissures relative to MRI, but still not 100% sensitive.
- Also, Dude, "Tear" is not the preferred nomenclature - "Fissure."

Schmorl Node: *Intravertebral Herniation*	Scheuermann's	Limbus Vertebra
This is a herniation of disc material through a defect in the vertebral body endplate into the actual marrow. Common - like 75% of people have them. Classic look is to favor the inferior endplate of the lower thoracic / upper lumbar spine. When they are acute they can have edema on T2 and be dark on T1 - mimicking osteomyelitis. Chronic versions will have a sclerotic rim. 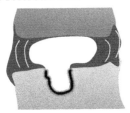	This is multiple levels (at least 3) of wedged vertebral bodies with associated Schmorl's nodes — 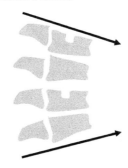 Most classically the thoracic spine of a teenager, resulting in kyphotic deformity (40 degrees in thoracic or 30 degrees in thoracolumbar). 25% of patients have scoliosis.	This is a fracture mimic that is the result of herniated disc material between the non-fused apophysis and adjacent vertebral body. 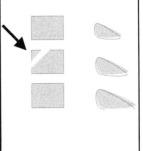

Disc Nomenclature:

In order to "improve accuracy" in the description of lumbar spine disc disease, a handful of elites gathered at an unknown location, ate caviar, drank wine, and then made a sacrifice to Moloch the Owl God - after which they issued a proclamation on what vocabulary words you are and are not allowed to use when describing degenerative disc herniation.

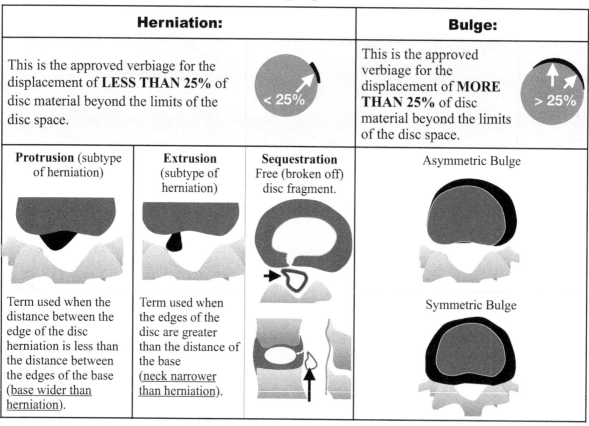

Herniation:			Bulge:
This is the approved verbiage for the displacement of **LESS THAN 25%** of disc material beyond the limits of the disc space.			This is the approved verbiage for the displacement of **MORE THAN 25%** of disc material beyond the limits of the disc space.
Protrusion (subtype of herniation)	**Extrusion** (subtype of herniation)	**Sequestration** Free (broken off) disc fragment.	Asymmetric Bulge
Term used when the distance between the edge of the disc herniation is less than the distance between the edges of the base (base wider than herniation).	Term used when the edges of the disc are greater than the distance of the base (neck narrower than herniation).		Symmetric Bulge

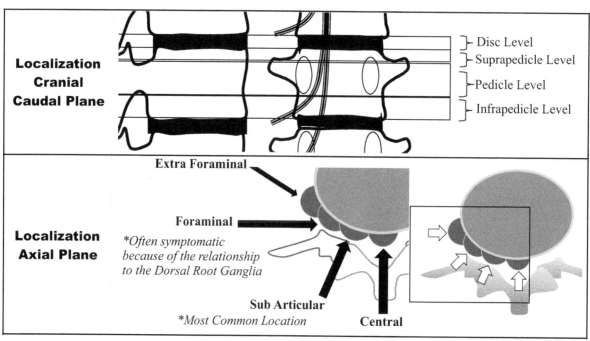

Localization Cranial Caudal Plane

- Disc Level
- Suprapedicle Level
- Pedicle Level
- Infrapedicle Level

Localization Axial Plane

Extra Foraminal

Foraminal
Often symptomatic because of the relationship to the Dorsal Root Ganglia

Sub Articular
Most Common Location

Central

Which Nerve is Compressed?

There are 31 pairs of spinal nerves, with each pair corresponding to the adjacent vertebra – the notable exception being the "C8" nerve. Cervical disc herniations are less common than lumbar ones.

The question is most likely to take place in the lumbar spine (the same spot most disc herniations occur). In fact more than 90% of herniations occur at L4-L5, and L5-S1.

A tale of two herniations. It was the best of times, it was the worst of times...

Scenario 1:

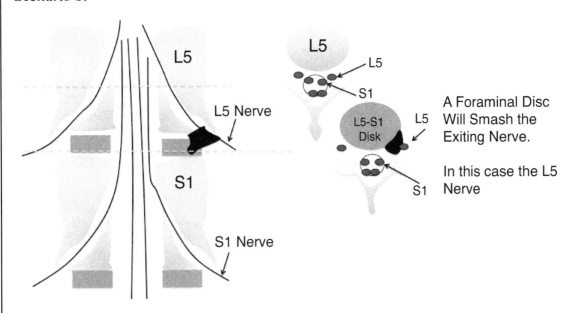

A Foraminal Disc Will Smash the Exiting Nerve.

In this case the L5 Nerve

Scenario 2:

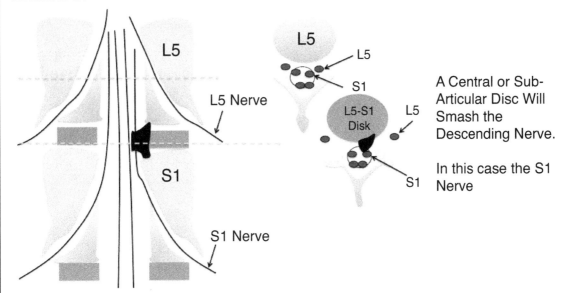

A Central or Sub-Articular Disc Will Smash the Descending Nerve.

In this case the S1 Nerve

LP / Myelogram Technique

Absolute Contraindications:
- Increased intracranial pressure or obstructed CSF flow
- Bleeding diathesis (<u>hypo</u>coagulability)
- *Myelogram Specific* — Iodinated contrast allergy

Relative Contraindications (vary per institution):
- Overlying infection, hematoma, or scarring
- *Myelogram Specific* - Recent myelogram (< 1 week)
- *Myelogram Specific* - History of seizures

Prior to the LP
(ACR-ASNR recommendations)

- STOP Coumadin 4-5 days
- STOP Plavix for 7 days
- Hold LMW Heparin for 12 hours
- Hold Heparin for 2-4 hours - document normal PTT
- Aspirin and NSAIDs are fine (not contraindicated)

Legit Indications for Fluoro Guided LP:
- Advanced degenerative spondylosis,
- Post-surgical changes,
- Patient is so fat ("a person of size"), when Dracula sucked his/her blood, he got diabetes.
- *Myelogram Specific* - MRI contraindication
- *Myelogram Specific* - Geriatric Professor Emeritus of Neurosurgery wants it, and it is better than doing the pneumoencephalogram he originally ordered.

NOT Legit Indications for Fluoro Guided LP — *all of which I've heard:*
- "The patient is crazy"
- "The patient is crazy & violent"
- "The patient is crazy, violent, and has high viral load HIV…. and Hep C"
- "The patient recently escaped a locked mental institution for the extremely violent and criminally insane, has both HIV and Hep C. He spits like a camel and has really terrible body odor."

Technical Overview

L2-L3 or L3-L4 are common entry points. A potential trick would be to show you imaging with a low lying conus (usually that thing stops at L1-L2).

Remember you need to be below the conus - so you might need to adjust down, depending on how low it is.

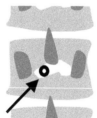

Target the interlaminar space, just off of midline.

Always aspirate before you inject anything.

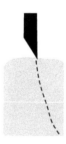

The needle will naturally steer toward the sharper side and away from the bevel. So, if you are directing the needle, you'll want the bevel side opposite the direction you are attempting to steer.

Myelogram Specific - Contrast should flow freely away from the needle tip, gradually filling the thecal sac. The outlining of the cauda equina is another promising sign that you did it right. If contrast pools at the needle tip or along the posterior or lateral thecal sac without free-flow, a subdural injection or injection in the fat around the thecal sac should be suspected.

Technical Strategies to Reduce the Incidence of Post Dural Puncture Headache (PDPH):

- Use a small needle (25 G), especially for epidural pain injections or myelography. You might have to use a 22G for a diagnostic LP or you are going to struggle to get enough fluid for a sample, and your opening pressures may not be accurate.
- Non-cutting "atraumatic" needle (diamond shaped tip) reduce incidence of PDPH
- Replace the stylet before you withdraw the needle. This isn't just for the 1 in a million chance that you suck a nerve root up in the needle. This has also been shown to reduce incidence of PDPH
- Direction of the bevel: This actually matters

You want to run the bevel parallel with the fibers to push them apart...not cut them.

Perpendicular is wrong. You are going to cut those fibers. Coming in at a crazy sideways angle is also not ideal (same reason).

<table>
<tr><th colspan="2" align="center">Blood Patch</th></tr>
</table>

Even a miniscule defect within the thecal sac post LP can allow leakage of spinal fluid resulting in intracranial hypotension and the dreaded chronic/debilitating post dural puncture headache. Classic PDPHs are bilateral, better laying down, and worse sitting up. They are also worse with coughing, sneezing, or straining to push out a large turd (from chronic opioid abuse). The procedure involves injecting between 3-20cc of the patients own blood into the epidural space near the original puncture site with the hope of sealing the hole.	• Most PDPHs start 24 hours after the puncture (between 24-48 hours) - larger leaks can present earlier. • Most people will wait 72 hours after the headache begins ("conservative therapy") prior to attempting the patch. • Most people will try at least twice before calling neurosurgery to sew to hole you carved out of the dura (you fucking psycho) • Severe atypical symptoms should prompt a CT (to exclude a subdural from severe hypotension).

"Failed Back Surgery Syndrome" (FBSS)

Another entity invented by NEJM to take down the surgical subspecialties. Per the NEJM these greedy surgeons generally go from a non-indicated spine surgery, to a non-indicated leg amputation, to a non-indicated tonsillectomy on an innocent child.

Text books will define it as recurrent or residual low back pain in the patient after disk surgery. This occurs about 40% of the time (probably more), since most back surgery is not indicated and done on inappropriate candidates. Causes of FBSS are grouped into early and late for the purpose of multiple choice test question writing:

Complications of Spine Surgery	
Recurrent Residual Disk	Will lack enhancement (unlike a scar – which will enhance on delays)
Epidural Fibrosis	Scar, that is usually posterior, and enhances homogeneously
Arachnoiditis	Buzzwords are *"clumped nerve roots"* and *"empty thecal sac"*, **Enhancement for 6 weeks post op is considered normal**. After 6 weeks may be infectious or inflammatory.
12,000 Square Foot Mansion Syndrome	As spine surgeons perform more and more unnecessary surgeries they need something to spend all that money on.

 THIS *vs* **THAT:** *Scar vs Residual Disc:*

T1 Pre Contrast they will look the same... like a bunch of mushy crap.
T1 Post Contrast the disc will still look like mushy crap, but the scar will enhance.

Conjoined Nerve Roots:

Two adjacent nerve roots sharing an enlarged common sleeve – at a point during their exit from the thecal sac. This can be a source of FBSS if it is the source of pain instead of a disc. Alternatively it could be misidentified as a disc preoperatively. In both cases, the Radiologist will be cast in the roll of "Scapegoat" during the malpractice suit.

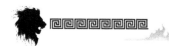
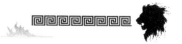
Odontoid Fracture Classification:

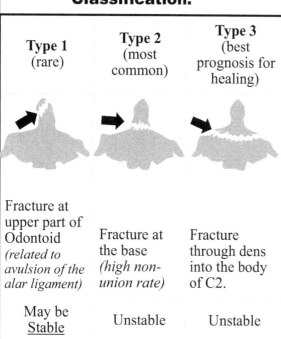

Type 1 (rare)	Type 2 (most common)	Type 3 (best prognosis for healing)
Fracture at upper part of Odontoid *(related to avulsion of the alar ligament)*	Fracture at the base *(high non-union rate)*	Fracture through dens into the body of C2.
May be <u>Stable</u>	Unstable	Unstable

Jefferson Fracture:

This is an axial loading injury (jumping into a shallow pool) – with the blow typically to the top of the head.

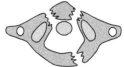

The anterior and posterior arches blow out laterally.

- About 30% will also have a C2 Fracture
- **Neurologic (cord) damage is rare**, because all the force is directed into the bones.

Could be shown on a plain film open mouth odontoid view.

Remember the C1 lateral masses shouldn't slide off laterally.

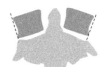

Normal Comparison

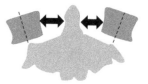

Increased distance between the lateral masses of C1 and odontoid peg

Os Odontoideum / Os Terminale:

These variants can mimic a type 1 Odontoid fracture. In both cases, you have an ossicle located at the position of the odontoid tip (the orthotopic position). The primary difference is that with an Os Odontoideum the base of the dens is usually hypoplastic.

- Prone to subluxation and instability.
- Associated with Morquio's syndrome.
- Orthotopic is the position on top of the dens.
- Dystopic is when it's fused to the clivus.

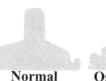
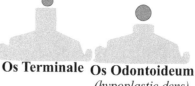

Normal   **Os Terminale**   **Os Odontoideum**
(hypoplastic dens)

Hangman's Fracture:

Seen most commonly when the chin hits the dashboard in an MVA ("direct blow to the face"). The **fracture is through the bilateral pars at C2** (or the pedicles – which is less likely). You will have anterior subluxation of C2 on C3 (> 2mm). Cord damage is actually uncommon with these, as the acquired pars defect allows for canal widening. There is often an associated fracture of the anterior inferior corner at C2 – from avulsion of the anterior longitudinal ligament. Traction is contraindicated.

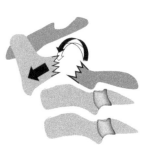

Flexion Teardrop:

This represents a teardrop shaped fracture fragment at the anterior-inferior vertebral body. Flexion injury is bad because it is associated with anterior cord syndrome (85% of patients have deficits). This is an unstable fracture, associated with posterior subluxation of the vertebral body.

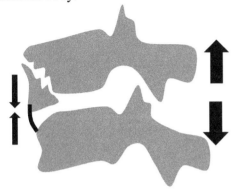

Extension Teardrop:

Another anterior inferior teardrop shaped fragment with avulsion of the anterior longitudinal ligament. This is less serious than the flexion type.

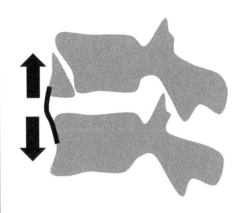

Flexion Teardrop	Extension Teardrop
Impaction Injury	Distraction Injury
Extremely Unstable	Stable in flexion (unstable in extension)
Hyperflexion	Hyperextension
Classic History: *"Ran into wall"*	Classic History *"Hit from behind"*

Clay-Shoveler's Fracture: This is an avulsion injury of a lower cervical / upper thoracic spinous process (usually C7). It is the result of a forceful hyperflexion movement (like shoveling).

The "ghost sign" describes a double spinous process at C6-C7 on AP radiograph.

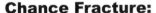

Chance Fracture:

These are flexion-distraction fractures that are classically associated with a lap-band seatbelt. There are 3 column (unstable) fractures.
Most commonly seen at the upper lumbar levels & thoracolumbar junction.
High association with solid organ trauma.

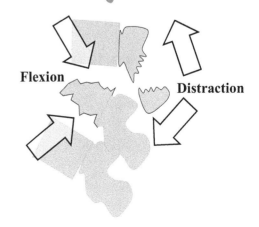

Flexion   Distraction

Facet Dislocation: This is a spectrum: Subluxed facets -> Perched -> Locked.

Unilateral: If you have unilateral locked facet (usually from hyperflexion and rotation) the superior facet slides over the inferior facet and gets locked. The unilateral is a stable injury. You will have the inverted hamburger sign on axial imaging on the dislocated side.

Bilateral: This is the result of severe hyperflexion. You are going to have disruption of the posterior ligament complex. When this is full on, you are going to have the dislocated vertebra displaced forward one –half the AP diameter of the vertebral body. This is <u>highly unstable</u>, and strongly associated with cord injury.

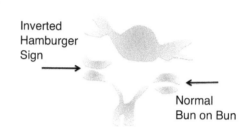

Inverted Hamburger Sign →

← Normal Bun on Bun

Atlantoaxial Instability:

The articulation between C1 and C2 allows for lateral movement (shaking your head no). The transverse cruciform ligament straps the dens to the anterior arch of C1. The distance between the anterior arch and dens shouldn't be more than 5 mm. The thing to know is the **association with Down syndrome and juvenile RA.**

Rotary subluxation can occur in children without a fracture, with the kid stuck in a "cock-robin" position – which looks like torticollis. Actually differentiating from torticollis is difficult and may require dynamic maneuvers on the scanner.

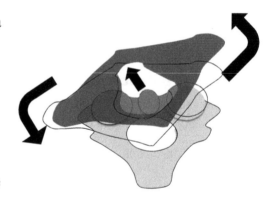

This never, ever, ever happens in the absence of a fracture in an adult (who doesn't have Downs or RA). Having said that, people over call this all the time in adults who have their heads turned in the scanner.

Pars Interarticularis Defect (Spondylolysis or Adult Isthmic Spondylolisthesis) : This is also discussed in the Peds chapter (vol 1, page 137). I'll make a few comments for the adult version. Defects in the pars interarticuaris are usually caused by repetitive micro-trauma (related to hyper-extension). It is nearly always at L5-S1 (90%). Pain is typically a L5 radiculopathy caused by <u>foraminal stenosis</u> at L5-S1. The term "pseudo-disc" is sometimes used to describe the deformed annular fibers seen in the setting of a related anterolithesis (forward slippage).

Instability

You will read different definitions of "instability" as it relates to spinal trauma. The one I prefer is something along the lines of *"lost capacity to withstand even a normal physiologic load without: potential damage to the spinal cord, nerve roots, or developing an incapacitating deformity that forces one to seek employment in a cathedral bell tower."*

For the purpose of multiple choice you will see the words *"stable"* or *"unstable"* associated with specific fracture types. There are also some radiologic "definitions" of instability which seem to vary depending on who you ask. In general, if you have acute segmental kyphosis greater than 11 degrees, acute anterolisthesis greater than 3-4 mm, or gross motion on flexion / extension imaging it is probably an unstable fracture. You will also hear people talk about a "power ratio" for occipitocervical instability, and a spinal column theory for the thoracolumbar injury.

Occipitocervical Instability

This can be traumatic (in which case the patient rarely lives because they rip their brainstem in half), or congenital (classically seen with Down Syndrome). Two popular methods for evaluating this:

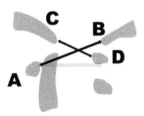

Powers Ratio = C-D: A-B
Ratio is greater than 1.0 = Ligamentous Instability

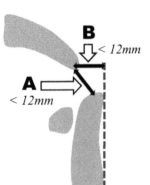

Harris Lines Rule of 12

Both the Basion-Dens (A) and Basion-Posterior Axial Distance (B) should be less than 12 mm.

Denis 3 Spinal Column Concept

Most often you will see this idea applied to thoracolumbar spinal fractures, although technically it has some validity in the lower cervical segments as well.

The idea is to divide the vertebral column into 3 vertical parallel columns , with <u>instability suggested when all 3 or 2 contiguous columns (anterior and middle column or middle and posterior column) are disrupted.</u>

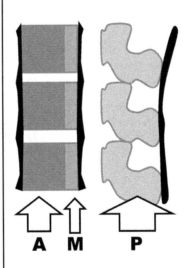

Anterior:
- Anterior Longitudinal Ligament
- Anterior 2/3 Vertebral Body

Middle:
- Posterior Longitudinal Ligament
- Posterior 1/3 Vertebral Body

Posterior:
- Posterior Ligaments
- Pedicles, Facets, Lamina, Spinous Process

The management does typically change with unstable fractures typically stabilized (either internal fusion or external bracing/reduction).

When Does a "Trauma" Indicate Imaging ?

Canadian C-Spine Rule:
- Age ≥65 years
- Paresthesias in extremities
- Dangerous mechanism:
- Fall ≥3 ft or 5 stairs
- Axial load to the head (empty swimming pool diving, piano fell on head - while chasing a road runner)
- High Speed MVA,
- Pedestrian vs Car
- Hulk Smash

Nexus Criteria:
- Focal neurologic deficit
- Midline spinal tenderness
- Altered level of consciousness
- Intoxication (you can't clear a drunk guys/girls c-spine while they are drunk).
- Distracting injury

THIS vs THAT: Stability

Unstable	Stable
Vertebral Overriding > 3mm ("Subluxation") Angulation > 11 Degrees	
Flexion Tear Drop	Extension Tear Drop (At least in Flexion)
Bilateral Facet Dislocation "Double-Locked"	Unilateral Facet Dislocation
Odontoid Fracture Type 2 and 3 *(most sources will say Type 2 & 3 or deploy the word "usually", but for sure if there is lateral displacement)*	Odontoid Fracture Type 1 *(usually stable - flex/extension films still usually done to exclude atlantooccipital instability)*
Two Contiguous Thoracolumbar Columns (anterior & middle or middle & posterior)	
Three Thoracolumbar Columns (Chance Fracture, Etc…)	Isolated Single Thoracolumbar Column Fracture
Jefferson Fracture	Clay Shoveler's Fracture
Hangman Fracture	Transverse Process Fracture
Atlanto-Occipital and Atlanto-Axial Dislocations	

Named Spine Fractures

Jefferson	Burst Fracture of C1	Axial Loading
Hangman	Bilateral Pedicle or Pars Fracture of C2	Hyperextension
Teardrop	Can be flexion or extension	Flexion (more common)
Clay-Shoveler's	Avulsion of spinous process at C7 or T1	Hyperflexion
Chance	Horizontal Fracture through thoracolumbar spine	"Seatbelt"

Trauma to the Cord:

There is a known correlation between spinal cord edema length and outcome. Having said that, you need to know the **most important factor for outcome is the presence of a hemorrhagic spinal cord injury** (these do very very badly).

Spinal Cord Syndromes			
Central Cord	Old lady with spondylosis or young person with bad extension injury.	Upper Extremity Deficit is worse than lower (corticospinal tracts are lateral in lower extremity)	
Anterior Cord	Flexion Injury	Immediate Paralysis	
Brown Sequard	Rotation injury or penetrating trauma	One side motor, other side sensory deficits	
Posterior Cord	Uncommon – but sometimes seen with hyperextension	Proprioception gone	

Anterior Cord Syndrome (The Really Bad One):

The anterior portion of the cord is jacked. Motor function and anterior column sensations (pain and temperature) are history. The dorsal column sensations (proprioception and vibration) are still intact.

This is the reason FLEXION injuries are so bad.

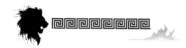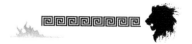
AVFs / AVMs:

There are 4 types. **Type 1 is by far the most common** (85%). **It is a Dural AVF**; the result of a fistula between the dorsal radiculomedullary arteries and radiculomedullary vein / coronal sinus – with the dural nerve sleeve. It is acquired and seen in older patients who present with progressive radiculomyelopathy. The most common location is the thoracic spine. If anyone asks, the "gold standard for diagnosis is angiography" , although CTA or MRA will get the job done. You will have T2 high signal in the central cord (which will be swollen), with serpentine perimedullary flow voids (which are usually dorsal).

\multicolumn{2}{c}{**Spinal AVM / AVFs**}	
Type 1	**Most Common Type** (85%). **Dural AVF** – with a single coiled vessel
Type 2	**Intramedullary Nidus** from anterior spinal artery or posterior spinal artery. Can have aneurysms, and can bleed. Most common presentation is SAH. Associated with HHT and KTS (other vascular syndromes).
Type 3	**Juvenile**, very rare, often complex and with a terrible prognosis
Type 4	Intradural **perimedullary** with subtypes depending on single vs multiple arterial supply. These tend to occur **near the conus.**

Foix Alajouanine Syndrome:

This is a <u>congestive myelopathy</u> associated with a Dural AVF. The classic history is a 45 year old male with lower extremity weakness and sensory deficits.

You have increased T2 signal (either at the conus or lower thoracic spine), with associated prominent vessels (flow voids). The underlying pathophysiology is venous hypertension - secondary to the vascular malformation.

Swollen High Signal Cord with <u>Serpentine flow voids</u> along the surface of cord

 Key Finding

The vascular malformation flow voids are - punctate, serpiginous, and serpentine.

They are NOT blob like - sorta like what you see with CSF pulsation signal loss.

Blob Like CSF Pulsation Artifacts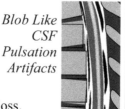

174

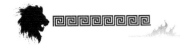 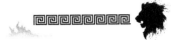

Syrinx – Also known as *"a hole in the cord"*. People use the word "syrinx" for all those fancy French / Latin words (hydromyelia, syringomyelia, hydrosyringomyelia, syringohydromyelia, syringobulbia etc…). They usually do this because they don't know what those words mean.

This is the simple version:

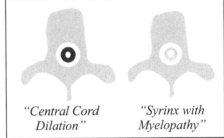

"Central Cord Dilation"   *"Syrinx with Myelopathy"*

- Hydromyelia = Lined by ependyma.
- Syringomyelia = NOT lined by ependyma

These is zero difference clinically - which is why everyone just says "syrinx." The distinction is strictly academic (i.e. multiple choice trivia).

Most (90%) cord dilations (healthy and sick ones) are congenital, and associated with Chiari I and II, as well as Dandy-Walker, Klippel-Feil, and Myelomeningoceles. The other 10% are acquired either by trauma, tumor, or vascular insufficiency.

In clinical practice, if there is perfectly central mid cord high signal dilation, surrounded by totally normal cord I call it "central cord dilation" or "benign central cord dilation." If there is the same thing but the cord around the dilation looks "sick" - grayish / high signal, or the cord is atrophic, then I use the word "**myelopathy**" or "myelopathic changes." <u>Myelopathy is a word for a diseased cord</u> - usually from disc/osteophyte compression. Although, you can have myelopathy for any number of neoplastic, post traumatic, or inflammatory processes.

Spinal Cord Infarct: - Cord infarct / ischemia can have a variety of causes. The most common cause is "idiopathic," although I'd expect the most common multiple choice scenario to revolve around treating an aneurysm with a stent graft, or embolizing a bronchial artery. Impairment involving the anterior spinal artery distribution is most common. With anterior spinal artery involvement you are going to have central cord / anterior horn cell high signal on T2 (because gray matter is more vulnerable to ischemia).

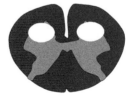

The "**owl's eye**" **sign** of anterior spinal cord infarct is a buzzword.

It's usually a long segment, (more than 2 vertebral body segments). <u>Diffusion</u> using single shot fast spin echo or line scan can be used with high sensitivity (to compensate for artifacts from spinal fluid movement).

Demyelinating (T2 / FLAIR Hyperintense):

Broadly you can think of cord pathology in 5 categories: Demyelinating, Tumor, Vascular, Inflammatory, and Infectious.

In the real world, the answer is almost always MS – which is by far the most common cause. The other three things it could be are Neuromyelitis Optica (NMO), acute disseminating encephalomyelitis (ADEM) or Transverse Myelitis (TM).

MS in the Cord: "Multiple lesions, over space and time." The lesions in the spine are typically short segment (< 2 vertebral segments), usually only affect half / part of the cord. The cervical cord is the most common location. There are usually lesions in the brain, if you have lesions in the cord (isolated cord lesions occur about 10% of the time). The lesions can enhance when acute – but this is less common than in the brain. You can sometimes see cord atrophy if the lesion burden is large.

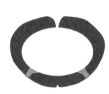

Transverse Myelitis: This is a focal inflammation of the cord. The causes are numerous (infectious, post vaccination – classic rabies, SLE, Sjogren's, Paraneoplastic, AV-malformations). You typically have at least 2/3 of the cross sectional area of the cord involved, and focal enlargement of the cord. Splitters will use the terms "Acute partial" for lesions less than two segments, and "acute complete" for lesions more than two segments. The factoid to know is that the "Acute partials" are at higher risk for developing MS.

ADEM: As described in the brain section, this is usually seen after a viral illness or infection typically in a child or young adult. The lesions favor the dorsal white matter (but can involve grey matter). As a pearl, the presence of cranial nerve enhancement is suggestive of ADEM. The step 1 trivia, is that the "anti-MOG IgG" test is positive in 50% of cases. Just like MS there are usually brain lesions (although ADEM lesions can occur in the basal ganglia and pons – which is unusual in MS).

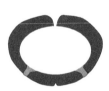

NMO (Neuromyelitis Optica): This is also sometimes called Devics. It can be monophasic or relapsing, and favors the optic nerves and cervical cord. Tends to be longer segment than MS, and involve the full transverse diameter of the cord (mild swelling). Brain lesions can occur (more commonly in Asians) and are usually periventricular. If any PhDs ask, the reason the periventricular location occurs is that the antibody (NMO IgG) attacks the Aquaporin 4 channels – which are found in highest concentration around the ventricles.

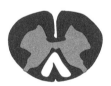

Subacute Combined Degeneration: This is a fancy way of describing the effects of a Vitamin B12 deficiency. The classic look is **bilateral, symmetrically increased T2 signal in the dorsal columns**, without enhancement. The appearance has been described as an "inverted V sign." The signal change typically begins in the upper thoracic region with ascending or descending progression.

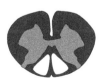

HIV Vacuolar Myelopathy: This is the most common cause of spinal cord dysfunction in untreated AIDS. Key word there is "untreated" - this is a late finding. Atrophy is the most common finding (thoracic is most common). The T2 high signal will be very similar to B12 (subacute combined degeneration) - symmetrically involving the posterior columns. It can only be shown 2 ways - (a) by telling you the patient has AIDS or risk factors such as unprotected anal sex at a truck stop with a man "bear" with a thick mustache while sharing IV drug needles, (b) not including B12 as an answer choice.

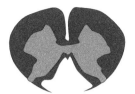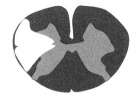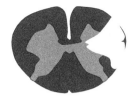

MS: Lesions favor the white matter of the cervical region. They tend to be random and asymmetric.

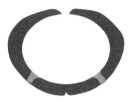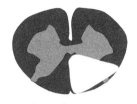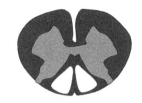

"Owl's Eye"
-Classic for **Ischemia** (Anterior)
-Also seen in **Polio**

-Ischemia
- More extensive anterior involvement.
-Also seen in **NMO**, **TM**, or **MS**

-Ischemia
-This time a posterior circulation pattern. These tend to be unilateral.
-**MS** can also look like this

Vitamin B12 (SCD) HIV

Posterior. Can look like an inverted "V"

MS	Usually Short Segment	Usually Part of the Cord	Not swollen, or Less Swollen	Can Enhance / Restrict when Acute
TM	Usually Long Segment	Usually involves both sides of the cord	Expanded, Swollen Cord	Can Enhance
NMO	Usually Long Segment	Usually involves both sides of the cord		Optic Nerves Involved
ADEM			Not swollen, or Less Swollen	
Infarct	Usually Long Segment			Restricted Diffusion
Tumor			Expanded, Swollen Cord	Can Enhance

Inflammatory / Infectious:

Arachnoiditis: This is a general term for inflammation of the subarachnoid space. It can be infectious but can also be post-surgical. **It actually occurs about 10-15% of the time after spine surgery, and can be a source of persistent pain / failed back.**

It's shown two ways:

(1) Empty Thecal Sac Sign – Nerve roots are adherent peripherally, giving the appearance of an empty sac.

(2) *Central Nerve Root Clumping.* This can range in severity from a few nerves clumping together, to all of them fused into a single central scarred band.

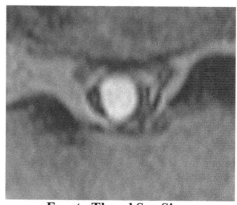

Empty Thecal Sac Sign

Guillain Barre Syndrome (GBS) - Also known as "Acute inflammatory demyelinating polyneuropathy" (AIDP). One of those weird auto-immune disorders that causes ascending flaccid paralysis. The step 1 trivia was **Campylobacter**, but you can also see it after surgery, or in patients with lymphoma or SLE.

The thing to know is **enhancement of the nerve roots of the cauda equina**.

Other pieces of trivia that are less likely to be asked are that the facial nerve is the most common cranial nerve affected, and that the anterior spinal roots enhance more than the posterior ones.

Chronic Inflammatory Demylinating Polyneuropathy (CIDP) - The chronic counterpart to GBS. Clinically this has a gradual and protracted weakness (GBS improves in 8 weeks, CIDP does not). The buzzword is thickened, enhancing, "onion bulb" nerve roots.

"Dreadlocks," "Locs," "Jaṭā" some people call them.

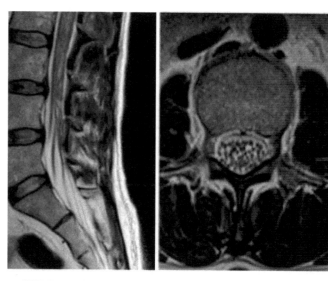

CIDP - Diffuse Thickening of the Nerve Roots

Tumor

The classic teaching with spinal cord tumors is to first describe the location of the tumor, as either (1) Intramedullary, (2) Extramedullary Intradural, or (3) Extradural. This is often easier said than done. Differentials are based on the location.

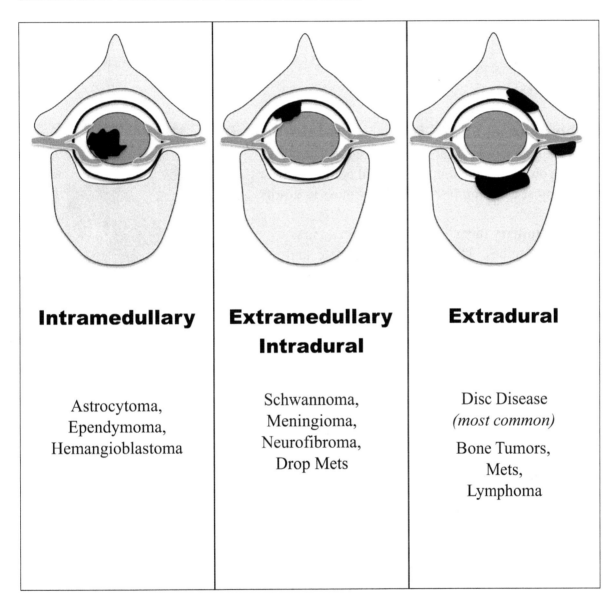

Intramedullary	Extramedullary Intradural	Extradural
Astrocytoma, Ependymoma, Hemangioblastoma	Schwannoma, Meningioma, Neurofibroma, Drop Mets	Disc Disease *(most common)* Bone Tumors, Mets, Lymphoma

Intramedullary:

Astrocytoma – This is the most common intramedullary tumor in peds. It favors the upper thoracic spine. There will be fusiform dilation of the cord over multiple segments. They are eccentric, dark on T1, bright on T2, and they enhance. They may be associated with rostral or caudal cysts which are usually benign syrinx(es).

Astrocytoma	Ependymoma
Most common in child	Most common in Adults
Eccentric	Central
Heterogenous Enhancement	Homogenous Enhancement
	More Often Hemorrhagic

Ependymoma – This is the most common primary cord tumor of the lower spinal cord and conus / filum terminale. You can see them in the cervical cord as well. This is the **most common intramedullary mass in adults**.

The "**myxopapillary form**" is exclusively found in the conus /filum locations. They can be hemorrhagic, and have a **dark cap on T2.** They have tumoral cysts about ¼ of the time. They are a typically long segment (averaging 4 segments).

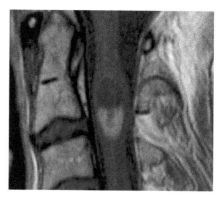
Ependymoma - Cervical Cord

Myxopapillary = Most commonly located in the Lumbar spine (conus/filum location)

Hemangioblastoma -

These are associated with Von Hippel Lindau (30%).

The thoracic level is favored (second most common is cervical).

The classic look is a wide cord with considerable edema. Adjacent serpinginous draining meningeal varicosities can be seen.

> **VHL Associations:**
> - Pheochromocytoma
> - CNS Hemangioblastoma *(cerebellum 75%, spine 25%)*
> - Endolymphatic Sac Tumor
> - Pancreatic Cysts
> - Pancreatic Islet Cell Tumors
> - Clear Cell RCC

Intramedullary Mets -

This is very very rare, but when it does happen it is usually lung (70%).

Extramedullary Intradural:

Schwannoma: This is the most common tumor to occur in the Extramedullary Intradural location. They are benign, usually solitary, usually arise from the dorsal nerve roots. They can be multiple in the setting of NF-2 and the Carney Complex. The appearance is variable, but the classic look is a dumbbell with the skinny handle being the intraforaminal component. They are T1 dark, T2 bright, and will enhance. They look a lot like neurofibromas. If they have central necrosis or hemorrhage, that favors a schwannoma.

Neurofibroma: This is another benign nerve tumor *(composed of all parts of the nerve: nerve + sheath)*, that is also usually solitary. There are two flavors: solitary and plexiform. The plexiform is a multilevel bulky nerve enlargement that is pathognomonic for NF-1. Their lifetime risk for malignant degeneration is around 5-10%. Think about malignant degeneration in the setting of rapid growth. They look a lot like schwannomas. If they have a hyperintense T2 rim with a central area of low signal – "target sign" that makes you favor neurofibroma.

Schwannoma	Neurofibroma
Does NOT envelop the adjacent nerve root	Does envelop the adjacent nerve root *(usually a dorsal sensory root)*
Solitary	Solitary
Multiple makes you think NF-2	Associated with NF -1 (even when single)
Cystic change / Hemorrhage	T2 bright rim, T2 dark center "target sign"
	Plexiform = Pathognomonic for NF-1

Meningioma: These guys adhere to but do not originate from the dura. They are more common in women (70%). They favor the posterior lateral thoracic spine, and the anterior cervical spine. They enhance brightly and homogeneously. They are often T1 iso to hypo, and slightly T2 bright. They can have calcifications.

Drop Mets: Medulloblastoma is the most common primary tumor to drop. Breast cancer is the most common systemic tumor to drop (followed by lung and melanoma). The cancer may coat the cord or nerve root, leading to a fine layer of enhancement ("zuckerguss").

Extradural:

Vertebral Hemangioma: These are very common – seen in about 10% of the population. They classically have thickened trabeculae appearing as parallel linear densities "jail bar" or "corduroy" appearance. In the vertebral body they are T1 and T2 bright, although the extraosseuous components typically lack fat and are isointense on T1.

Osteoid Osteoma: This is also covered in the MSK chapter, but as a brief review focusing on the spine, they love to involve the posterior elements (75%), and are rare after age 30. They tend to have a nidus and surrounding sclerosis. The nidus is T2 bright and will enhance. The classic story is night pain, improved with aspirin. Radiofrequency ablation can treat them (under certain conditions).

Osteoblastoma: This is similar to an Osteoid osteoma but larger than 1.5 cm. Again, very often in the posterior elements – usually of the cervical spine.

Aneurysmal Bone Cyst: These guys are also covered in the MSK chapter. They also like the posterior elements and are usually seen in the first two decades of life. They are expansile (as the name implies) and can have multiple fluid levels on T2. They can get big and look aggressive.

Giant Cell Tumor: These guys are also covered in the MSK chapter. These are common in the sacrum, although rare anywhere else in the spine. You don't see them in young kids. If they show this, it's going to be a **lytic expansile lesion in the sacrum with no rim of sclerosis.**

Chordoma: This is **most common in the sacrum** (they will want you to say clivus – that is actually number 2). The thing to know is that a vertebral primary tends to be more aggressive / malignant than its counter parts in the clivus or sacrum. The classic story in the vertebral column is "involvement of two or more adjacent vertebral bodies with the intervening disc. " Most are **very T2 bright**.

Leukemia: They love to show it in the spine. You have loss of the normal fatty marrow – so it's going to be homogeneously dark on T1. More on this in the MSK chapter.

Mets: The classic offenders are prostate, breast, lung, lymphoma, and myeloma. Think **multiple lesions with low T1 signal**. Cortical breakthrough or adjacent paravertebral components are also helpful.

Vertebra Plana:
The pancake flat vertebral body. Just say Eosinophilic Granuloma in a kid (could be neuroblastoma met), and Mets / Myeloma in an adult. 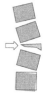

Blank for Scribbles:

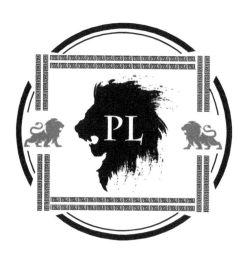

11

MUSCULOSKELETAL

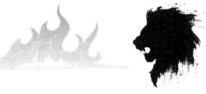

PROMETHEUS LIONHART, M.D.

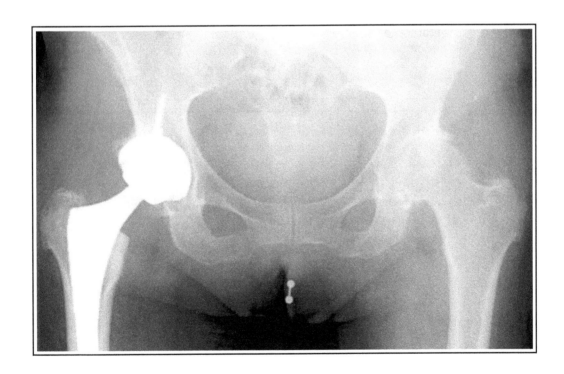

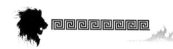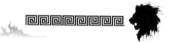
Fracture Vocab

		Pathologic Fracture:	Open Fracture (*Compound Fracture*):
Stress Fracture = Fracture resulting from the mismatch of bone strength and *chronic* mechanical force. They come in two flavors (A) Fatigue, and (B) Insufficiency.		You will sometimes hear people use this term synonymously with "Insufficiency Fracture". However, for the purpose of multiple choice this term will most likely refer to a <u>fracture through a lytic bone lesion.</u>	A fracture associated with an open wound. Typically these will go to the OR for reduction and washout - given the obvious risk for infection.
Fatigue Fracture (sometime simply called a "*stress fracture*"). Abnormal stress on <u>*Normal Bone*</u>. *Classic Scenario -* Insane (but kinda hot) Type A Female Cross Country Runner - literally runs until her legs & feet break in half.	**Insufficiency Fracture** Normal stress on <u>*Abnormal bone*</u>. *Classic Scenario -* Old lady with horrible osteoporosis breaks her back (compression fracture) by walking down a few steps. She blames Obama for the fracture.	These lytic lesions can be mets or be benign primary bone lesions (like an ABC, or Bone Cyst).	Tuft Fractures (finger tip fracture) with disruption of the nail plate are considered "open" fractures - and although the typically won't go to the OR they do get antibiotics (whereas an intact nail bed often won't).

Phases of Fracture Healing:

Physiology PhDs will describe 3 phases of bone healing (Inflammatory, Reparative, and Remodeling). From a Radiologist's perspective the most important thing to understand about this process is that around 7-14 days granulation tissue will be forming between the bone fragments. This results in an increased lucency of the fracture site related to bone resorption.

In other words, a healing fracture will be MORE LUCENT at 7-14 days.

This explains the disclaimer cowardly Radiologists throw out when they are afraid they missed a fracture *"Consider Repeat in 7-10 days,"* The idea is that in 7-10 days, you should be able to see the fracture line , if one is present , because of the increase in bone lucency that occurs normally in the healing process.

Fracture Healing Continued -

In general, bones heal in about 6-8 weeks, but is location dependent. Healing is the fastest in the phalanges (around 3 weeks), and the slowest is either the tibia or femoral neck/shaft - depending on what you read (around 2-3 months).

> Phalanges = Heal Fast (3 Weeks)
> Tibia = Heal Slow (10 Weeks)
> Everything Else = 6-8 weeks

Abnormal Healing Vocab

Delayed Union	Non-Union	Mal-Union
fracture not healed within the expected time period (but still might). Some sources will say "twice as long as expected"	fracture is not going to heal without intervention. Some sources will say "6-9 months." The classic locations are the scaphoid, anterior tibia, and lateral femoral neck.	This is union in poor anatomic position (healed crooked as a politician).

Risk Factors For Abnormal Healing (Delayed and Non-Union)

(these are the ones I think are most testable):

Vitamin D Deficiency	Gastric Bypass	Drugs / Meds
Vitamin D plays a vital role in calcium uptake and metabolism. Vitamin D deficiency is actually the most common vitamin deficiency in America (supposedly).	Having your gut rewired results in altered calcium absorption (causes secondary hyperparathyroid and stripping of calcium from bones) and therefore higher rates of non-union.	Tobacco (Smoking or Chewing) NSAIDS Prednisone (steroids)

unfused spinous process - failure to fuse the neural arch.
- well defined cortical margin

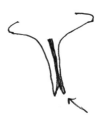

THIS *vs* THAT - Compressive Side vs Tensile Side:

This comes up in two main areas - the femoral neck and the tibia.

• Fractures of the **C**ompressive side are constantly pushed back together - these do well.

• Fractures of the **T**ensile side are constantly pulled apart - these are a pain in the ass to heal.

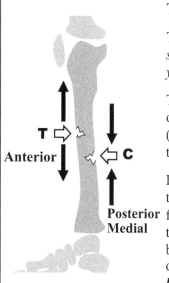

Tibial Stress Fracture:

This is the *most common site of a stress fracture in young athletes*.

These are most common on the compressive side (posterior medial) in either the proximal or distal third.

Less common are the tensile side (anterior) fractures, and these favor the mid shaft. They are bad news and don't heal - often called "***dreaded black lines***."

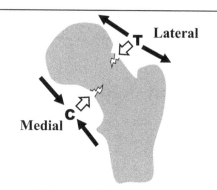

Femoral Stress Fracture:

Fractures along the compressive (medial) side are more common, typically seen in a younger person along the inferior femoral neck.

Fractures along the tensile (lateral) side are more common in old people.

SONK (Spontaneous Osteonecrosis of the Knee):

This is totally named wrong, as it is another type of insufficiency fracture. You see this in old ladies with the classic history of "sudden pain after rising from a seated position." Young people can get it too (much less common), usually seen after a meniscal surgery.

 Key Factoids:
• It's an insufficiency fracture (NOT osteonecrosis) think SINK not SONK
• Favors the medial femoral condyle (area of maximum weight bearing)
• Usually unilateral in an old lady without history of trauma
• Associated with meniscal injury

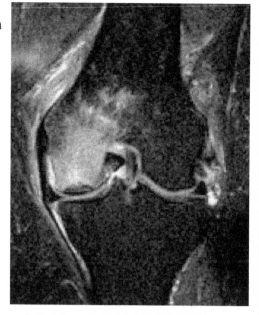

SONK — LOTS OF EDEMA
- Subchondral Deformity (arrows)

Navicular Stress Fracture – You see these in runners who run on hard surfaces. The thing to know is that just like in the wrist (scaphoid), the navicular is high risk for AVN.

March Fracture: This is a metatarsal stress fracture which is fairly common. Classically seen in military recruits that are marching all day long.

Calcaneal Stress Fracture – The calcaneus is actually the most fractured tarsal bone. The fractures are usually intra-articular (75%). The stress fracture will be seen with the fracture line perpendicular to the trabecular lines.

You'll rue the day you crossed me Trebek—ular Lines.

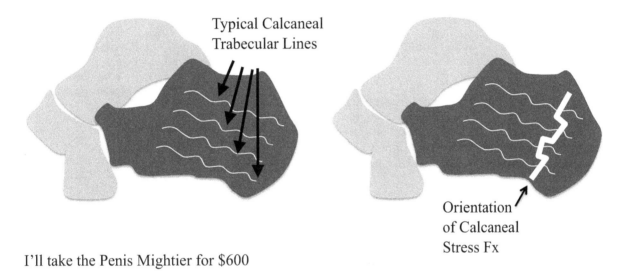

Typical Calcaneal Trabecular Lines

Orientation of Calcaneal Stress Fx

I'll take the Penis Mightier for $600

THIS vs THAT : High Risk vs Low Risk Stress Fractures:	
You can sort these based on the likelihood of uncomplicated healing when treated conservatively.	
High Risk	**Low Risk**
Femoral Neck (tensile side)	Femoral Neck (compressive side)
Transverse Patellar Fracture	Longitudinal Patellar Fracture
Anterior Tibial Fracture (midshaft)	Posterior Medial Tibial Fracture
5th Metatarsal	2nd and 3rd Metatarsal
Talus	Calcaneus
Tarsal Navicular	
Sesamoid Great Toe	

Scaphoid Fracture

Most common carpal bone fracture.

Typical age group is an adolescents and young adults (Grandma is more likely to get a distal radial fracture with a similar mechanism — fall).

Distal Pole /

Scaphoid Tubercle

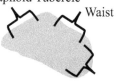

Waist

Proximal Pole

Blood flow is "retrograde" (distal to proximal). This is because the scaphoid surface is almost entirely (80%) covered with cartilage.

As such, the proximal pole most susceptible to **AVN and Non-Union**.

The first sign of AVN = Sclerosis (the dead bone can't turn over / recycle)

Most common (70 %) fracture site = waist

Displacement of > 1mm will likely get a fixation screw to pull the fragments together.

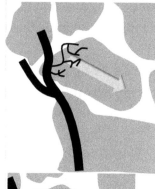

"Retrograde" (distal to proximal) via the Dorsal Carpal Branch of Radial Artery

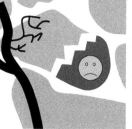

Proximal Pole is at Risk for AVN / Mal-Union

Trans-Scaphoid Perilunate Dislocation

Capitate

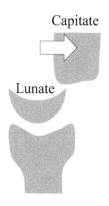

Lunate

Perilunate dislocation (discussed later in the chapter) have a high association (60%) with a scaphoid fracture

Scapholunate Ligament Disruption

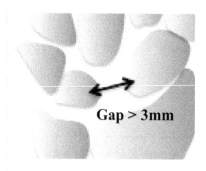

Gap > 3mm

Seen with 10-30% of distal radius and/or carpal fractures

The SL ligament is composed of 3 parts (volar, dorsal, and middle), with the dorsal band being the most important for carpal stability *(opposite of luno-triquetral which is volar)*.

Disruption of the ligament predisposes for DISI deformity (discussed later in the chapter in greater depth).

Humpback Deformity

This deformity results from angulation of the proximal and distal fragments - in the setting of a waist fracture.

Can progress to progressive collapse and non-union.

Associated with DISI

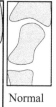

Normal

Humpback shown on lateral view

AVN

As above the proximal pole is at greatest risk.

The first sign of AVN = Sclerosis (the adjacent bones will demineralize, but the avascular bone will not). Later the bone will fragment.

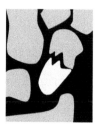

MRI = T1 Dark

Trivia: **"Prieser Disease"** is an atraumatic AVN of the scaphoid

SLAC and SNAC Wrists

Both are potential complications of trauma, with similar mechanisms.

SLAC Wrist (Scaphoid-Lunate Advanced Collapse) occurs with injury (or degeneration via CPPD) to the S-L ligament.

SNAC Wrist (Scaphoid Non-Union Advanced Collapse) occurs with a scaphoid fracture.

Just remember that the scaphoid always wants to rotate in flexion - the scaphoid-lunate ligament is the only thing holding it back. If this ligament breaks it will tilt into flexion, messing up the dynamics of the wrist. The radial scaphoid space will narrow, and the capitate will migrate proximally.

Treatment depends on the occupation/needs of the wrist. Wrist fusion will maximize strength, but cause a loss of motion. Proximal row carpectomy will maximize ROM, but cause a loss of strength.

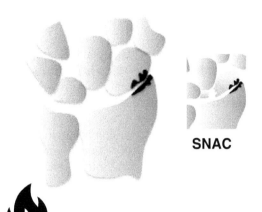

SNAC

- Radioscaphoid joint is first to develop degenerative changes

- Capitate will migrate proximally and there will eventually be a **DISI deformity**

Scapholunate Ligament Tear:

The Terry Thomas look (gap between the scaphoid and lunate) on plain film.

There are actually 3 parts (volar, dorsal, and middle), with the <u>dorsal band being the most important</u> for carpal stability. If they tear the carpals will migrate away from each other.

Predisposed for DISI deformity and all that crap I talked about earlier. More on this complex carpal instability on the next page.

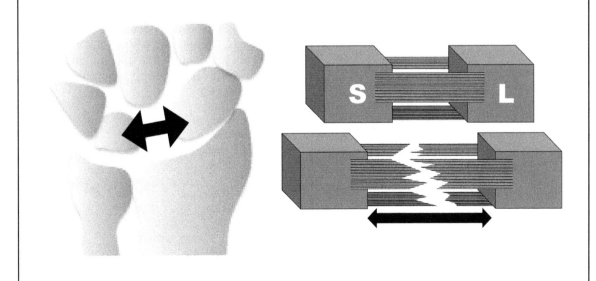

⚖️ THIS vs **THAT** - **DISI** vs **VISI**

This topic can be very confusing. Here is the way I like to think about it.

I imagine two people (Lunate and Scaphoid) standing on opposite sides of a very steep hill. At the apex of the hill is a man named "Scapholunate Ligament" - I agree, it's a strange name. His parents were probably vegetarians.

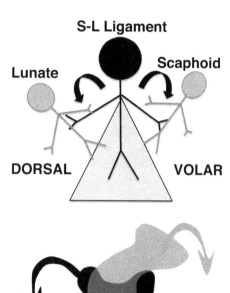

This hill is very steep, so Scapholunate Ligament has grabbed each of the people (Lunate and Scaphoid) by the hand - he was worried they might fall. In fact, the only thing keeping these two people from tumbling down the hill is the insane grip strength of Scapholunate Ligament (rumor has it he can close a #3 Captain of Crush - which would certify him as an official Captain of Crush).

By using this analogy perhaps you can infer that if you have carpal ligament disruption, the carpal bones will rotate the way they naturally want to (down the hill). The reasons for their rotational desires are complex but basically have to do with the shape of the fossa they sit on.

Just remember the scaphoid wants to flex (rock volar) and the lunate wants to extend (rock dorsal). The only thing holding them back is their ligamentous attachment to each other.

DISI (Dorsal Intercalated Segmental Instability) - I like to call this *dorsiflexion instability* because it helps me remember what's going on. After a "Radial sided injury" (scapholunate side), the lunate becomes free of the stabilizing force of the scaphoid and rocks dorsally. Remember SL ligament injury is common, so this is <u>common</u>.

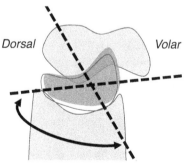

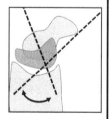

Normal Scaphoid-Lunate Angle is 30-60 degrees

DISI: Widening of the SL angle - with dorsiflexion of the lunate.

Angle > 60
(some sources say 80)

VISI (Volar Intercalated Segmental Instability) - I like to call this *volar-flexion (palmar-flexion) instability* because it helps me remember what's going on. After a "Ulnar sided injury" (lunotriquetral side), the lunate no longer has the stabilizing force of the lunotriquetral ligament and gets ripped volar with the scaphoid (*remember the scaphoid stays up late every night dreaming of tilting volar*). Remember LT ligament injury is not common, so this is not common. It's so uncommon in fact that if you see it - it's probably a normal variant due to wrist laxity.

VISI: Narrowing of the SL angle - with volar-flexion of the lunate & scaphoid.

Angle < 30 (this acute angle looks like a V to me - "V" for "V")

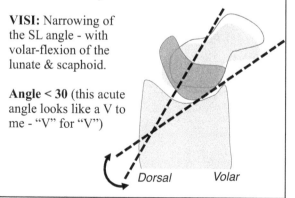

Carpal Dislocations - *A spectrum of severity*

Least Severe → **Most Severe**

Capitate

Lunate

V   D

Scapho-Lunate Dissociation	Peri-Lunate Dislocation	Mid-Carpal Dislocation	Lunate Dislocation
• SL- Wider Than 3 mm • Clenched Fist View can worsen it *(would make a good next step question)* • Chronic SL dissociation can result in a SLAC wrist	Trivia to Know = Note that the Lunate stays put - it's the carpal bones around the lunate ("peri-lunate bones") that move. 60% associated with Scaphoid Fractures	Trivia to Know = Both Lunate and Capitate lose radial alignment. Associated with Triquetro-Lunate interosseous ligament disruption Associated with a <u>Triquetral Fracture</u>	Trivia to Know = Lunate moves, others stay It happens with a Dorsal radiolunate ligament injury "Most Severe"

Vulnerable Zones Theory

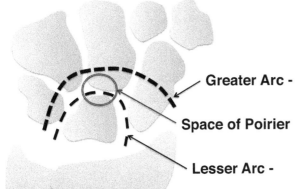

Greater Arc -

Space of Poirier

Lesser Arc -

Dislocations around the lunate are described in two flavors

Lesser Arc: Pure Ligament Injury (No Fractures)

Greater Arc: Associated with fractures. Described by saying "trans" the name of the fracture then the dislocation. Example "Trans-scaphoid, peri-lunate dislocation"

Space of Poirier - Ligament free ("**poor**") area, that is a site of weakness

Anatomic Trivia Regarding the Spaces of the Wrist:

Which synovial spaces normally communicate ?

The answer is **pisiform recess and radiocarpal joint**. I can think of two ways to ask this (1) related to fluid – the bottom line is that excessive fluid in the pisiform recess should not be considered abnormal if there is a radiocarpal effusion, and (2) that either space can be used for wrist arthrography.

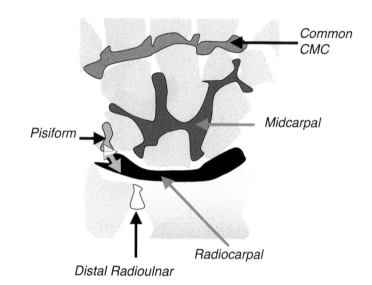

Other joint spaces in the body, easily lending to multiple choice testing:

Glenohumeral Joint and Subacromial Bursa	Should NOT communicate. Implies the presence of a full thickness rotator cuff tear.
Ankle Joint and Common (lateral) Peroneal Tendon Sheath	Should NOT communicate. Implies a tear of the calcaneofibular Ligament.
Achilles Tendon and Posterior Subtalar Joint	Should NOT communicate. The Achilles tendon does NOT have a true tendon sheath.
Pisifrom Recess and Radiocarpal Joint	Should normally communicate.

Anatomic Trivia - Triangular Fibrocartilage Complex — TFCC

I'll begin by saying that this is arguably the most complex anatomy in the entire body (maybe second only to the posterior lateral corner). A detailed understanding is well beyond the scope of the exam (probably…). Having said that, the TFC is specifically mentioned on the official study guide, so we need to at least talk about it.

The TFCC functions as the primary stabilizer and shock absorber of the distal radial ulnar joint (DRUJ). The TFCC is critical for a range of activities (doing a pushups , punching General Zod, etc…).

Anatomic Trivia - Triangular Fibrocartilage Complex — TFCC - Continued

It looks crazy complicated - but you really only need to know at most 5 structures,

Of the 5, the Hand Surgeon only really gives a shit about the **Articular Disc** and **Radioulnar Ligaments.**

TFCC 5 Components:

1. Triangular Fibrocartilage (Articular Disc)
2. Volar & Dorsal Radioulnar Ligaments
3. Meniscus Homologue
4. UCL
5. Tendon Sheath of the UCU

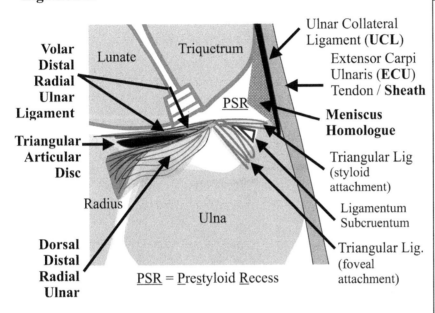

Volar Distal Radial Ulnar Ligament

Lunate

Triquetrum

Ulnar Collateral Ligament (**UCL**)

Extensor Carpi Ulnaris (**ECU**) Tendon / **Sheath**

Meniscus Homologue

PSR

Triangular Articular Disc

Radius

Ulna

Triangular Lig (styloid attachment)

Ligamentum Subcruentum

Triangular Lig. (foveal attachment)

Dorsal Distal Radial Ulnar

PSR = Prestyloid Recess

MR Signal:

"TFC Proper" (Articular Disc) will be dark on every sequence.

- The ulnar attachment often looks intermediate in signal, this is normal related to loose connective tissue in the region.

- The radial attachment will also have intermediate signal, but this is from the normal articular cartilage.

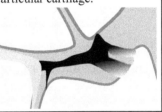

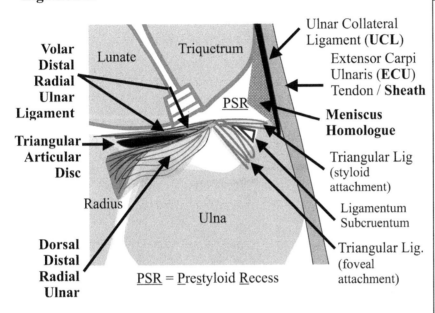
(lower left diagram)

Dorsal Distal Radial Ulnar Ligament

Prestyloid Recess

Extensor Carpi Ulnaris (**ECU**) **Sheath** and Tendon

Lunate Fossa of the Radius

Triangular Articular Disc

UCL

Meniscus Homologue

Volar Distal Radial Ulnar Ligament

TFCC Injuries:

You can group these into:

"Class 1" Acute Injuries: Usually via fall onto extended wrist.

"Class 2" Chronic Degeneration: These are more common, and associated with positive ulnar variance and ulnar impaction.

Central perforations are common - and might even be "expected" on an old person.

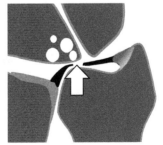

Central Tear, with Ulnar Positive Variance and Abutment (cystic change in the lunate) - more on next page.

TFC Vasculature & Healing

Similar to how the knee meniscus has "red" and "white" zones - the ulnar side of the TFC is vascular and more likely to heal. Radial sided injuries are relatively avascular and less likely to heal.

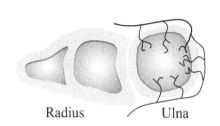
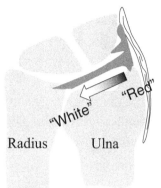

Ulnar Variance / Impaction

Ulnar Variance -

This is determined by comparing the lengths of the ulna and distal radius.

These length differences can occur congenitally, or be acquired from impaction / fracture deformity.

Neutral

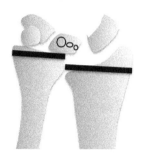

Positive Variance:

Association:
- Ulnar Impaction Syndrome

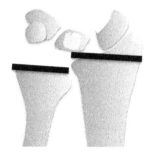

Negative Variance:

Association:
- AVN of the Lunate ("Kienbock")

Ulnar Impaction Syndrome (Ulnar Abutment):

Seen with positive ulnar variance.

Essentially the distal ulna smashes into the *lunate*, degenerating it (cystic change / geodes etc…) and *tears up the TFCC.*

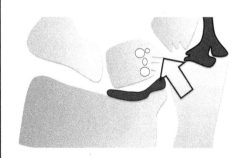

Kienbocks:

AVN of the lunate, seen in people in their 20s-40s. The most likely testable trivia is the association with negative ulnar variance. It's going to show signal drop out on T1.

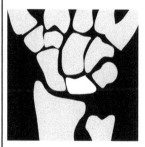
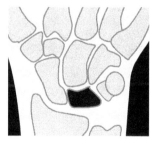

Sclerotic on Plain Film   Low Signal on T1

Distal Radius / Wrist Fractures:

There are 3 named fractures of the distal radius / wrist worth knowing.

Distal Radius

Radial Rim

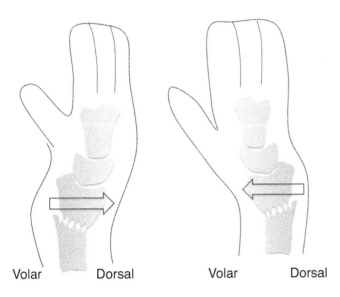

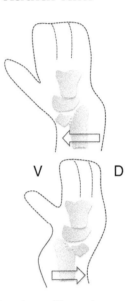

Colles' Fracture
(Outward)
"Collie Dogs" Like it Outside

- Distal Metaphysis Fx
- **Dorsal** Angulation
- Old Lady Fracture
- Ulnar Styloid Fx is Commonly Associated

Smith Fracture
(Inward)

- Distal Metaphysis Fx
- **Volar** Angulation
- Younger Patient
- Ulnar Styloid Fx is Commonly Associated

Barton Fracture
(Dorsal or Volar)

- Radial Rim Fx
- **Volar is More Common**
- Radial-Carpal Dislocation is the "hallmark"
- Typically Surgical (they have a high rate of re dislocation / mal-union)

Radial Tilt

- There is a **normal volar tilt** of around 11 degrees
- With distal radial fractures this can get fucked up
- Most Orthopods won't accept anything past neutral
- A TRUE lateral is necessary to measure it

How do you know your lateral is "true"?

The volar cortex of the pisiform overlies the central 1/3 of the interval between the scaphoid and capitate

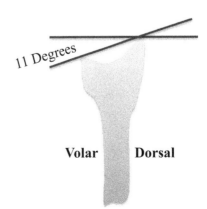

Wrist Tendon Anatomy Review:

With regard to the extensor tendons, there are four things to know:

- There are 6 extensor compartments (5 fingers + 1 for good luck).

- First compartment (APL and EPB) are the ones affected in de Quervain's

- Third compartment has the EPL which courses beside Lister's Tubercle.

- The sixth compartment (Extensor Carpi Ulnaris) – can get an early tenosynovitis in rheumatoid arthritis.

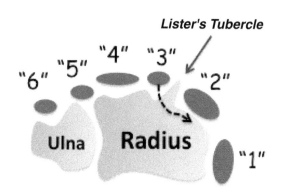

Carpal Tunnel: They could show you the carpal tunnel, but only to ask you about anatomy.

What goes through the carpal tunnel (more easily asked as *"what does NOT go through")?*

Knowing what is in (and not in) the carpal tunnel is high yield for multiple choice testing. The tunnel lies deep to the palmaris longus, and is defined by 4 bony prominences (pisiform, scaphoid tubercle, hook of hamate, trapezium tubercle), with the transverse carpal ligament wrapping the contents in a fibrous sheath.

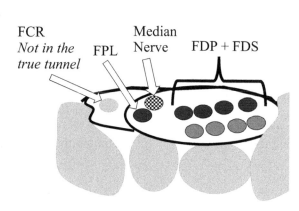

The tunnel contains 10 things

- 4 Flexor D. Profudus (FDP)

- 4 Flexor D. Superficials (FDS)

- 1 Flexor Pollicis Longus (FPL), and

- 1 Median Nerve

The Flexor Carpi Radialis (FCR) is NOT truly in the tunnel. The extensor tendons are on the other side of the hand. Note that Flexor Pollicis Longus (FPL) goes through the tunnel, but Flexor Pollicis Brevis does not (it's an intrinsic handle muscle). Palmaris longus (if you have one) does NOT go through the tunnel.

Does NOT go through the tunnel

-Flexor Carpi Radialis

-Flexor Carpi Ulnaris

-Palmaris Longus (if you have one)

-Flexor Pollicis BREVIS

Carpal Tunnel Syndrome (CTS):

- Median Nerve Distribution (thumb-radial aspect of 4th digit), often bilateral, and may have thenar muscle atrophy.
- On Ultrasound, enlargement of the nerve is the main thing to look for
- It's usually from repetitive trauma,
- *Trivia* = **Association with <u>Dialysis</u>**, Pregnancy, DM, and HYPOthyroidism

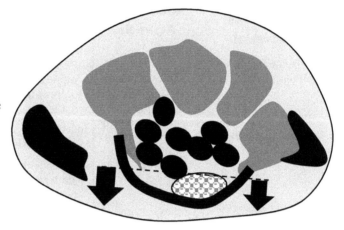

Classic Findings:
- Increased Signal in the Median Nerve
- The Nerve May Also Be Swollen or Look Smashed / Flattened
- <u>Bowing of the Flexor Retinaculum</u>

Guyon's Canal Syndrome:

- Entrapment of the ulnar nerve as it passes through Guyon's canal (formed by the pisiform and the hamate – and the crap that connects them).
- Classically caused by handle bars *"handle bar palsy."*
- Fracture of the hook of the hamate can also eat on that ulnar nerve.

Sub-Sheath Tear / Dislocation

This refers to a traumatic dislocation to the extensor carpi ulnaris (ECU - compartment 6) out of its normal groove at the level of the distal ulna. This dislocation / subluxation implies rupture of the overlying sheath.

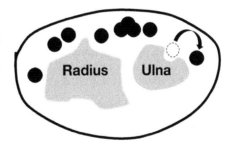

Trivia - the direction of dislocation is medial.

Tenosynovitis:

This is an inflammation of the tendon, with increased fluid seen around the tendon. This will be shown on MRI (or US).

DIFFUSE		FOCAL	
Tuberculous or Nontuberculous Mycobacterial	**Rheumatoid Arthritis:**	**Penetrating Infection** (can be focal or diffuse)	**Overuse**
Hand and wrist are the most common tendons affected	Multiple Flexor Tendons or Isolated Extensor Carpi Ulnaris if early *(ECU = Compartment 6)*	Tenosynovitis of any flexor tendon is a surgical emergency as it can spread rapidly to the common flexors of the wrist.	This is going to be classic locations like 1st extensor compartment for De Quervains — discussed more below.
Diffuse exuberant tenosynovitis that spares the muscles.		Increased pressure in the sheath can cause necrosis of the tendons.	
		Patients with delayed treatment tend to do terrible	
Usually occurs in patients who are immunocompromised.	Tenosynovitis can present as an early RA findings (before bone findings).		
Discrete filling defects in the fluid filled sheaths ("rice bodies") is a classic TB finding.		Myocobacterium Marinum is usually direct infection in a fisherman or sushi chef.	

De Quervain's Tenosynovitis:

So called "Washer Woman's Sprain" or "Mommy Thumb."
Occurs from repetitive activity / overuse.
The classic history is "new mom - holding a baby."

First Extensor Compartment (Extensor Pollicis Brevis and Abductor Pollicis Longus

Ultrasound: Increased fluid within the first extensor tendon compartment

MRI: increased T2 signal in the tendon sheath

Finkelstein Test = Pain on passive ulnar deviation.

The presence or absence of an intratendinous septum (between the EPB and APB) - tendons on the is a prognostic factor. If its absent, this will nearly always resolve with conservative treatment alone.

Intersection Syndrome:

A repetitive use issue (classically *seen in rowers*),

Occurs where the first extensor tendons, "intersects" the second extensor compartment tendons. The result is extensor carpi radialis brevis and longus tenosynovitis.

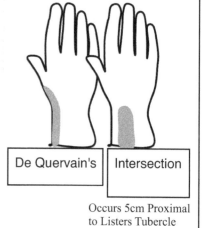

De Quervain's | Intersection

Occurs 5cm Proximal to Listers Tubercle

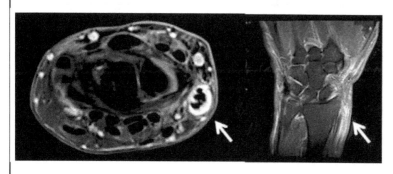

Bennett and Rolando Fractures:

- They are both fractures at the base of the first metacarpal
- The Rolando fracture is comminuted (Bennett is not)
- *Trivia:* The pull of the *Abductor Pollicis Longus (APL)* tendon is what causes the dorsolateral dislocation in the Bennett Fracture

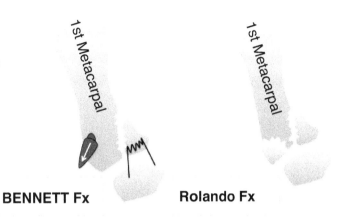

BENNETT Fx   **Rolando Fx**

Gamekeeper's Thumb (Skier):

- Avulsion fracture at the base of the proximal first phalanx associated with <u>ulnar collateral ligament disruption.</u>
- The frequently tested association is that of a **"Stener Lesion."** A Stener Lesion is when the Adductor tendon aponeurosis gets caught in the torn edges of the UCL. The displaced ligament won't heal right, and will need surgery.
- It makes a "yo-yo" appearance on MRI - supposedly...
- *Next Step* - Don't do "stress views" that can cause a stener. <u>MRI</u> is the more appropriate test.

DO NOT perform radiographic stress views for Gamekeepers Thumbs

UCL

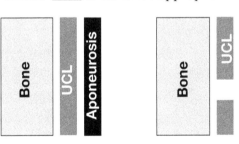

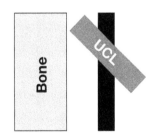

Stener

Ulnar collateral ligament is retracted and displaced superficial to the adductor aponeurosis.

Trigger Finger:
The idea is the overuse / repetitive trauma causes scarring in the flexor tendon sheath. The fancy word is "stenosing tenosynovitis." This is most commonly shown with ultrasound. If they should you a hand ultrasound think about this.

Another common area of "stenosing tenosynovitis" is at the ankle specifically the flexor hallucis longus tendon around the ankle in patients with the os trigonum syndrome.

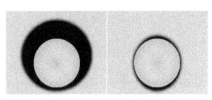

Thick Sheath   Normal for Comparison

Site-Specific Entities - Elbow & Forearm

General Trivia:

- Radial Head Fracture is most common in adults (supracondylar is most common in PEDs)
- *Sail sign* - elevation of the fat pads from a joint effusion. Supposedly a sign of occult fracture. The testable trivia is (1) the posterior fat pad is more specific (*posterior is positive*), and (2) the posterior fat pad can appear falsely elevated (false positive) if the lateral isn't a true 90 degree flexed lateral. *"Posterior Positive, Posterior Position Dependent"*
- Capitellum fractures are associated with posterior dislocation

Forearm Fractures / Eponyms:

Forearm fractures are "ring" or "pretzel" type fractures, similar to the pelvis or mandible. Think about breaking a pretzel, it always snaps in two spots (not just one). So forearm fractures are often two fractures, or a fracture + dislocation.

There are 3 French sounding (therefore high yield) fractures of the forearm which follow this ring / pretzel principal.

Monteggia Fracture (MUGR):

Fracture of the proximal ulna, with anterior dislocation of the radial head.

Dislocation of the radial head follows the angulation of the Ulnar Fx.

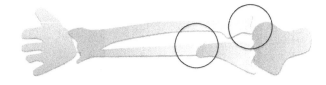

Galeazzi Fracture (MUGR)

Radial shaft fracture, with anterior dislocation of the ulna at the DRUJ.

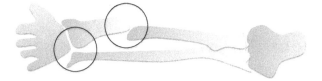

Essex-Lopresti

Fracture of the radial head + Anterior dislocation of the distal radial ulnar joint.

Unstable fracture - With *rupture of the interosseous membrane*

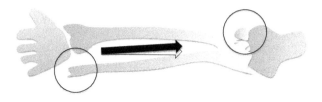

Cubital Tunnel Syndrome

There are several causes - the most common in the real world is probably repetitive valgus stress. The most common shown on multiple choice is probably an accessory anconeus.

WTF is an "Anconeus"? It a piece of shit muscle that does nothing but get in the way of an orthopedic scope. It's normally on the lateral side the elbow. You can have an *"Accessory Anconeus"* - also called an *"Anconeus Epitrochlearis"* - on the medial side which will exert mass effect on the ulnar nerve.

Anatomic Trivia: The site where the ulnar nerve passes beneath the cubital tunnel retinaculum also known as the epicondylo-olecranon ligament or Osborne's ligament.

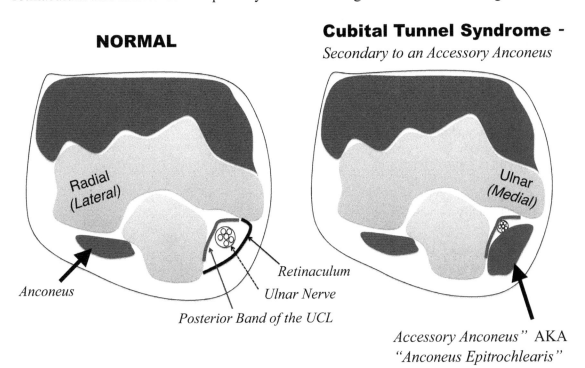

NORMAL

Cubital Tunnel Syndrome - *Secondary to an Accessory Anconeus*

Radial (Lateral)

Ulnar (Medial)

Retinaculum
Ulnar Nerve
Posterior Band of the UCL
Anconeus

Accessory Anconeus" AKA "Anconeus Epitrochlearis"

Lateral Epicondylitis *(more common than medial) – seen in Tennis Players -*
- Extensor Tendon Injury (classically extensor carpi radialis brevis)
- Radial Collateral Ligament Complex – Tears due to varus stress

Medial Epicondylitis *(less common than lateral) – seen in golfers*
- Common flexor tendon and ulnar nerve may enlarge from chronic injury

Partial Ulnar Collateral Ligament Tear:

For the exam all you really need to know is that throwers (people who valgus overload) hurt their ulnar collateral ligament (which attaches on the medial coronoid - *sublime tubercle*). The ligament has three bundles, and the **anterior bundle is by far the most important**. If you get any images it is most likely going to be of the partial UCL tear, described as the **"T sign,"** with contrast material extending medial to the tubercle.

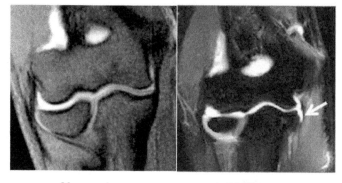

Normal   **T-Sign**
                "UCL Partial Tear"

Little Leaguer Elbow

The children of insecure men who sucked at sports in high school are most susceptible to this injury. The mechanism is repetitive micro-trauma from endless hours of training (necessary to finally rectify the injustice which beset their family when dad was benched senior year from the junior varsity baseball squad).

We are talking about a repetitive chronic injury to the medial epicondyle. When I say injury I mean stress fracture, avulsion, or delayed closure of the medial epicondylar apophysis. This is usually associated with UCL injury.

Children aren't the only ones who can fuck up their elbows pursuing the kind of immortality that is only offered to those worthy enough to step foot on the field at Yankee stadium. There is a well described **"valgus overload syndrome"** seen in throwers, consisting of a triad of lateral compression, medial tension, and posterior sheer. This mechanism results in UCL injury (often anterior band), Arthritis at the Posterior Humerus / Ulna, and the development of an OCD at the capitellum.

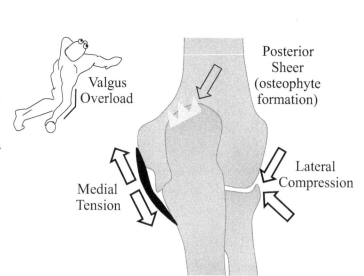

Valgus Overload

Posterior Sheer (osteophyte formation)

Lateral Compression

Medial Tension

Epitrochlear Lymphadenopathy – This is a classic look for cat-scratch disease.

Dialysis Elbow: This is the result of olecranon bursitis from constant pressure on the area, related to positioning of the arm during treatment.

Biceps Tear

Tears can be partial or complete. When complete the tear typically occurs in shoulder with the tendon avulsing off the labrum (or at the level of the bicipital groove).

Common mechanism is incorrect deadlift form (while doing cross fit like an ape on cocaine). If you plan on going nuts slinging that shit around consider switching to a double over grip. If you want to use over under grips - you need strict form (keep your arms locked out dummy). There are tons of highlight reals on youtube of people tearing biceps while deadlifting - notice every single one is using an over under grip, and not maintaining straight arm technique.

 Partial Biceps Tear – Gamesmanship
-Partial tears often are associated with bicipitoradial bursitis

Patients present with a painful mass in the antecubital fossa (rolled up muscle) - with the classic history of "trying to impress the girl in the pink spandex sports bra with my deadlift." This rolled up muscle is sometimes referred to as the "Popeye Deformity" - in reference to my childhood hero - a heavily muscled blue collar worker, who smokes, and solves his all of his problems with violence.

Sneaky: Injury to the bicep is associated with median nerve symptoms

Tricep Rupture

The tricep tendon has the honorable distinction of being the LEAST common tendon in the body to rupture. Even tendinopathy is fairly uncommon relative to other nearby structures. When it does tear you should be thinking about **salter harris II fractures of the olecranon** - that is the classic scenario.

I think because this is so uncommon that mimics would be more likely on the exam. So, I'd be aware of two things: (1) the normal striated appearance of the insertion at the olecranon, and (2) the common entity of olecranon bursitis - which you should think of first if you see a bunch of fluid signal in the posterior elbow.

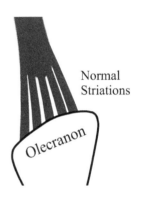

Normal Striations

Olecranon

Elbow Dislocation

This is the second most common joint dislocated in the adult. The associated fractures are usually the radial head and the coronoid process.

Instability in the elbow (so called **Posterior Rotary Instability**) is described in a pattern starting in the posterior lateral corner with tearing of the lateral UCL.

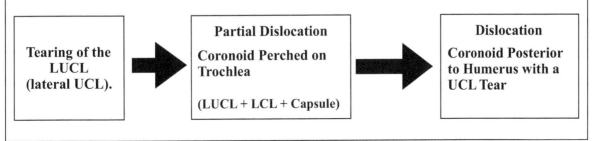

| Tearing of the LUCL (lateral UCL). | → | Partial Dislocation Coronoid Perched on Trochlea (LUCL + LCL + Capsule) | → | Dislocation Coronoid Posterior to Humerus with a UCL Tear |

Site-Specific Entities - Shoulder

Dislocation:

- *Anterior inferior* (subcoracoid) are by far the most common (like 90%).
    - **Hill-Sachs is on the Humerus.**
    - Hill-Sachs is on the posterior lateral humerus, and *best seen on internal rotation view.*
    - Bankart – anterior inferior labrum
    - Greater tuberosity avulsion fracture occurs in 10-15% of anterior dislocations in patient's over 40.
- *Posterior Dislocation*: uncommon – probably from seizure or electrocution
    - *Rim Sign* – no overlap glenoid and humeral head
    - *Trough Sign* – reverse Hill Sachs, impaction on anterior humerus
    - *"Light Bulb Sign"* - Arm may be locked in internal rotation on all views
- *Inferior Dislocation (luxatio erecta humeri)* – this is an uncommon form, where the arm is sticking straight over the head. The thing to know is 60% get neurologic injury (usually the axillary nerve).

Hill-Sachs	Posterolateral humeral head impaction fracture (anterior dislocation)	
Bankart	Anterior Glenoid Rim (anterior dislocation)	
Trough Sign	Anterior humeral head impaction fracture (posterior dislocation)	
Reverse Bankart	Posterior Glenoid Rim (posterior dislocation)	

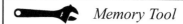 *Memory Tool*

I remember that hip dislocations are posterior - from the straight leg dashboard mechanism.

Then I just remember that shoulders are the opposite of that (the other one, is the other one).

Shoulder = Usually Anterior

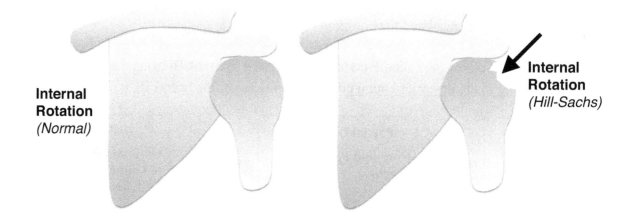

Internal Rotation *(Normal)*

Internal Rotation *(Hill-Sachs)*

Proximal Humerus Fracture:

This is usually in an old lady falling on an out stretched arm. Orthopods use the Neer classifications (how many parts the humerus is in ?). Three or four part fractures tend to do worse.

The Post Op Shoulder (Prosthesis)

There are 4 Main Types: Humeral Head Resurfacing, Hemi-Arthroplasty, Total Shoulder Arthroplasty, and the Reverse Total Shoulder Arthroplasty.

What is this "reverse total shoulder" ?
A conventional total shoulder mimics normal anatomy. A reserve total shoulder is the bizarro version; with a plastic cup on the humeral head and metallic sphere on the glenoid.

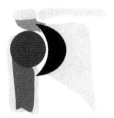 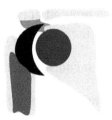

Conventional   *Reverse*

Who gets what? -

The surgical choice depends on two main factors:

(1) Is the Cuff Intact?
(2) Is the Glenoid Trashed ?

	Cuff-Intact	Cuff- Deficient
Glenoid Intact	Resurfacing or Hemi	Hemi or Reverse
Glenoid Deficient	TSA	Reverse

Complications / Trivia:

—Total Shoulder Most Common Complication = Loosening of the Glenoid Component
—Total Shoulder Complication - *"Anterior Escape"* - This describes anterior migration of the humeral head after subscapularis failure.

—Reverse Total Shoulder Does NOT require an intact rotator cuff - patient rely heavily on the deltoid.
—Reverse Shoulder Complication - *Posterior Acromion Fracture* - from excessive deltoid tugging.

Impingement / Rotator Cuff Tears:

This is a high yield / confusing subject that is worth talking about in a little more detail. In general, rotator cuff pathology is the result of overuse activity (sports) or impingement mechanisms. There are two types of impingement with two major sub-divisions within those types. Like many things in Radiology, if you get the vocabulary down, the pathology is easy to understand.

External: This refers to impingement of the rotator cuff overlying the bursal surfaces (superficial surfaces) that are adjacent to the coracoacromial arch. As a reminder, the arch is made up of the coracoid process, acromion, and coracoacromial ligament.

Primary External Causes (Abnormal Coracoacromial Arch) :

- The **hooked acromion** (type III Bigliani) is more associated with external impingement than the curved or flat types.

- **Subacromial osteophyte formation** or thickening of the coracoacromial ligament

- **Subcoracoid impingement**: Impingement of the subscapularis between the coracoid process and lesser tuberosity. This can be secondary to congenital configuration, or a configuration developed post traumatically after fracture of the coracoid or lesser tuberosity.

Secondary External Causes (Normal Coracoacromial Arch):

- "**Multidirectional Glenohumeral Instability**" – resulting in micro-subluxation of the humeral head in the glenoid, resulting in repeated micro-trauma. The important thing to know is this is *typically seen in patients with generalized joint laxity*, often involving <u>both</u> shoulders.

Internal: This refers to impingement of the rotator cuff on the undersurface (deep surface) along the glenoid labrum and humeral head.

- **Posterior Superior:** This is a type of impingement that occurs when the posterior superior rotator cuff (junction of the supra and infraspinatus tendons) comes into contact with the posterior superior glenoid. Best seen in the ABER position, where these tendons get pinched between the labrum and greater tuberosity. This is seen in athletes who make overhead movements (throwers, tennis, swimming).

- **Anterior Superior:** This is internal impingement that occurs when the arm is in horizontal adduction and internal rotation. In this position, the undersurface of the biceps and subscapularis tendon may impinge against the anterior superior glenoid rim.

Impingement Continued...

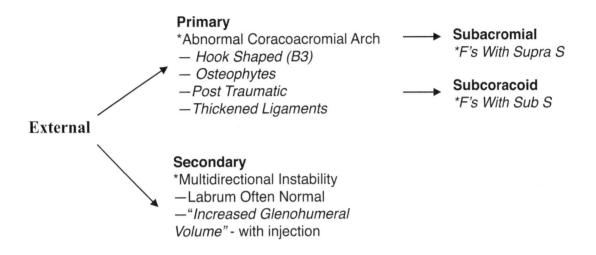

External

Primary
*Abnormal Coracoacromial Arch
— *Hook Shaped (B3)*
— *Osteophytes*
— *Post Traumatic*
— *Thickened Ligaments*

→ **Subacromial**
*F's With Supra S

→ **Subcoracoid**
*F's With Sub S

Secondary
*Multidirectional Instability
—Labrum Often Normal
—*"Increased Glenohumeral Volume"* - with injection

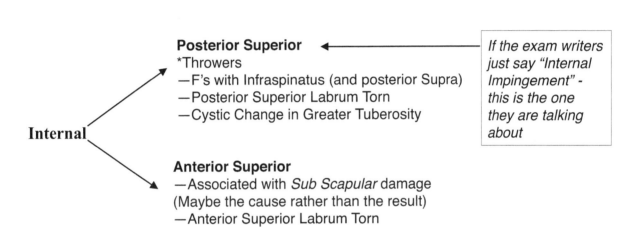

Internal

Posterior Superior
*Throwers
—F's with Infraspinatus (and posterior Supra)
—Posterior Superior Labrum Torn
—Cystic Change in Greater Tuberosity

Anterior Superior
—Associated with *Sub Scapular* damage
(Maybe the cause rather than the result)
—Anterior Superior Labrum Torn

> If the exam writers just say "Internal Impingement" - this is the one they are talking about

High Yield Trivia Points on Impingement	
Subacromial Impingement – most common form, resulting from attrition of the coracoacromial arch.	Damages **Supraspinatus Tendon**.
Subcoracoid Impingement – Lesser tuberosity and coracoid do the pinching.	Damages **Subscapularis** *(remember the coracoid is anterior - and so is the subscapularis)*.
Posterior Superior "<u>Internal</u>" Impingement – Athletes who make overhead movements. Greater tuberosity and posterior inferior labrum do the pinching.	Damages **Infraspinatus** (and posterior fibers of the supraspinatus).

Rotator Cuff Tears:

People talk about these tears as either "**B**ursal Sided" (meaning the top part), or "**A**rticular Sided" (meaning the undersurface).

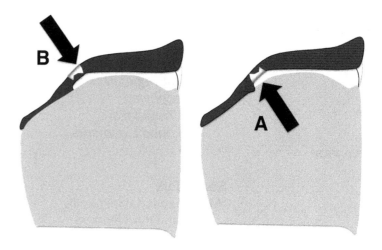

A tear of the articular surface is more common (3x more) than the bursal surface. The underlying mechanism is usually degenerative, although trauma can certainly play a role.

The **most common of the four muscles to tear is the Supraspinatus** - with most tears occurring at the *"critical zone"* - 1-2 cm from the tendon footprint. This relatively avascular "critical zone" is also the most common location for Calcium Hydroxyapatite (HADD) - or "calcific tendinitis." The Teres Minor is the least common to tear.

A partial tear that is > 50% often results in a surgical intervention.

"Massive rotator cuff tear" - refers to at least 2 out of the 4 rotator cuff muscles.

A final general piece of trivia is that a tear of the fibrous rotator cuff interval (junction between anterior fibers of the Supraspinatus and superior fibers of the subscapularis), is still considered a rotator cuff tear.

How do you know it's a full thickness tear? You will have high T2 signal in the expected location of the tendon. On T1 you will have **Gad in the bursa.**

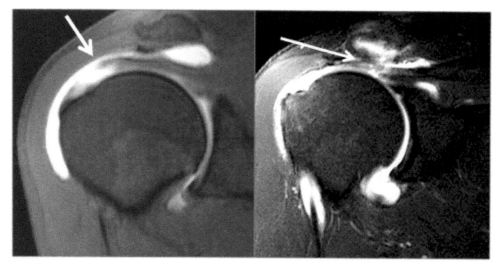

Full Thickness Tear

- With Gad crossing over the cuff into the bursa.

Adhesive Capsulitis "Frozen Shoulder"

An inflammatory condition characterized by a global decrease in motion. You can have primary types, but a multiple choice key would be a history of trauma or surgery.

It most commonly effects the rotator cuff interval - and that is the most likely spot they will show it. The classic look is a T1 (or non-fat sat T2) in the sagittal plane showing _loss of fat in the rotator cuff interval_ (the spot with the biceps tendon - between the Supra S, and the Sub Scap).

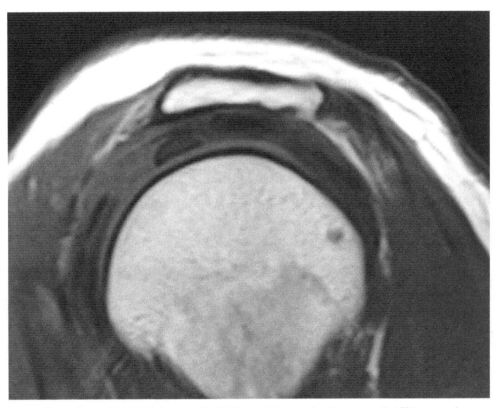

Grey Smudgy Shit Instead of Clean Fat in the Rotator Cuff Interval

BUZZWORD: _"Decreased Glenohumeral Volume"_ - with injection

** Remember in Multi-Directional Instability the volume was increased.

BUZZWORDS: _"Thickened Inferior and Posterior Capsule"_

"Enhancement of the Rotator Cuff Interval" - Post gad

Injury to the Labrum:

SLAP: Labral tears favor the <u>superior</u> margin and track anterior to posterior. As this tear involves the labrum at the insertion of the long head of the biceps , injury to this tendon is associated and part of the grading system (type 4).

Things to know about SLAP tears:

- When the SLAP extends into the biceps anchor (type 4), the surgical management changes from a debridement to a debridement + biceps tenodesis.

- The mechanism is usually an over-head movement (classic = swimmer)

- People over 40 usually have associated Rotator Cuff Tears

- **NOT associated with Instability** *(usually)*

SLAP Mimic - The Sublabral Recess. This is essentially a normal variant where you have incomplete attachment of the labrum at 12 o'clock. The 12 o'clock position on the labrum has the shittiest blood flow - that's why you see injury there and all these development variants.

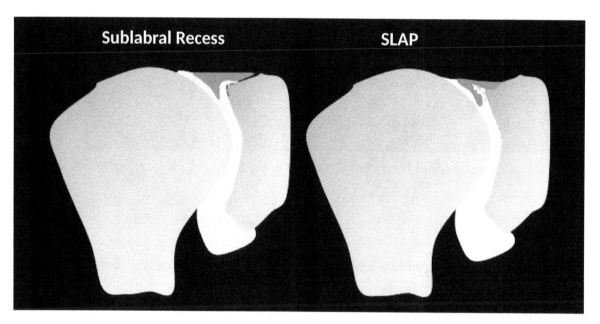

Sublabral Recess	SLAP
Follows Contour of Glenoid	Extends Laterally
SMOOTH Margin	Ratty Margin
Located at Biceps Anchor	Located at Biceps Anchor & Posteriorly

Labral Tear Mimic - The Sublabral Foramen
- This is an unattached (<u>but present</u>) portion of
the labrum - located at the anterior-superior
labrum   (1 o'clock to 3 o'clock).

As a rule it should NOT extend below the
equator (3 o'clock position).

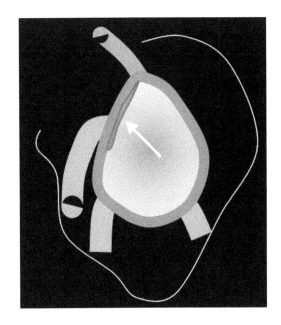

Labral Tear Mimic - The Buford Complex - A commonly tested (and not infrequently
seen) variant is the Buford Complex. It's present in about 1% of the general population. This
consists of an <u>**absent**</u> **anterior/superior labrum** (1 o'clock to 3 o'clock)**, along with a
thickened middle glenohumeral ligament**.

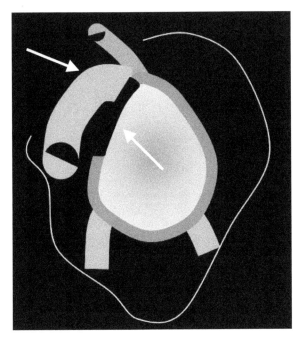

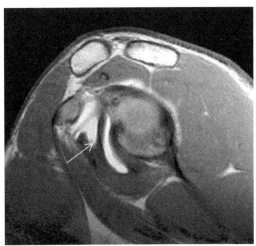

Buford Complex:
- Thick Middle GH Ligament
- Absent Anterior Superior Labrum

Bankart Lesions:

There is an alphabet soup of Bankart (anterior dislocation) related injuries.

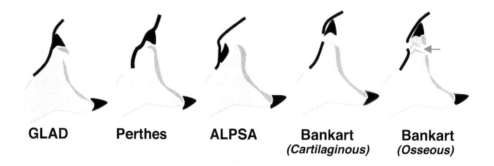

GLAD   Perthes   ALPSA   Bankart *(Cartilaginous)*   Bankart *(Osseous)*

GLAD = Glenolabral Articular Disruption. It's the most mild version, and it's basically a superficial anterior inferior labral tear with associated articular cartilage damage ("impaction injury with cartilage defect"). Not typically seen in patients with underlying laxity. It's common in sports. **No instability** *(aren't you GLAD there is no instability)*

Perthes = Detachment of the anteroinferior labrum (3-6 o'clock) with medially stripped but *intact periosteum*.

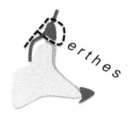

Memory Aid:
-The detached labrum sorta looks like a "**P**"

ALPSA = Anterior Labral Periosteal Sleeve Avulsion. Medially displaced labroligamentous complex with absence of the labrum on the glenoid rim. *Intact periosteum*. It scars down to glenoid.

True Bankart: Can be cartilaginous or osseous. *The periosteum is disrupted*. There is often an associated Hill Sach's fracture.

GLAD	Perthes	ALPSA	True Bankart
Superficial partial labral injury with cartilage defect	Avulsed anterior labrum (only minimally displaced). Inferior GH complex still attached to periosteum	Similar to perthes but with "bunched up" medially displaced inferior GH complex	Torn labrum
No instability	Intact Periosteum (lifted up)	Intact Periosteum	*Periosteum Disrupted*

Posterior Glenohumeral Instability

As I mentioned previously, anterior shoulder dislocations are way more common than posterior shoulder dislocations. Therefore the Bankart, ALPSA, Perthes, etc... are the ones you typically think of as the stigmata of prior dislocation.

However, all that shit can happen in reverse with a posterior dislocation.

Reverse Osseous Bankart:

A fracture of the <u>posterior inferior</u> rim of the glenoid.

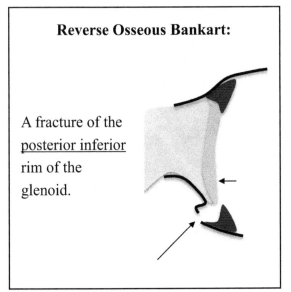

POLPSA:

This is the bizarro version of the ALPSA, where the posterior labrum and the posterior scapular <u>periosteum</u> <u>(still intact)</u> are stripped from the glenoid resulting in a recess that communicates with the joint space.

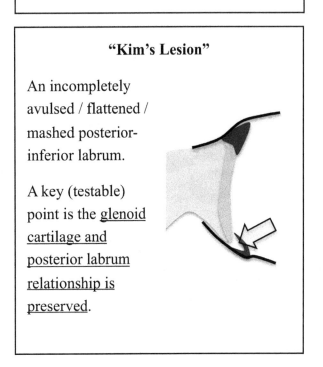

"Bennett Lesion"

An <u>extra-articular curvilinear calcification</u> - associated with <u>posterior labral tears</u> (maybe the POLPSA).

It's related to injury of the posterior band of the inferior glenohumeral ligament.

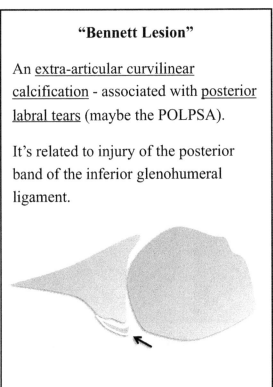

"Kim's Lesion"

An incompletely avulsed / flattened / mashed posterior-inferior labrum.

A key (testable) point is the <u>glenoid cartilage and posterior labrum relationship is preserved</u>.

HAGL:

A non-Bankart lesion that is frequently tested is the **HAGL** (Humeral avulsion glenohumeral ligament). This is an **avulsion of the inferior glenohumeral ligament**, and is most often the result of an anterior shoulder dislocation (just like all the above bankarts). The "J Sign" occurs when the normal U-shaped inferior glenohumeral recess is retracted away from the humerus, appearing as a J.

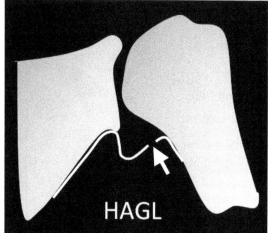 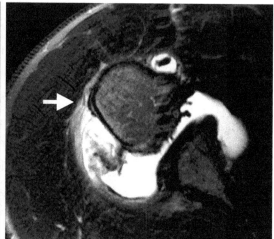

Axial MR - Showing the IGHL
Torn at its Humeral Attachment

Subluxation of the Biceps Tendon: The subscapularis attaches to the lesser tuberosity. It sends a few fibers across the bicipital groove to the greater tuberosity , which is called the "transverse ligament". A tear of the subscapularis opens these fibers up and allows the biceps to dislocate (usually medial). **Subscapularis Tear = Medial Dislocation of the Long Head of the Biceps Tendon.**

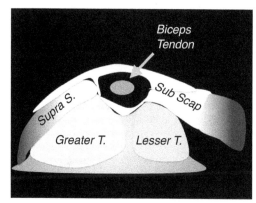 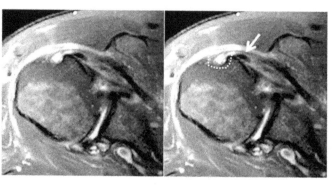

Sub Scap Tendon - Forming portions of the *"Transverse Ligament"* that holds the biceps tendon in the groove

Subluxation of the Biceps Tendon
Occurs with a Tear of the Subscapularis

Nerve Entrapment: *High Yield Trivia:*

Suprascapular Notch vs Spinoglenoid Notch: A cyst at the level of the suprascapular notch will affect the supraspinatus and the infraspinatus. At the level of the spinoglenoid notch, it will only affect the infraspinatus.

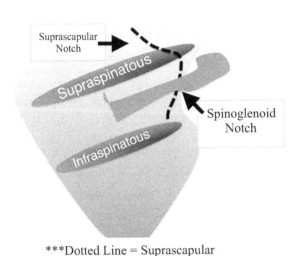

***Dotted Line = Suprascapular

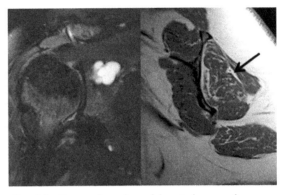

Cyst in the spinoglenoid notch causing fatty atrophy of the Infraspinatous

Quadrilateral Space Syndrome: Compression of the Axillary Nerve in the Quadrilateral Space (usually from fibrotic bands). They will likely show this with **atrophy of the teres minor**. Another classic question is to name the borders of the quadrilateral space: Teres Minor Above, Teres Major Below, Humeral neck lateral, and Triceps medial.

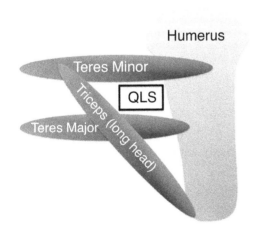

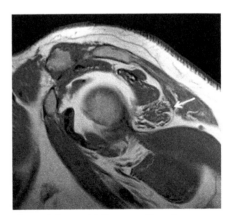

Quadrilateral Space Syndrome -Atrophy of Teres Minor

Parsonage-Turner Syndrome: This is an idiopathic involvement of the brachial plexus. Think about this when you see muscles affected by pathology in two or more nerve distributions (suprascapular and axillary etc..).

Site-Specific Entities - Hip / Femur / Sacrum

Femoral Shaft Fractures:

- On the inside (**medial**) is the classic **stress** fracture location

- On the outside (**lateral**) is the classic **bisphosphonate** related fx location. As shown in the image, you see cortical thickening (white arrow) along the lateral femur, eventually progressing into a fracture.

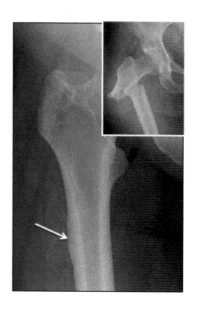

Hip Fracture / Dislocation:

You see these with dash board injuries. The **posterior dislocation** (almost always associated with a fracture as it's driven backwards) is much more common than the anterior dislocation.

BUZZWORD:

"Foot in __internal__ rotation"

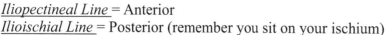

Ilioischial

Iliopectineal

Anterior Column vs Posterior Column - the acetabulum is supported by two columns of bone that merge together to form an "inverted Y"

Iliopectineal Line = Anterior
Ilioischial Line = Posterior (remember you sit on your ischium)

The both column fracture by definition divides the ilium proximal to the hip joint, so you have no articular surface of the hip attached to the axial skeleton (that's a problem).

Corona Mortis: The anastomosis of the inferior epigastric and obturator vessels sometimes rides on the superior pubic ramus. During a lateral dissection - sometimes used to repair a hip fracture - this can be injured. I talk about this more in the vascular chapter.

Hip Fracture Leading to AVN: The location of the fracture may predispose to AVN. It's important to remember that, since the femoral head gets vascular flow from the circumflex femorals, a **displaced intracapsular fracture could disrupt this blood supply – leading to AVN.** **Testable Point:** Degree of fracture displacement corresponds with risk of AVN.

Avulsion Injury:

This is seen more in kids than adults. Adult bones are stronger than their tendons. In kids it's the other way around. One pearl is that if you see an **isolated "avulsion" of the lesser trochanter in a seemingly mild trauma / injury in an adult - query a pathologic fracture.** Now, to discuss what I believe to be one of the highest yield topics in MSK, *"where did the avulsion come from?"*

The easiest way to show this is a plain film pelvis (or MRI) with a tug/avulsion injury to one of the muscular attachment sites. The question will most likely be *"what attaches there?"* or *"which muscle got avulsed?"*

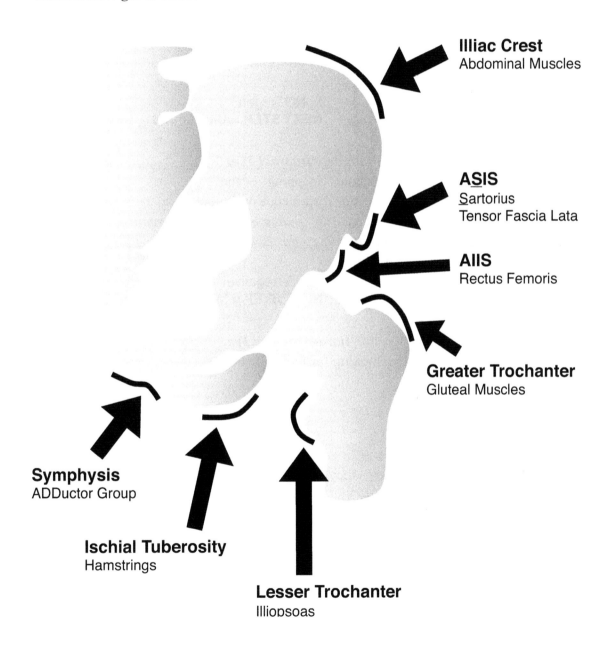

Illiac Crest
Abdominal Muscles

ASIS
Sartorius
Tensor Fascia Lata

AIIS
Rectus Femoris

Greater Trochanter
Gluteal Muscles

Symphysis
ADDuctor Group

Ischial Tuberosity
Hamstrings

Lesser Trochanter
Illiopsoas

Snapping Hip Syndrome:

The clinical sensation of "snapping" or "clicking" with hip flexion and extension. The key point is that it is clinical. This is the way people work this thing up:

Clinical Eval for the *"External Type"*
(IT band "snapping" over the Greater Trochanter)

This is to evaluate for the *"Intra-Articular Type"*
Looking for Hip Degen / Loose Bodies, Etc

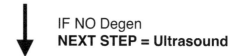

IF NO Degen
NEXT STEP = Ultrasound

This is to look for the *"Internal Type"*
Look for Dynamic "Snapping" of the
Iliopsoas over the Iliopectineal eminence or femoral head
This has to be shown with a CINE - because the finding is a dynamic moving of a tendon
If you see a hip ultrasound for snapping - this is what they are going for

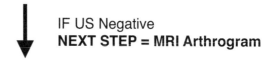

IF US Negative
NEXT STEP = MRI Arthrogram

This is to evaluate for the *"Intra-Articular Type"* … Again
This time looking for Labral Tears

Trivia:

- "Snapping Hip" is a "clinical sensation" - they have to tell you that patient feels "snapping"
- The 3 Types, and the Work-Up Algorithm Above:
- Types:
  - External (most common) = Iliotibial Band over Greater Trochanter
  - Internal = Iliopsoas over Iliopectineal eminence or femoral head
  - Intra-Articular = Labral tears / joint bodies

IT Band Syndrome

This is a repetitive stress syndrome seen most classically in runners. The key finding is **fluid on both sides of the IT band**, extending posterior and lateral.

Fluid in the joint does not exclude the diagnosis, but for the purpose of multiple choice if you see fluid around the band and none in the joint you can be fairly certain this is the pathology the question writer is after.

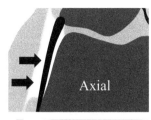

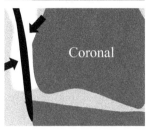

Hip Labrum

This is complicated and I'm not going to go into depth talking about all the little bumps and variants. I would just know a few things:

1: Anterior-Superior Tears (white arrows) are by far the most common.

2: Paralabral Cysts (black arrow) are associated with tears and likely a hint that a tear is present.

3: Just like a shoulder intra-articular contrast will increase your sensitivity.

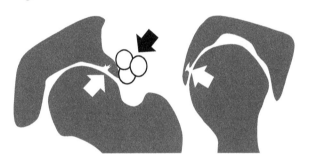

Coronal View   **Sagittal View**
-Showing the classic anterior superior cleft of a tear

Iliopsoas Bursa

Gamesmanship: A fluid signal "mass" with anterior to the femur (adjacent to the psoas tendon) at the level of the ischial tuberosity is likely Iliopsoas Bursitis

- Largest bursa of the entire body.

- Communicates with the joint in 15% of the population

- Seen Anterior to the hip

- Trivia: The illiospsoas tendon runs anterior to the labrum on axial and can mimic a tear.

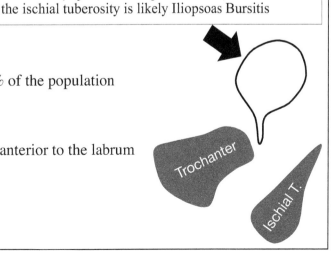

Femoroacetabular Impingement (FAI): This is a syndrome of painful hip movement. It's based on hip / femoral deformities, and honestly might be total BS. Supposedly it can lead to early degenerative changes.   There are two described subtypes: (A) Cam and (B) Pincher (technically there is a mixed type - but I anticipate multiple choice to make it more black and white).

CAM Type: This is an osseous "bump" along the femoral head-neck junction.

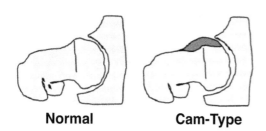

Normal   **Cam-Type**

> ***Memory Aid***
>
> I remember that the femoral one (cam-type) is more common in men because the femoral head kinda looks like a penis.
>
> Be honest, you were thinking that too.

Pincer Type: Whereas the CAM type is a deformity of the femur, the pincer type represents a deformity of the acetabulum. Whereas the CAM type is more common in a young athletic male, the pincer is more common in a middle aged woman *(insert sexist joke here)*.

The most classic way to show or ask this is the so-called **"cross over sign"**, where the acetabulum is malformed - causing the posterior lip to "Cross over" the anterior lip. A Key point is that the coccyx needs to be centered at the symphysis pubis to even evaluate this (rotation fucks things up).

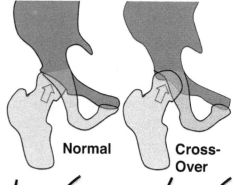

Normal   **Cross-Over**

The other associated finding(s) of the pincer subtype worth knowing are the acetabular over coverage buzzwords (Coxa Profunda and Protrusio), and the Ischial Spine Sign:

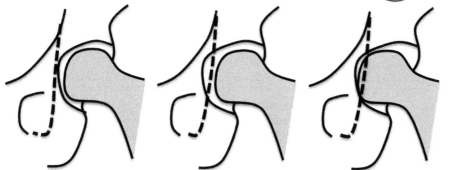

Normal

Coxa Profunda
(Acetabulum projects medial to the ilioischial line)

Acetabular Protrusion
(Femur projects medial to the ilioischial line)

Prominent Ischial Spine

Classic FAI Association:

- Os Acetabuli (40%)
- Labral Tears
- Early Arthritis

Os Acetabuli

This is an unfused secondary ossification center. It's actually normal in kids (should fuse by adult hood). It has several testable associations including FAI and Labral Tears

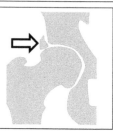

Total Hip Arthroplasty

Bone Remodeling / Stress Shielding:
The stress is transferred through the metallic stem, so the bone around it is not loaded. Orthopods call this "Wolff's Law" – where the unloaded bone just gets resorbed.

Happens more with uncemented arthroplasty. To some degree this is a normal finding - but when advanced can predispose to fracture.

Potentially Asymptomatic Complications of Hip Arthroplasty:

- Stress Shielding
- Aggressive Granulomatosis

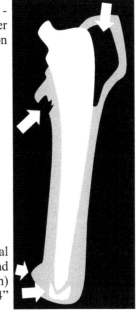

Proximal stress shielding - greater trochanter bone resorption

Calcar Resoption

Distal stress loading: cortical thickening & pedestral (around the bottom) "Zone 4"

Heterotopic Ossifications: This is very common (15-50%). It's usually asymptomatic. The trivia regarding multiple choice tests is that "hip stiffness" is the most common complaint.
Also in Ank Spon patients, because they are so prone to heterotopic ossifications, they sometimes give them low dose prophylactic radiation prior to THA.

Aseptic Loosening: This is the most common indication for revision. The criteria on x-ray is **> 2 mm at the interface** (suggestive). If you see **migration of the component,** you can call it *(migration includes varus tilting of the femoral stem).*

Subsidence: Basically an arthroplasty that is sliding downward. This is a described reason for early failure of THA. You see this most often in arthroplasty implants <u>without a collar</u>.

Greater than **1 cm** along the femoral component , or progression after 2 years are indications of loosening.

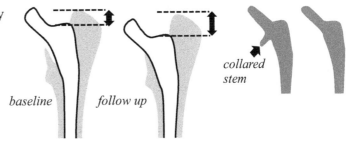

baseline *follow up* *collared stem*

Distance from the tip of the greater trochanter to the superolateral shoulder of the stem is increased relative to baseline.

Wear Patterns: It is normal to have a little bit of thinning in the area of weight bearing – this is called "Creep." It is not normal to see wear along the superior lateral aspect.

- Wear = Pathologic

- Creep = Normal

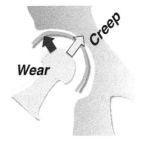

Creep

Wear

Particle Disease (Aggressive Granulomatosis): Any component of the device that sheds will cause an inflammatory response. The more wear that occurs the more particles — <u>wear is the primary underlying factor.</u> Macrophages will try and eat the particles and spew enzymes all over the place. This process can cause <u>progressive lytic focal regions around the replacement and joint effusions</u>.

Things to know about particle disease (in THA):

- Most commonly seen in non-cemented hips
- Tends to occur 1-5 years after surgery — "late complication"
- X-ray shows "smooth" endosteal scalloping (distinguishes from infection)
- Aseptic - ESR & CRP will be normal
- Produces no secondary bone response — no sclerosis
- Can be seen around screw holes (particles are transmitted around screws)

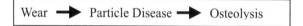

Wear ➡ Particle Disease ➡ Osteolysis

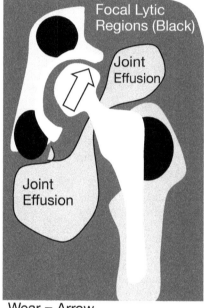

Focal Lytic Regions (Black)

Joint Effusion

Joint Effusion

Wear = Arrow

Sacrum:

You can get fractures of the sacrum in the setting of trauma, but if you get shown or asked anything about the sacrum it's going to be either (a) SI degenerative change - discussed later, (b) unilateral SI infection, (c) a chordoma - discussed later, (d) sacral agenesis, or (e) an insufficiency fracture. Out of these 5 things, the insufficiency fracture is probably the most likely.

Sacral Insufficiency Fracture - The most common cause is postmenopausal **osteoporosis.** You can also see this in patients with renal failure, patients with RA, **pelvic radiation**, **mechanical changes after hip arthroplasty**, or extended steroid use. They are often (usually) occult on plain films.

They will have to show this either with a bone scan, or MRI. The classic "**Honda Sign**" from the "H" -shaped appearance is probably the most likely presentation on a multiple choice test.

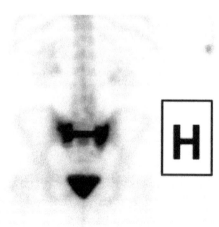

"Honda Sign"
Sacral Insufficiency Fx

Segond Fracture:

This is a fracture of the **Lateral** Tibial Plateau (*common distractor is medial tibia*). The thing to know is that it is **associated with ACL tear (75%)**, and occurs with **internal rotation.**

Reverse Segond Fracture:

This is a fracture of the **Medial** Tibial Plateau. The thing to know is that it is **associated with a PCL tear,** and occurs with **external rotation.** There is also an associated **medial meniscus** injury.

Arcuate Sign:

This is an avulsion of **proximal fibula** (insertion of arcuate ligament complex). The thing to know is that **90% are associated with cruciate ligament injury (usually PCL)**

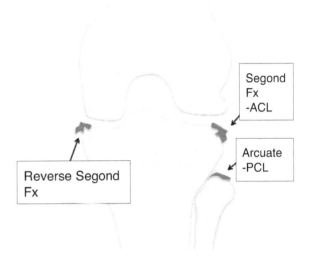

Deep Intercondylar Notch Sign:

This is a depression of the <u>lateral</u> femoral condyle (terminal sulcus) that occurs secondary to an impaction injury. This is **associated with ACL tears.**

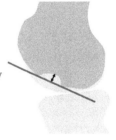

Deep Lateral Femoral Notch
- ACL Insufficiency
- Acute ACL Tear

Anatomy Blitz:

Ligaments:

- ACL: Composed of two bundles (anteromedial & posterolateral). The tibial attachment is thicker then the femoral attachment. Both the ACL and PCL are intra-articular and extrasynovial.

- PCL: The strongest ligament in the knee (you don't want a posterior dislocation of your knee resulting in dissection of your popliteal artery).

- MCL: The MCL fibers are laced into the joint capsule at the level of the joint, with connection to the medial meniscus. Unlike the ACL and PCL, the MCL is an extra-articular structure.

- Conjoint Tendon: Formed by the biceps femoris tendon and the LCL.

ACL & PCL are extrasynovial and intra-articular. The synovium folds around the ligaments. This is why a torn ACL won't heal on its own (usually).

The ligament can be torn even if the synovium is intact - this is why the "taunt" angle of the ligament is a key feature of integrity - more on that later

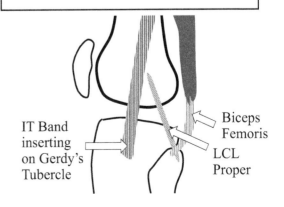

Magic Angle Phenomenon

The PCL and Patellar tendon may have foci of intermediate signal intensity on sagittal images with short echo time (TE) sequences where the tendon forms an angle of 55 degrees with the main magnetic field (*magic angle phenomenon*).

This will NOT be seen on T2 sequences (with long TE). This phenomenon is reduced at higher field strengths due to greater shortening of T2 relaxation times.

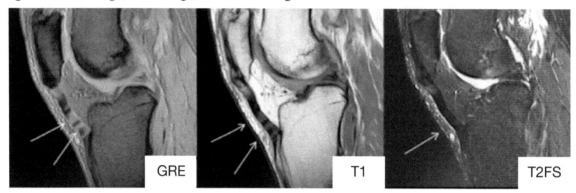

Magic Angle: You see it on short TE sequences (T1, PD, GRE). It goes away on T2

ACL Tear: ACL tears happen all the time, usually in people who are stopping and pivoting.

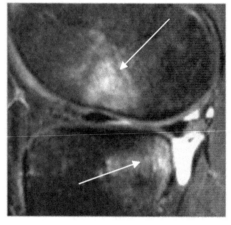

- Associated with Segond Fracture (lateral tibial plateau) and tibial spine avulsion
- ACL Angle lesser than Blumensaat's Line
- **O'donoghue's Unhappy Triad: ACL Tear, MCL Tear, Medial Meniscal Tear**
- *Classic Kissing Contusion Pattern:* The lateral femoral condyle (sulcus terminals) bangs into the posterior lateral tibial plateau. This is 95% specific in adults.
- *Anterior Drawer Sign* = Ortho Physical Exam Finding suggesting ACL Tear.

ACL Tear
-Kissing Contusion Pattern

ACL Mucoid Degeneration:

This can mimic acute or chronic partial tear of the ACL. There will be no secondary signs of injury (contusion etc..). It predisposes to ACL **ganglion cysts**, and they are usually seen together. The **T2/STIR buzzword is "celery stalk"** because of the striated look. The **T1 buzzword is "drumstick"** because it looks like a drum stick.

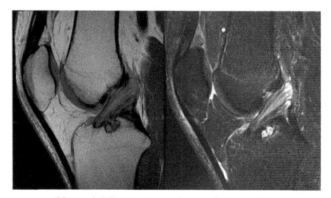

Mucoid Degeneration of the ACL
- "Drumstick / Celery Stick"

ACL Repair:

ACL can be repaired with two primary methods. Method 1: Using the middle one-third of the patellar tendon, with the patella bone plug attached to one end and tibial bone plug attached at the other. Method 2: Using a graft made of the semitendinosus or gracilis tendon, or both. The graft is then attached with all sorts of screws, bolts, etc… There is a lower reported morbidity related to harvest site using this method.

Graft Evaluation:

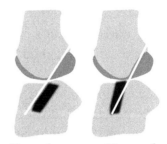

Normal Tibial Tunnel   *ABnormal Steep & Anterior to B Line (both are bad)*

There are two tunnels (tibial and femoral) between which the graft runs. Here are the testable pearls:

Tibial Tunnel: Should parallel the roof of the femoral intercondylar notch. Too Steep = Impinged by femur on extension. Too Flat = Lax & won't provide stability. Too Far Anterior ("Intersection with Blumensaat line") = Can lead to pinching at the anterior inferior intercondylar roof. Buzzword "Roof Impingement."

Femoral Tunnel: Supposedly the primary factor for maintaining length and tension during range of motion. This is referred to as "maintained isometry."

Femoral Tunnel = Maintains Isometry. Tibial Tunnel = Roof Impingement.

"Arthrofibrosis" Can be focal or diffuse (focal is more common). The focal form is the so called **"Cyclops" lesion** – so named because of its arthroscopic appearance. It's gonna be a low signal mass-like scar in Hoffa's fat pad. It's bad because it limits extension.

Buzzword "palpable audible clunk"

Seen around 16 weeks – it obviously won't occur immediately post op because you have to build up your scar.

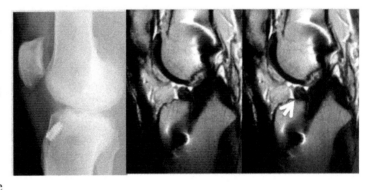

Cyclops Lesion - Scar Associated with Ventral Graft

"Graft Tear" - Usually Ortho can just pull on his fucking leg is see if the graft is trashed (anterior drawer sign). For imaging, the simple way to understand this: "flat angle = tear." The ACL should parallel the roof of the intercondylar notch. If the angle becomes flat, a tear is likely.

Trivia: The graft is most susceptible to tear in the remodeling process (4-8 months post op).

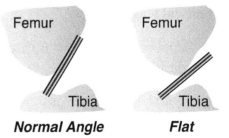

Normal Angle   **Flat**

Trivia: Other signs of graft tear: grossly high T2 signal (some is ok), fiber discontinuity, uncovering of the posterior horn of the lateral meniscus (secondary sign), anterior tibial translation (secondary sign).

Posterior Lateral Corner (PLC): The most complicated anatomy in the entire body. My God this posterior lateral corner! Just think about the LCL, the IT band, the biceps femoris, and the popliteus tendon. The most likely way to show this on a single image (multiple choice style) is **edema in the fibular head.**

Who cares? Missed PLC injury is a very common cause of ACL reconstruction failure.

PCL Tear: The posterior collateral ligament is the strongest ligament in the knee. A tear is actually uncommon, it's more likely to stretch and appear thickened (> 7 mm). PCL tears should make you think about posterior dislocation as the mechanism of injury..

Next Step / Association = If you see a PCL Tear - look at the popliteal flow void. If the knee dislocated posterior, a dreaded consequence is vascular compromise. Depending on the wording of the question they might need a run-off (watch your back).

Meniscal Anatomy:

The meniscus is "C shaped", thick along the periphery and thin centrally.

Medial meniscus is thicker posteriorly.

Lateral meniscus has equal thickness between anterior and posterior portion.

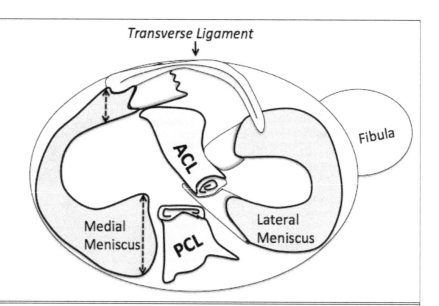

Meniscal Healing

The Peripheral "Red Zone" is vascular and might heal.

The Central "white zone" is avascular and will not heal. The blood supply comes from the geniculate arteries (which enter peripherally).

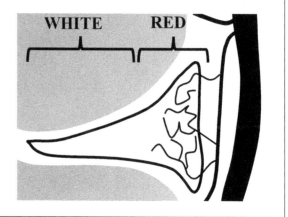

Meniscal Tears:

As stated, the peripheral meniscus (red zone) has better vasculature than the inner 2/3s (white zone) and might heal on its own. In general, you can group tears based on their general direction (as seen on a sagittal section MRI - i.e. the triangles and bowties) - as either vertical (top-to-bottom) or horizontal (front-to-back). You can then sub-group them depending how they look on subsequent sections.

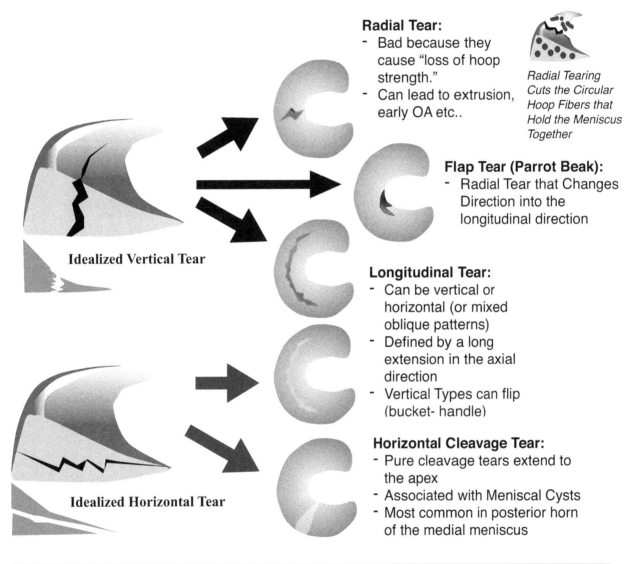

Radial Tear:
- Bad because they cause "loss of hoop strength."
- Can lead to extrusion, early OA etc..

Radial Tearing Cuts the Circular Hoop Fibers that Hold the Meniscus Together

Idealized Vertical Tear

Flap Tear (Parrot Beak):
- Radial Tear that Changes Direction into the longitudinal direction

Longitudinal Tear:
- Can be vertical or horizontal (or mixed oblique patterns)
- Defined by a long extension in the axial direction
- Vertical Types can flip (bucket-handle)

Idealized Horizontal Tear

Horizontal Cleavage Tear:
- Pure cleavage tears extend to the apex
- Associated with Meniscal Cysts
- Most common in posterior horn of the medial meniscus

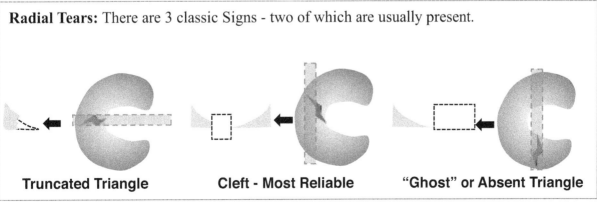

Radial Tears: There are 3 classic Signs - two of which are usually present.

Truncated Triangle   **Cleft - Most Reliable**   **"Ghost" or Absent Triangle**

Discoid Meniscus:

This is a normal variant of the **lateral meniscus** that is **prone to tear.** It's not C-shaped, but instead shaped like a disc. In other words, it's too big (too many bowties!).

Gamesmanship - "Pediatric Patient with Meniscal Tear".

Trivia - There are three types, with the most rare and most prone to injury being the *Wrisberg Variant*.

Gamesmanship "Bow Ties" If shown on sagittal they have to show you 3 or more "bow ties" / double triangles.

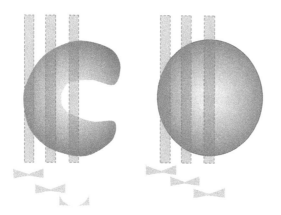

Normal Meniscus will have 2 bowtie shapes in the sagittal plane - assuming 3mm slices with 1mm gap.

Discoid Meniscus will have 3 or more bowties

Gamesmanship: If shown on coronal they need to show you a meniscus stretching into the notch.

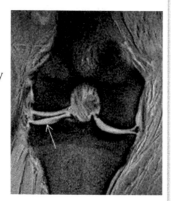

Discoid Meniscus
-Extending into Notch

Bucket Handle Tear:

This is a torn meniscus (usually **medial** - 80%) vertical longitudinal sub-type, that flips medially to lie anterior to the PCL.

Gamesmanship - Most likely shown as the classic Aunt Minnie appearance of a "**double PCL.**"

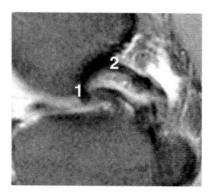

Buckle Hand Tear
-Double PCL Sign

Gamesmanship - Can also be shown as "not enough bowties," the opposite of the "too many bowties" look of a discoid meniscus.

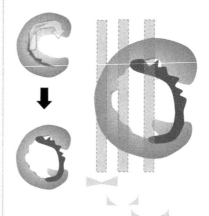

Only 1 bowtie - instead of the normal 2.

The middle of the second bowtie is flipped medially.

Trivia: The appearance of a double PCL can **only occur in the setting of an intact ACL**, otherwise it won't flip that way. Just know it sorta indirectly proves the ACL is intact (I can just see some knucklehead asking that).

Meniscal Cysts:

Most often seen near the lateral meniscus and are <u>often associated with horizontal cleavage tears</u>.

Meniscocapsular Separation:

This is a rare (in real life - maybe not on exams) injury. The idea is that the deepest layer of the **MCL** complex (capsular ligament) is relatively weak and is the first to tear. This deep tearing may result in the separation of the meniscus and the MCL. I've never seen it occur in isolation (theoretically it can). The important things to remember are probably (1) it happens more with proximal MCL tears, and (2) this is a serious injury — requires immobilization or surgery.

Meniscal Ossicle:

This is a focal ossification of the posterior horn of the medial meniscus, that can be secondary to trauma or simply developmental. They are <u>often associated with radial root tears.</u>

Meniscofemoral Ligaments:

There are 2 (Wrisberg, Humphry) which can be mimics of meniscal tears. Wrisberg is in the back (*"humping Humphry"*). You could also remember that "H" comes before "W" in the alphabet.

Meniscal Flounce: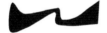

This an uncommon finding of a **"ruffled"** appearance of the meniscus that mimics a tear.

It's <u>NOT associated with an increased incidence of tear</u> - but can look like one, if you don't have any idea what one looks like.

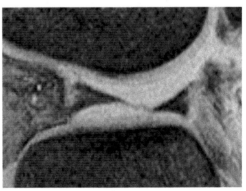

"Flounce"
Ruffled = Not a Tear

Patella Dislocation:

Dislocation of the patella is usually lateral because of the shape of the patella and femur. The contusion pattern is classic.

- It's Lateral
- Contusion Pattern - Classic
- Associated <u>tear of the MPFL</u> (medial patellar femoral ligament)
- Associated with *"Trochlear Dysplasia"* - the trochlea is too flat.

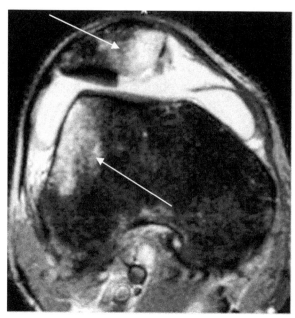

Patellar Dislocation
Classic Contusion Pattern (arrows)

Patella Alta / Baja:

The patella will move up or down in certain traumatic situations. If the quadricep tendon tears you will get unopposed pull from the patellar tendon resulting in a low patella (Baja). If the patella tendon tears you will get unopposed quadriceps tendon pull resulting in a high patella (Alta).

The "classic" association with patellar tendon tear (Alta) is **SLE**, (also can see in elderly, trauma, athletics, or RA).

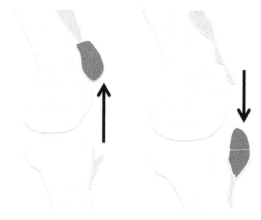

Patella Alta   **Patella Baja**

 "Bilateral patellar rupture" is a buzzword for chronic steroids.

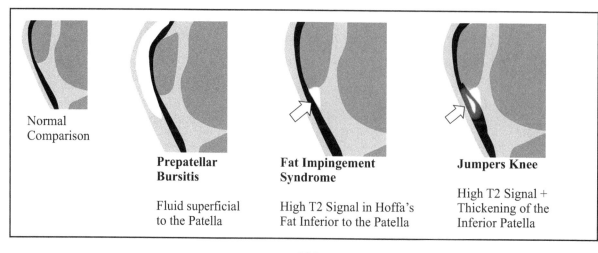

Normal Comparison

Prepatellar Bursitis

Fluid superficial to the Patella

Fat Impingement Syndrome

High T2 Signal in Hoffa's Fat Inferior to the Patella

Jumpers Knee

High T2 Signal + Thickening of the Inferior Patella

Tibial Plateau Fracture: This injury most commonly occurs from axial loading (falling and landing on a straight leg). The **lateral plateau is way more common than the medial**. If you see medial, it's usually with lateral. Some dude named Schatzker managed to get the classification system named after him, of which type 2 is the most common (split and depressed lateral plateau).

Pilon Fracture (Tibial plafond fracture): This injury also most commonly occurs from axial loading, with the talus being driven into the tibial plafond. The fracture is characterized by comminution and articular impaction. About 75% of the time you are going to have fracture of the distal fibula.

Tibial Shaft Fracture: This is the most common long bone fracture. It was also *listed as the most highly tested subject in orthopedic OITE exam (with regard to trauma)*, over the last 8 years. Apparently there are a bunch of ways to put a nail or plate in it. It doesn't seem like it could be that high yield for the CORE compared to other fractures with French or Latin sounding names. I will point out that the tibia is one of the slowest healing bones in the body *(10 weeks)*.

Tillaux Fractures: **This a Salter-Harris 3,** through the anterolateral aspect of the distal tibial **epiphysis**.

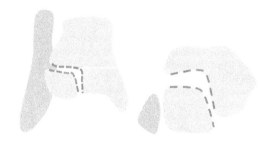

Trivia: This pattern requires an open physis along the lateral distal tibia. This is why you see this fracture pattern in the window between the start of medial physis fusion and the complete fusion of the lateral physis (lateral physis typically closes around 12-15).

Trivia: The distal tibial growth plate closes from medial to lateral (medial first).

Triplane Fracture: This is a **Salter-Harris 4**, with a vertical component through the **epiphysis,** horizontal component through the physis, **and** oblique through the **metaphysis**.

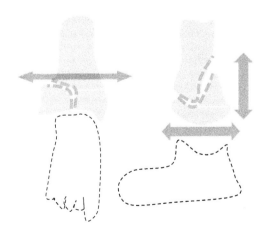

*The addition of the fracture plane in the posterior distal tibial metaphysis (coronal plane) distinguishes this from the Tillaux.

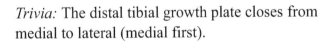

Maisonneuve Fracture:

This is an unstable fracture involving the medial tibial malleolus and/or **disruption of the distal tibiofibular syndesmosis**.

 The most common way to show this is to first show you the ankle with the widened mortis, and *"next step?"* get you to ask for the proximal fibula - which will show the **fracture of the proximal fibular shaft**.

This fracture pattern is unique as the forces begin distally in the tibiotalar joint and then ride up the syndesmosis to the proximal fibula.

 Trivia: The fracture **does not extend into the hindfoot.**

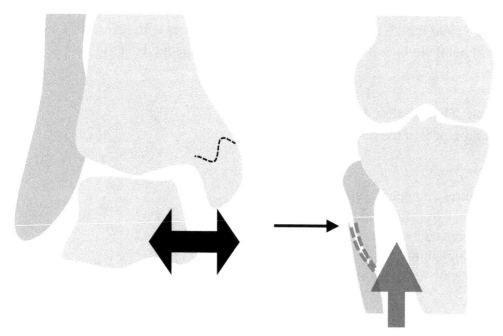

Wide Medial Malleolus
(+/- Medial Malleolus Fracture)
— Distal Tibiofibular syndesmosis
+/- Deltoid Lig Injury

Proximal Fibula Fracture
— From upward force extension
("the rippin and the tearin") via the syndesmosis

Site-Specific Entities - Ankle (the rest of it) / Foot

Casanova Fracture – If you see bilateral calcaneal fractures, you should *"next step?"* look at the spine (T12-L2) for a compression or burst fracture. These tend to occur in axial loading patterns (possibly from jumping out a window to avoid an angry husband).

Trivia:
- Peroneal tendons can become entrapped with lateral calcaneal fractures.
- Calcaneal fractures are the most common (60%) Tarsal Bone Fx
- Fractures of the calcaneus are either extra-articular or intra-articular - *depends on subtalar joint involvement.* Intra-articular fractures will have a fracture line through the *"critical angle of Gissane"*

Bohler's Angle – The line drawn between the anterior and posterior borders of the calcaneus on a lateral view. An angle less than 20 degrees, is concerning for a fracture.

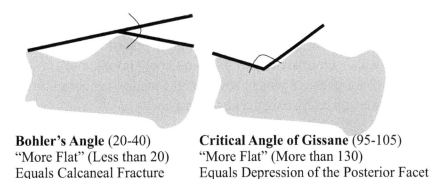

Bohler's Angle (20-40)
"More Flat" (Less than 20)
Equals Calcaneal Fracture

Critical Angle of Gissane (95-105)
"More Flat" (More than 130)
Equals Depression of the Posterior Facet

Stress Fracture of the 5th Metatarsal:
This is considered a high risk fracture (hard to heal).

Jones Fracture: This is a fracture at the base of the fifth metatarsal, 1.5cm distal to the tuberosity. These are placed in a non-weight bearing cast (may require internal fixation- because of risk of non-union.

Avulsion Fracture of the 5th Metatarsal:
This is more common than a jones fracture. The classic history is a dancer. It may be **secondary to tug from the lateral cord of the plantar aponeurosis or peroneus brevis** (this is controversial).

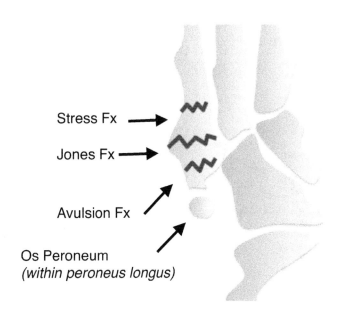

Stress Fx ➝

Jones Fx ➝

Avulsion Fx ➚

Os Peroneum
(within peroneus longus)

Painful Os Peroneus Syndrome (POPS)

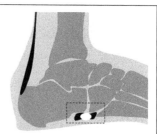

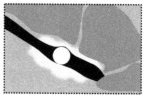

• Os Peroneus (accessory ossicle) is within the Peroneus LONGUS

• This ossicle is seen in about 10% of gen pop

• Stress reaction and pain can progress to tendon disruption = POPS

MR Key Findings: Edema in the os peroneus just before the peroneus longus tendon enters the cuboid tunnel

Lisfranc Injury: This is the **most common dislocation of the foot**. The Lisfranc joint is the articulation of the tarsals and metatarsal bases. This joint is recessed creating a "keystone" locking mechanism, and would make a good place to amputate if you were a surgeon assisting in the Napoleonic invasion of Russia. The Lisfranc ligament connects the medial cuneiform to the 2nd metatarsal base on the plantar aspect.

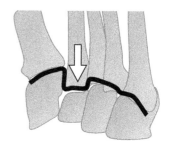

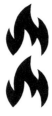
• Can't exclude it on a non-weight bearing film
• Associated fractures are most common at the base of the 2nd MT - *"Fleck Sign"*
• Fracture non-union and post traumatic arthritis are gonna occur if you miss it (plus a lawsuit).

"Fleck Sign" - This is a small bony fragment in the Lisfranc Space (between 1st MT and 2nd MT) - that is associated with an avulsion of the LF ligament.

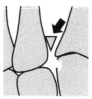

A **"fleck"** of bone near the base of the 2nd MT can sometimes be the only clue.

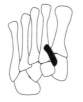 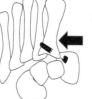 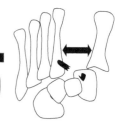

Normal   Homo-Lateral   Divergent

Mechanism =
Extreme Plantar Flexion + Axial Load

3 Ligaments make up the complex between the medial cuneiform and 2nd MT.

The plantar band is the strongest

Medial

2nd MT

236

Anatomic Trivia

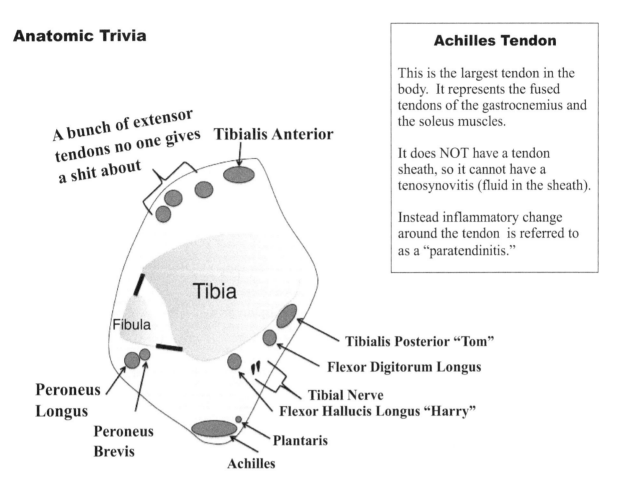

A bunch of extensor tendons no one gives a shit about

Tibialis Anterior

Tibia

Fibula

Peroneus Longus

Peroneus Brevis

Achilles

Plantaris

Flexor Hallucis Longus "Harry"

Tibial Nerve

Flexor Digitorum Longus

Tibialis Posterior "Tom"

> **Achilles Tendon**
>
> This is the largest tendon in the body. It represents the fused tendons of the gastrocnemius and the soleus muscles.
>
> It does NOT have a tendon sheath, so it cannot have a tenosynovitis (fluid in the sheath).
>
> Instead inflammatory change around the tendon is referred to as a "paratendinitis."

The Mythical **Master Knot of Henry** - This has a funny sounding name, therefore it's high yield. This is where Dick (FDL) crosses over Harry (FHL) at the medial ankle.

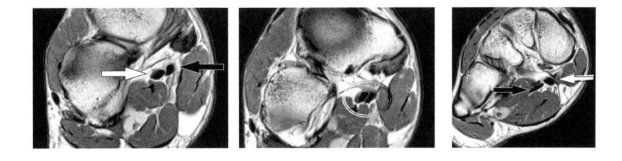

Harry (white) starts out lateral relative to Dick (black). They cross at the "master knot" and then Harry (white) ends up medial on it's way to the big toe (Harry = Hallucis).

What is the Master Knot of Henry? It's a "Harry Dick"

Ligamentous Injury: The highest yield fact is that the **anterior talofibular ligament is the weakest ligament and the most frequently injured** (usually from inversion).

Posterior Tibial Tendon Injury / Dysfunction: This results in a progressive flat foot deformity, as the PTT is the primary stabilizer of the longitudinal arch. When chronic, the tear is most common behind the medial malleolus (this is where the most friction is). When acute, the tear is most common at the insertion into the navicular bone. **Acute Flat Arch should make you think of PTT tear.**

You will also have a hindfoot valgus deformity (from unopposed peroneal brevis action). The other point of trivia to know is that the spring ligament is a secondary supporter of the arch (it holds up the talar head), and it will thicken and degenerate without the help of the PTT. Don't get it twisted though, the spring ligament is very thick and strong and almost never ruptures in a foot/ankle trauma.

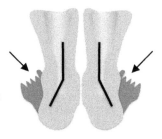

Hindfoot Valgus
"Too Many Toes"

I Say Acute Flat Foot, You Say Posterior Tibial Tendon Injury

Sinus Tarsi Syndrome: **Never make this diagnosis in the setting of acute trauma*

The space between the lateral talus and calcaneus. The sinus tarsi is not just a joint space. It is an important source of proprioception and balance. Fucking it up has consequences (if your goal is to make prima ballerina assoluta).

The "syndrome" is caused by hemorrhage or inflammation of the synovial recess with or without tears of the associated ligaments (talocalcaneal ligaments, inferior extensor retinaculum). There are associations with rheumatologic disorders and abnormal loading (flat foot in the setting of a posterior tibial tendon tear).

MRI finding is obliteration of fat in the sinus tarsi space, and replacement with scar.

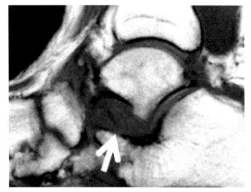

Loss of Normal T1 Bright Fat (arrow)

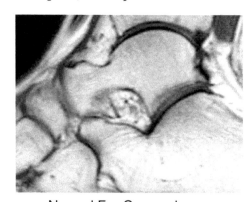

Normal For Comparison

Plantar Fasciitis:

This is an inflammation of the fascia secondary to either repetitive trauma (overuse via endless rounding on fat diabetic, smokers as a medicine intern), abnormal mechanics (pes cavus, etc), or arthritis (Reiters, etc…).

The pain is localized to the origin of the plantar fascia, and worsened by dorsiflexion of the toes. This is usually a clinical diagnosis.

Buzzword is *"most severe in the morning."*

As a rapid anatomy review, the plantar fascia consists of 3 bands with the central / lateral part normally thicker than the medial part the thinnest.

Coronal T1 diagram through the heel

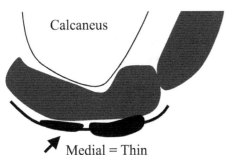

Plain film might show heel spurs (which are not specific), but could be a hint. A bone scan may show increased tracer in the region of the calcaneus (from periosteal inflammation).

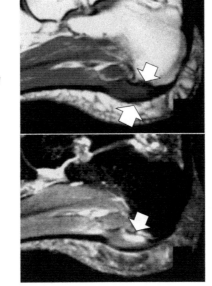

MRI may show:

a thickened fascia (> 4mm) , most often the central band

with increased T2 signal, most significant near its insertion at the heel.

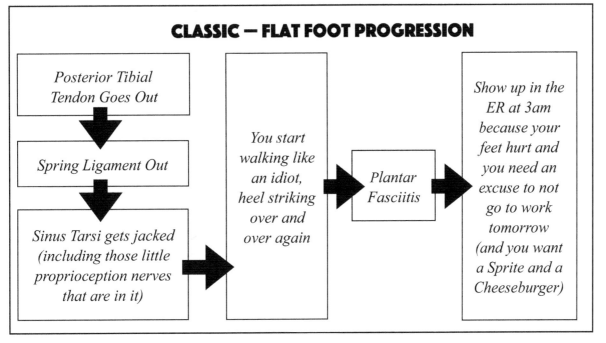

CLASSIC — FLAT FOOT PROGRESSION

Posterior Tibial Tendon Goes Out → *Spring Ligament Out* → *Sinus Tarsi gets jacked (including those little proprioception nerves that are in it)* → *You start walking like an idiot, heel striking over and over again* → *Plantar Fasciitis* → *Show up in the ER at 3am because your feet hurt and you need an excuse to not go to work tomorrow (and you want a Sprite and a Cheeseburger)*

Split Peroneus Brevis:

You can see longitudinal splits in the peroneus in people with inversion injuries. The history is usually "chronic ankle pain".

The tendon will be C shaped or **boomerang shaped** with central thinning and partial envelopment of the peroneus longus. Alternatively, there may be 3 instead of 2 tendons. The tear occurs at the lateral malleolus.

There is a strong (80%) association with lateral ligament injury.

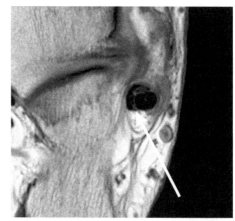

Split Peroneus Brevis
-*Boomerang*

Anterolateral Impingement Syndrome:

Injury to the anterior talofibular ligaments and tibiofibular ligaments (usually from an inversion injury) can cause lateral instability, and chronic synovial inflammation.

You can eventually produce a "mass" of hypertrophic synovial tissue in the lateral gutter.

The **MRI finding is a "meniscoid mass" in the lateral gutter of the ankle**, which is a balled up scar (**T1 and T2 dark**).

Tarsal Tunnel Syndrome:

Pain in the distribution of the posterior tibial nerve (first 3 toes) from compression as it passes through the tarsal tunnel (behind the medial malleolus).

It's usually unilateral (unlike carpal tunnel which is usually bilateral), unusually "idiopathic" although pes planus (hindfoot valgus) can predispose by tightening the retinaculum.

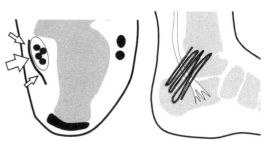

Tarsal tunnel is a covered by the flexor retinaculum (arrows) and includes tom, dick, harry the posterior tibial artery and nerve.

You can see atrophy of multiple foot muscles (not just minimi as seen with "Baxter").

Having said that, any mass lesion (ganglion cysts, neurogenic tumors, varicosities, lipomas, severe tenosynovitis, and accessory muscles) can cause compression of the nerve in the tunnel.

Morton's Neuroma: Soft tissue mass (tear drop shaped) shown between the 3rd and 4th metatarsal heads (third intermetatarsal space) is most likely a Morton's Neuroma (especially on multiple choice tests). The proposed pathology results from compression / entrapment of the plantar digital nerve in this location by the intermetatarsal ligament. Over time this results in thickening and development of perineural fibrosis.

 "Mulder's Sign" - is a physical exam (a sonographic sign) where you squeeze the patients foot and reproduce the pain (or see the scar pop out under ultrasound).

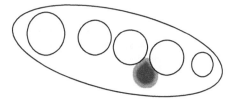

Trivia: Morton's Neuroma is NOT a Neuroma (a tumor). It's a scar.

Classic Look: It is a scar, so it's gonna be dark on T1 and T2 (usually). It is tear drop shaped and projects downward.

People make a big deal about this thing staying below the plantar ligament.

Mortons: T1 Dark Below the Plantar Ligament

The reason is that your primary differential is **intermetatarsal bursitis** - which will extend above the transverse ligament, be fluid signal, and have a more cystic look. Small bursa in this location can be normal as long as the stay smaller than 3mm.

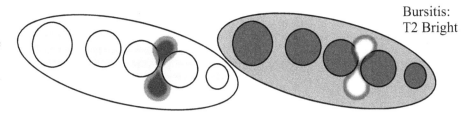

Bursitis: Above the Ligament (dumbbell shaped)

Bursitis: T2 Bright

Haglund's Syndrome / Deformity

This is also called the "Mulholland deformity" for the purpose of fucking with you. Depending on what you read there are either 3 or 4 classic features:

- Retro-Achilles bursitis, /
- Retrocalcaneal bursitis,
- Thickening of the distal Achilles tendon (insertional portion)
- Calcaneal Bony Prominence "prominent posterior superior os calcis"

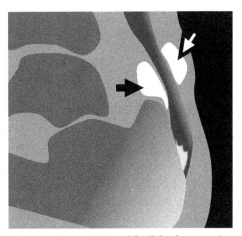

The <u>deformity is the "bump."</u> The "syndrome" is the bursitis and Achilles tendon thickening. They call this thing the "pump bumps," because wearing high-heeled shoes is supposedly a predisposing factor

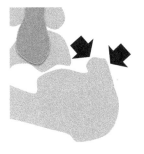

Retrocalcaneal Bursitis (black arrow)
Retro-Achilles / Adventitial Bursitis (white arrow)

Os Trigonum Syndrome

The idea is that the Os Trigonum (accessory ossicle) puts the smash on the FHL ("Harry") during extreme ankle flexion — toe pointing shit ("Pointe technique") that ballet dancers do… or other repetitive micro trauma.

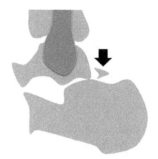

Classic findings are going to be

(1) "Stenosing" tenosynovitis / collection of fluid around the FHL, and

(2) edema within the Os Trigonum and across the synchondrosis between the Os and the Posterior Talus.

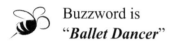 Buzzword is **"Ballet Dancer"**

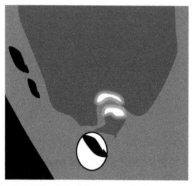

Axial T2 - Fluid Around the FHL Edema in the Os and Posterior

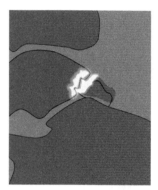

Sag T2 - Edema in the Os and Posterior Talus

Achilles Tendon Injury:

Acute rupture is usually obvious with a fluid filled gap. The gap size will determine treatment (big gaps need surgery). The tear is usually 4 cm above the calcaneal insertion and the classic history is an unconditioned middle aged fake athlete ("weekend warrior") with acute pain and loss of the ability to plantar flex.

Without a large gap these things can be very hard to tell apart from a **Xanthoma** (both can just look like a very thick tendon). There are a few differences that can be used to differentiate - per my chart.

Achilles Tendon Tear (partial / small gap)	Xanthoma
Thick Tendon (> 7mm)	Thick Tendon (> 7mm)
Unilateral	Bilateral (usually)
Associated with being a fake athlete	Associated with having very high cholesterol
Step 1 Trivia: Fluoroquinolone antibiotics	

Plantaris Rupture

("Tennis Leg"): This is usually presented as the classic trick: "Achilles tendon ruptured but can still plantar flex." Remember not everyone has this tendon (it's absent in 10% of the population). The classic look on MRI is focal fluid collection between the soleus and the medial head of the gastrocnemius. There is an association with ACL tears.

Avulsions of the Calcaneal Tuberosity:

This is sort of an Aunt Minnie with the back of the bone totally ripped off via the Achilles. The classic association is *diabetes*. When you see this you have to think *diabetes.*

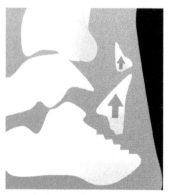

Calcaneal Avulsion

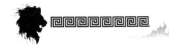 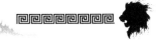

Osteopenia: This just means increased lucency of bones. Although this is most commonly caused by osteoporosis, that is not always the case.

Osteomalacia: This is a soft bone from excessive uncalcified osteoid. This is typically related to vitamin D issues (either renal causes, liver causes, or other misc causes). It generally looks just like diffuse osteopenia. For the purpose of multiple choice you should think about 4 things: Ill-defined trabeculae, Ill-defined corticomedullary junction, bowing, and "Loosers Zones."

Looser Zones: These things are wide lucent bands that transverse bone <u>at right angles</u> to the cortex. These things can happen in lots of different locations - but the classic two are the *femoral neck* and the *pubic rami*. Typically there is sclerosis surrounding the lucency. You should think two things: **osteomalacia** and **rickets**. Less common is OI. The other piece of trivia is to understand **they are a type of insufficiency fracture**.

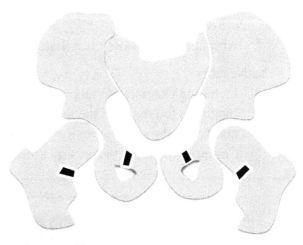

Looser Zones
— Raise your suspicion for this shit when you see (1) Symmetric Findings
(2) The "90 Degree" to the cortex line

Osteoporosis: The idea is that you have low bone density. Bone density peaks around 30 and then decreases. It decreases faster in women during menopause. The imaging findings are a thin sharp cortex, prominent trabecular bars, lucent metaphyseal bands, and spotty lucencies.

Causes: Age is the big one. Medications (steroids, heparin, dilantin), Endocrine issues (cushings, hyperthryoidism), Anorexia, and Osteogenesis Imperfecta.

Complications: Fractures – Most commonly of the spine (2nd most common is the hip, 3rd most common is the wrist).

DEXA:

This is a bone mineral density test and an excellent source of multiple choice trivia.

General Things to know about DEXA
- T score = Density relative to young adult
- T score defines osteopenia vs osteoporosis
- T score > -1.0 = Normal, -1.0 to -2.5 = Osteopenia, < **-2.5 Osteoporosis**
- Z score = Density relative to age-matched control "to **Za Zame** Age"
- False negative / positive (see below)

False Positive / Negative on DEXA: DEXA works by measuring the density. Anything that makes that higher or lower than normal can fool the machine.

False Positive:
- Absent Normal Structures: Status post laminectomy

False Negative:
- Including excessive Osteophytes, dermal calcifications, or metal
- Including too much of the femoral shaft when doing a hip - can elevate the number as the shaft normally has denser bone.
- Compression Fx in the area measured

FRAX:

The **F**racture **R**isk **A**ssessment **T**ool is a clinical risk tool used to predict fractures by using clinical risk factors (age, sex, race, BMI, family history, personal fracture history, prior steroid use, where the patient lives, etc...) with or without femoral neck bone density. The fracture risk is calculated as a ten year fracture probability.

Trivia:

- FRAX calculates fracture risk at a **10 year probability**
- FRAX adds "value" by helping to identify the subset of osteopenic patients who are at a higher risk for fracture - and might benefit from pharmacologic intervention
- FRAX is NOT supposed to be used in patient who have already been placed on meds for osteoporosis. The entire point of the FRAX is to make big pharma more money... I mean help identify those who would benefit most from pharmacologic intervention - those already on meds don't need identified.
- FRAX is applicable for men and women
- FRAX is recommended to calculate 10 year fracture risk in patients with a T-Score between -1 and -2.5.
- Some guidelines suggest pharmacologic intervention for patients with a FRAX calculated 10 year hip fracture risk of > 3% or major fracture risk of > 20%

Reflex Sympathetic Dystrophy (RSD):

Also called *"Complex Regional Pain Syndrome"* — which makes it sound like some Rheumatology Psycho-somatic bullshit (i.e. fibromyalgia).

Also called *"Sudeck Atrophy"* - which makes it sound serious - like some incurable neurodegenerative death sentence.

The classic clinical vignette is a history of trauma or infection.

On plain film, it can cause severe osteopenia (like disuse osteopenia). Some people say it **looks like unilateral RA, with preserved joint spaces**. Hand and shoulder are the most common sites of involvement.

It's one of the many causes of a 3 phase hot bone scan. In fact, *intra-articular uptake* of tracer on bone scan is typically seen (on multiple choice) in patients with RSD (secondary to the increased vascularity of the synovial membrane), and this is somewhat characteristic.

Transient Osteoporosis:

There are two types of presentations.:

Transient osteoporosis of the hip: For the purpose of multiple choice tests, by far you should expect to see the **female in the 3ʳᵈ trimester of pregnancy** with involvement of the left hip. Having said that, it's actually more common in men in whom it's usually bilateral. The joint space should remain normal. It's self limiting (hence the word transient) and resolves in a few months. *Plain film shows osteopenia, MRI shows Edema, Bone scan shows increased uptake focally.*

Regional migratory osteoporosis - This is an idiopathic disorder which has a very classic history of **pain** in a joint, which gets better and then shows up in another joint. It's associated with osteoporosis – which is also self-limiting. It's more common in men.

Hip Edema - Strategy Session — This vs That - Transient Osteoporosis vs AVN vs Fx

On radiograph, transient osteoporosis and AVN look totally different. Transient Osteoporosis is super lucent - so lucent that sometimes you can barely see the femoral head. AVN on the other hand, will have patchy areas of sclerosis.

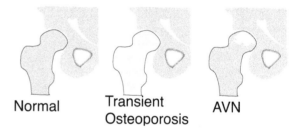

On MRI, the story is different. These things can look similar. They both have edema on STIR, and they are both are dark on T1. The difference is that AVN should be shown with a serpiginous dark line (double line if you are lucky) - that represents infarct core. Joint effusions can be seen in both - so this isn't helpful.

Now - if these assholes want to take it to the twilight zone, they can add "insufficiency fracture" to the list of distractors. This is really a dirty trick as both Transient Osteoporosis and AVN are susceptible to this. The distinction is that this fracture line should be less serpiginous and instead parallel the subchondral bone of the femoral head.

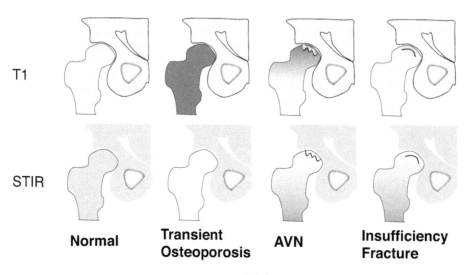

Osteoporotic Compression Fracture: Super Common. On MR you want to see a *"band like"* fracture line - which is typically T1 dark (T2 is more variable). The non-deformed portions of the vertebral body should have normal signal.

Neoplastic Compression Fracture: Most vertebral mets don't result in compression fracture until nearly the entire vertebral body is replaced with tumor. If you see abnormal marrow signal (not band like) with involvement of the posterior margin you should think about cancer.

> ### *What is this "Abnormal Marrow Signal" ?*
>
> Normally (in an adult) the marrow of the spine is fatty - so it should be T1 bright. The internal control is an adjacent normal disc (not a desiccated disk).
>
> If you see dark stuff - it might just be red marrow. BUT if it is darker than the adjacent (normal) disc, you have to assume that it's a bad thing.

 Next Step ? - Look at the rest of the spine - mets are often multiple.

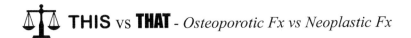 **THIS** vs **THAT** - *Osteoporotic Fx vs Neoplastic Fx*

If I was going to show a Neoplastic vs Osteoporotic Fracture case, this is how I would do it. I would have 2 sequences, a T1 and a STIR. The STIR would be positive (bright on both). The Osteoporotic Fracture would have a T1 dark line. The Neoplastic Fracture would be diffusely low T1 signal and blobby - and I would stick a few lesions in other vertebral bodies.

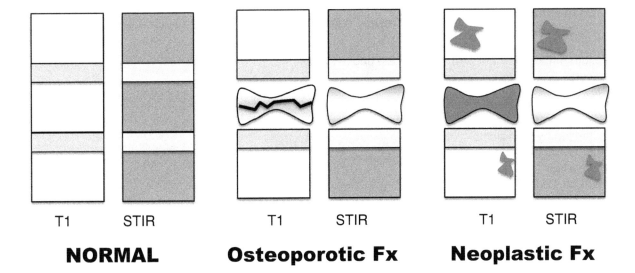

T1 STIR	T1 STIR	T1 STIR
NORMAL	**Osteoporotic Fx**	**Neoplastic Fx**

OCDs/ OCLs

Osteochondritis Dissecans (OCD):

The new terminology is actually to call these "OCLs" (the "L" is for Lesion). This a spectrum of aseptic separation of an osteochondral fragment which can lead to gradual fragmentation of the articular surface and secondary OA. Most of the time it is secondary to trauma, although it could also be secondary to AVN.

> **OCD Trivia:**
>
> Most common in males under 18
>
> Most common in the lateral aspect of the medial femoral condyle

Where it happens: Classic locations include the femoral condyle (most common site in the knee), patella, talus, and capitellum.

Staging: There is a staging system, which you probably need to know exists.

- Stage 1: Stable – Covered by intact cartilage, Intact with Host Bone
- Stage 2: Stable on Probing, Partially not intact with host bone.
- Stage 3: Unstable on Probing, Complete discontinuity of lesion.
- Stage 4: Dislocated fragment

Treatment / Who cares? If the fragment is unstable you can get secondary OA. You want to **look for high T2 signal undercutting the fragment from the bone to call it unstable** (edema can force a false positive). Thus, the absence of high T2 signal at the bone fragment interface is a good indicator of osseous bridging and stability. Granulation tissue at the interface (which will enhance with Gd), does not mean it's stable.

THIS vs THAT: Capitellum Lesions		
Osteochondritis Dissecans	**Panner's Disease**	**Pseudo-Lesion**
Capitellum of the dominant arm in throwers	Also in the capitellum of throwers	
Anterior convex margin of the capitellum. Unstable lesions are characterized by high signal fluid that encircles the osteochondral fragment on T2W image	Entire Capitellum is abnormal in signal (low T1, high T2)	Posterior Capitellum
Can lead to intra-articular loose bodies	Loose body formation is NOT seen (usually)	A coronal image through the posterior capitellum can mimic a defect. This occurs because the most posterior portion of the capitellum has an abrupt slope.
Slightly older patients (12-16 years)	5 to 10 years old *"Peter Pan wanted to stay young"*	

Osteochondroses:

These are a group of conditions (usually seen in childhood) that are characterized by involvement of the epiphysis, or apophysis with findings of collapse, sclerosis, and fragmentation – suggesting osteonecrosis.

Kohlers	Tarsal Navicular	Boys 4-6. Treatment is not surgical.
Freiberg Infraction	Second Metatarsal Head	Adolescent Girls – can lead to secondary OA
Sever's	Calcaneal Apophysis	Some say this is a normal "growing pain"
Panner's	Capitellum	Kid 5-10 "Thrower"; does not have loose bodies.
Perthes (LCP)	Femoral Head	White kid; 4-8.
Kienbock	Carpal Lunate	Associated with negative ulnar variance. Seen in adults 20-40.
Scheuermann	Thoracic Spine	Causes kyphosis. 3 adjacent levels with wedging, plus a thoracic kyphosis of > 40 degrees (normal 20-40)
Osgood-Schlatter Disease (OSD)	Tibial Tubercle	Adolescents (10-15) who jump and kick. Need Fragmentation + Soft Tissue Swelling.
Sinding-Larsen-Johansson (SLJ)	Inferior Patella	Adolescents (10-15) who jump.

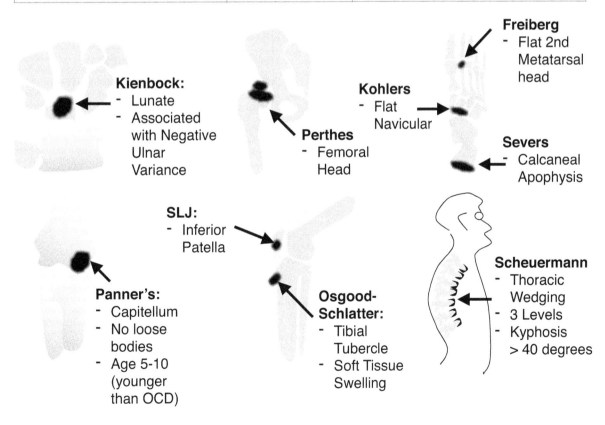

Kienbock:
- Lunate
- Associated with Negative Ulnar Variance

Perthes
- Femoral Head

Kohlers
- Flat Navicular

Freiberg
- Flat 2nd Metatarsal head

Severs
- Calcaneal Apophysis

SLJ:
- Inferior Patella

Panner's:
- Capitellum
- No loose bodies
- Age 5-10 (younger than OCD)

Osgood-Schlatter:
- Tibial Tubercle
- Soft Tissue Swelling

Scheuermann
- Thoracic Wedging
- 3 Levels
- Kyphosis > 40 degrees

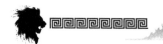 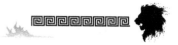
With regard to osteomyelitis, radiographs will be normal for 7-10 days. Essentially, osteomyelitis can have any appearance, occur in any location, and occur at any age. Children have hematogenous spread usually hitting the long bones (metaphysis). Adults are more likely to have direct spread (in diabetic).

However, you can have hematogenous spread in certain situations as well (IV Drugs).

I Say **This**, You Say **THAT**
Osteomyelitis in Spine = IV Drug User
Osteomyelitis in Spine with Kyphosis (Gibbus Deformity) = TB
Unilateral SI joint = IV Drug User
Psoas Muscle Abscess = TB

General Rule: Septic joints more common in adults. Osteomyelitis more common in kids.

Classic Look: Hallmarks are destruction of bone and periosteal new bone formation.

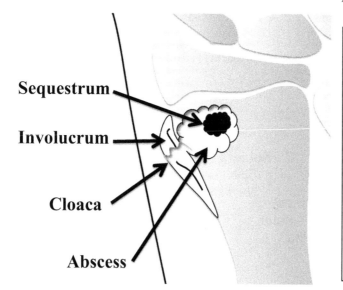

Vocab:

Sequestrum = Piece of necrotic bone surround by granulation tissue

Involucrum = Thick sheath of periosteal bone around sequestrum

Cloaca = Defect in the periosteum (bone skin) caused by infection

Sinus Tract: A channel from the bone to the skin (lined with granulation tissue).

Chronic Osteomyelitis: This is defined as osteomyelitis lasting longer than 6 weeks. Some trivia worth knowing:
- Draining sinus tracts are a risk factor for squamous cell CA
- Most specific sign of active chronic osteomyelitis is the presence of a sequestrum (best shown with computed tomography)
- MRI diagnosis of healed osteomyelitis is based on the return of normal fatty marrow

Acute Bacterial Osteomyelitis can be thought of in three different categories: 1) hematogenous seeding (*most common in child*), 2) contiguous spread, and 3) direct inoculation of the bone either from surgery or trauma.

Acute hematogenous osteomyelitis has a predilection for the long bones of the body, specifically the metaphysis, which has the best blood flow and allows for spreading of the infection via small channels in the bone that lead to the subperiosteal space.

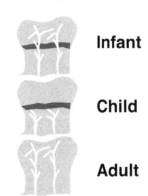

- Age < 1 month = Multi-centric involvement, **often with joint involvement.** Bone scan often negative (75%) at this age

- Age < 18 months = Spread to epiphysis through blood

- Age 2-16 years = Trans-physeal vessels are closed (primary focus is metaphysis).

In the slightly older baby (<18 months) these vessels from the metaphysis to the epiphysis atrophy and the growth plate stops the spread (although spread can still occur). This creates a "septic tank" effect. This same thing happens with certain cancers (leukemia); the garbage gets stuck in the septic tank (metaphysis). Once the growth plates fuse, this obstruction is no longer present.

MRI findings of osteomyelitis: Low signal in the bone marrow on T1 imaging adjacent to an ulcer or cellulitis is diagnostic.

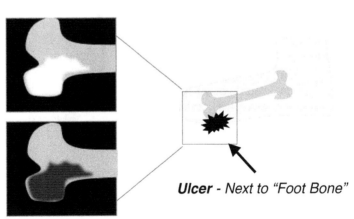

STIR - High Signal in Bone Adjacent to Ulcer *(more sensitive sign)*

T1 - Corresponding Low Signal *(more specific sign)*

Ulcer *- Next to "Foot Bone"*

The Ghost Sign: *Neuropathic Bone vs Osteomyelitis in a Neuropathic Bone*
A bone that becomes a ghost (poor definition of margins) on T1 imaging, but then re-appears (more morphologically distinct) on T2, or after giving IV contrast, is more likely to have osteomyelitis.

Discitis / Osteomyelitis:

Mechanism (Adult)

Infection of the disc and infection of the vertebral body nearly always go together.

The reason has to do with the route of seeding; which typically involves

(1) Seeding of the vertebral endplate (which is vascular)

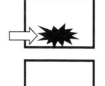

(2) Eruption and crossing into the disc space

(3) Eventual involvement of the adjacent vertebral body

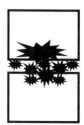

Typical Look & Trivia

Early:
- Plain Film: Hard to see
- MRI: Paraspinal and Epidural inflammation, T2 bright disc signal, and disc enhancement.

Later Plain Film:
- Adjacent irregular endplate destruction.
- Disc Space Narrowing

Later MR:
- T1 - Dark Marrow
- T2 - Bright Marrow
- Post Contrast Enhancement

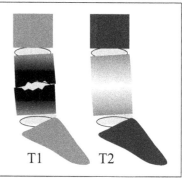

T1   T2

Trivia:
- Adults: the source is usually from a recent surgery, procedure, or systemic infection.
- Children (younger than 5) it's usually from hematogenous spread.
- Step 1 trivia: Staph A is the most common bug, and always think about an IV drug user.
- Almost always (80% of the time) the ESR and CRP are elevated.
- Gallium is superior to WBC scan in the spine.

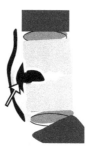

Paraspinal Abscess

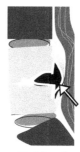

Epidural Abscess

Epidural Abscess

This is an infected collection between the dura and periosteum.

Classic Appearance:
- T1 Dark, T2 Bright,
- Peripheral Enhancement, &
- Restricted Diffusion.

Classic Scenario:
- HIV patient
- Bad Diabetic.

Pediatric Discitis / Osteomyelitis

Children have direct blood supply to the intervertebral disc, so they can get isolated discitis. Isolated Discitis is basically never seen in adults. The classic scenario is: kid (younger than 4) with a upper respiratory infection, now with back pain — usually lumbar.

TB

This is a special topic (high yield) with regard to MSK infection. It's not that common, with < 5% of patients with TB having MSK involvement. Although on multiple choice tests, I think you'll find it appears with a high frequency.

Pott Disease
(tuberculosis of the spine)

The vertebral body is involved with sparing of the disc space until late in the disease (very different than more common bacterial infections).

*It tends to **spare the disc space***
It tends to have multi-level thoracic "skip" involvement
Buzzword "Large paraspinal abscess
Buzzword "Calcified Psoas Abscess"
Buzzword "Gibbus Deformity" – which is a destructive focal kyphosis

Mimic - Brucellosis (unpasteurized milk from an Amish Person) , can also have disc space preservation.

"Gibbus Deformity"

This is a focal kyphosis seen in "Pott Disease" , among many other thing

---

"Tuberculosis Dactylitis" (Spina Ventosa)

Typically seen in kids with involvement of the short tubular bones of the hands and feet.

It is often a smoldering infection without periosteal reaction.

Classic look is a **diaphyseal expansile lesion** with soft tissue swelling.

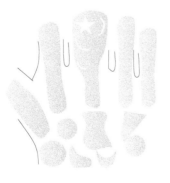

"Rice Bodies"

These are sloughed, infarcted synovium seen with end stage RA, and TB infection of joints.

Septic Arthritis

You see this the most in large joints which have an abundant blood supply to the metaphysis (shoulder, hip, knee).

IV drug users will get it in the SI joint, and sternoclavicular joint.

Conventional risk factors include being old, having AIDS, RA, and prosthetic joints.

On plain film you might see a joint effusion, or MRI will show synovial enhancement. If untreated this will jack your joint in less than 48 hours.

Pneumoarthrogram Sign
If you can demonstrate air within a joint - you can exclude a joint effusion.
No joint effusion
=
No septic joint

Necrotizing Fasciitis:

This is a very bad actor that kills very quickly. The good news is that it's pretty rare, typically only seen in HIVers, Transplant patients, diabetics, and alcoholics. It's usually polymicrobial (the second form is Group A Strep).

Gas is only seen in a minority of cases, but if you see gas in soft tissue this is what they want. Diffuse fascial enhancement is what you'd see if the ER is dumb enough to order cross sectional imaging (they often are).

Fournier Gangrene is what they call it in the scrotum ("testes satchel").

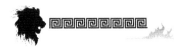 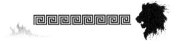
There are tons of primary osseous malignancies, the most common are myeloma/plasmacytoma (27%), Osteosarcoma (20%) and Chondrosarcoma (20%). I'll discuss myeloma/plasmacytoma later in the chapter when I get to lucent lesions. This discussion will focus more on the bone forming aggressive tumors.
I guess before I do that though, I should review what "aggressive" means. In the real world, dealing with bone lesions is simple - it's either aggressive, not aggressive, or not sure. Even though multiple choice is very different than actual clinical radiology, that first mental calculus of - *aggressive vs not aggressive* - may still be useful in eliminating distractors.

What makes a lesion *"aggressive"* ?

According to Helms, the **wide zone of transition is the best sign that a lesion is aggressive.** This is actually a useful pearl. The simplest way to conceptualize this is to ask yourself if you can trace the edges of the lesion with a pencil. If you can the lesion is probably benign. If the edges are blurry or there is a gradient to the edge - this is a more likely an aggressive lesions.

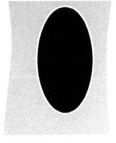 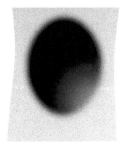

Narrow Zone -
Benign

Wide Zone -
Aggressive

The reason is that margins reflect the growth the lesion. Bones are dumb. They really only know how to do two things - make bone and destroy bone. The margins are the reflection of bone formation. If the margins are sharp and sclerotic, this means the bone has time to adjust to the irritation and lay down a coat of mature bone. If the margins are not distinct (zone of transition is wide) this indicates a faster growing lesion and therefore a higher probability of malignancy (or infection).

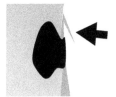

If the tumor grows rapidly enough it can break through the cortex and destroy the newly formed bone capsule / lamellated bone. When this happens you end up with a triangular structure - called the **Codman triangle** (as shown in diagram).

When we think about bone lesions, we often imagine lytic holes or bone destruction. Bone destruction occurs from complex methods best understood as either direct obliteration via the tumor or pissed off osteoclasts enraged by the uninvited tumor / hyperemia. Trabecular bone loss occurs more rapidly (relative to cortical bone), but is noticed later because cortical bone is more smooth and organized. Supposedly you need to destroy 70% of the trabecular bone before it is noticed radiographically.

Bone destruction that occurs in a uniform geographic pattern (especially with a sharp well defined border) is more suggestive of a benign slow growing lesion. A moth-eaten (cluster of small lytic holes) or permeative (ill-defined tiny oval or streak like lucencies) suggests rapid infiltrative tumor growth — as seen in myeloma, lymphoma, and Ewings sarcoma. It is worth noting that osteomyelitis and hyperparathyroidism can also demonstrate these aggressive patterns - pre-test probably is always important.

Geographic　**Moth Eaten**　**Permeative**

Osteosarcoma:

There are a bunch of subtypes, but for the purpose of this discussion there are 4. Conventional Intramedullary (85%), Parosteal (4%), Periosteal (1%), Telangiectatic (rare). All the subtypes produce bone or osteoid from neoplastic cells. Most are idiopathic but you can have secondary causes (*usually seen in elderly*) XRT, Pagets, Infarcts, etc...

Conventional Intramedullary: More common, and higher grade than the surface subtypes (periosteal, and parosteal). Primary subtypes typically occur in young patients (10-20). The most common location is the femur (40%), and proximal tibia (15%).

 Buzzwords include various types of aggressive periosteal reactions:

- *"Sunburst"*- periosteal reaction that is aggressive and looks like a sunburst
- *Codman triangle* - With aggressive lesions, the periosteum does not have time to ossify completely with new bone (e.g. as seen in single layer and multi-layered periosteal reaction), so only the edge of the raised periosteum will ossify – creating the appearance of a triangle.
- *Lamellated* (onion skin reaction) – multi layers of parallel periosteum, looks like an onion's skin.

 Trivia:

- Osteosarcoma met to the lung is a "classic" cause of occult pneumothorax.

"Reverse Zoning Phenomenon" – more dense mature matrix in the center, less peripherally (*opposite of myositis ossificans*).

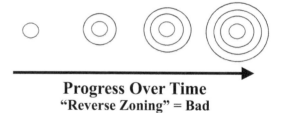

Progress Over Time
"Reverse Zoning" = Bad

Parosteal Osteosarcoma: Generally low grade, **BULKY** parosteal bone formation. Think Big… just say Big. This guy loves the posterior distal femur (*because of this location it can mimic a cortical desmoid "tug lesion" early on*). The lesion is metaphyseal 90% of the time. The buzzword is "***string sign***" – which refers to a radiolucent line separating the bulky tumor from the cortex.

Periosteal Osteosarcoma:

Worse prognosis than parosteal but better than conventional osteosarcoma. Tends to occur in the diaphyseal regions, classic medial distal femur.

THIS vs THAT	
Parosteal	**Periosteal**
Early Adult / Middle Age	Age Group (15-25)
Metaphyseal (90%)	Diaphyseal
Likes Posterior Distal Femur	Likes Medial Distal Femur
Marrow extension (50%)	Usually no marrow extension
Low Grade	Intermediate Grade

Telangiectatic Osteosarcoma:

About 15% have a narrow zone of transition. Fluid-Fluid levels on MRI is classic. They are High on T1 (from methemoglobin). Can be differentiated from ABC or GCT (maybe) by tumor nodularity and enhancement.

FLUID-FLUID LEVELS DDx:

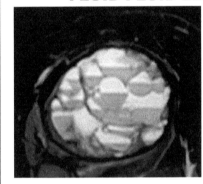

Telangiectatic
Osteosarcoma
Aneurysmal Bone Cyst
Giant Cell Tumor

Parosteal	Periosteal	Telangiectatic	Classic (Intramedullary)	Secondary OS
4%	1%	*Rare As Fuck*	85%	*Started off as Pagets*

More Evil than Skeletor →

Metaphyseal Posterior Distal Femur

Diaphyseal Medial-Distal Femur

Cystic on Plain Film
Fluid Levels on MR

Femur - 40%
Tibia - 15%

Other Bad Actors

Chondrosarcoma:

Usually seen in older adults (M>F). Likes flat bones, limb girdles, proximal tubular bones. Can be central (intramedullary) or peripheral (at the end of an osteochondroma). Most are low grade.

Risk Factors: Pagets, and anything cartilaginous (osteochondromas, Maffucci etc…)

Gamesmanship: If you want to say chondroblastoma but it's an <u>adult</u> think <u>clear cell chondrosarcoma</u>

Gamesmanship:

If shown with CT - they have to show you some "chondroid matrix" - "arcs and rings"

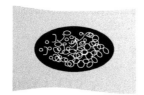

THIS *vs* THAT
Enchondroma vs Low Grade Chondrosarcoma
Factors Favoring Chondrosarcoma:
<u>Pain</u> Cortical Destruction Scalloping of > 2/3 of the cortex >5cm in Size "Changing Matrix"

Ewings:

 Permeative lesion in the <u>diaphysis</u> of a child = Ewings
(could also be infection, or EG).

Extremely rare in African-Americans. Likes to met bone to bone *(skip lesions are more common in Ewings, relative to Osteosarcoma).* Does NOT form osteoid from tumor cells, but can mimic osteosarcoma because of its marked sclerosis *(sclerosis occurs in the bone only, not in the soft tissue – which is NOT the case in osteosarcoma).*

Chordoma:

Usually seen in adults (30-60), usually slightly younger in the clivus and slightly older in the sacrum. Most likely questions regarding the chordoma include location (**most common sacrum**, second most common clivus, third most common vertebral body), and the fact that they are **very T2 bright**.

Chordoma Most Commons:
* Most common primary malignancy of the spine.
* Most common primary malignancy of the sacrum.
* When involving the spine, most common at C2.

I Say Chordoma, *You Say "Midline, Midline, Midline!"*
Why is it always midline? It's made of cells left over from the "notochord" (some embryology bullshit that was involved in making MIDLINE structures).
Chordomas are NEVER EVER seen off the midline (NEVER in the hip, leg, arm, hand, etc…).

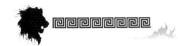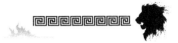
FEGNOMASHIC is a "useful" mnemonic for lucent bone lesions made popular by Clyde Helms. As it turns out, you can rearrange the letters of FEGNOMASHIC to form a word FOGMACHINES. I find it a lot easier to remember a mnemonic if it actually forms a real word. Having said that, the whole idea of memorizing a list of 11 or 12 barely related things is stupid. You would never give a differential that included all of those, as they occur in different places, in different ages, and often look very different.

Differentials (for people who know what they are looking at) are usually never deeper than 3 or 4 things. If you are giving a differential of 12 things, just say you don't know what it is. Seriously in the real world bone lesions only come in 3 flavors: 1 - Bad (cancer or infection), 2 - Obviously benign (not sure I'll waste saliva mentioning it in my report) , 3 - Ehh hard to tell - get a follow up. This is actually pretty much true of lesions everywhere in the body. Realizing this allows for the following paradigm shift:

Eyeball: Oh Shit! A lesion that has non-aggressive features. I wonder what it is…. Neuron 1: We better look it up and give it a name. Neuron 2: Maybe we should give a list of possible names. Then people will read our report and think we are smart. Bystander Neurons: Initiate Waffle Protocol	Eyeball: Oh Shit! A lesion that has non-aggressive features. I wonder what it is…. Lion Neuron 1: Who gives a shit? It's benign… next case. Lion Neuron 2: This is an ortho study. Literally no one will ever read this report. Bystander Neurons: Bro… can we finish this fucking list already? We need to look at that new Tesla Roadster, 0-60 is sub 2 seconds.

But… we aren't training for real life. The realm of multiple choice is obviously different.

For multiple choice, when you encounter a lucent bone lesion you can expect one of two questions (1) *what is it ?* or (2) *what is it associated with ?* In either case you are going to need to figure out what it is. In the real world you would probably have to give a short differential, but in the world of multiple choice you will have to come up with one answer. Don't fret, they have to give you clues so you can pick just one. A useful mental exercise when eliminating multiple choice distractors is to ask yourself "why is it NOT this?" It's an exercise that is often not performed at the workstation - but very valuable in the test environment - especially for these types of questions.

Here is my suggested method:

(1) Age of the patient? - If you are lucky they will tell you. If you are less lucky you will have to guess. Growth plates open = kid. Growth plates closed with no degenerative change = young adult. Growth plates closed with degenerative changes = older than 40.

Age - Key Facts
• < 30 = EG, ABC, NOF, Chondroblastoma, and Solitary Bone Cysts   • Any Age = Infection   • > 40 = Mets and Myeloma (unless it's neuroblastoma mets).

(2) Location of the lesion ? Metaphysis, Epiphysis, Diaphysis? Is this an epiphyseal equivalent discussion (see the next page for discussion).

(3) Classic Locations and Looks ? See my summary at the end of this section

Location:

Epiphysis:

In general, only a few lesions tend to arise in the epiphysis. The "four horseman of the (e)apophysis" is the mnemonic I like to use, and I think about the company AIG that was involved in some scandal a few years ago. **AIG** "the evil" **C**ompany.

ABC, **I**nfection, **G**iant Cell, and **C**hondroblastoma.
The caveat is that ABC is usually metaphyseal but after the growth plate closes it can extend into the epiphysis.

For the purpose of multiple choice tests, it is important to not forget about the malignant tumor at the end of the bone (epiphysis) – Clear Cell Chondrosarcoma. This guy is slow growing, with a variable appearance (lytic, calcified, lobulated, ill defined, etc...). Just remember **if they say malignant epiphyseal you say Clear Cell Chondrosarcoma.**

Epiphyseal Equivalents:
(bones that will have the same lesions as the epiphysis)
Carpals, Patella, Greater Trochanter, Calcaneus

Metaphysis

The metaphysis is the fastest growing area of a bone, with the best blood supply. This excellent blood supply results in an increased predilection for Mets and Infection. Most of the cystic bone lesions can occur in the metaphysis.

Diaphysis

Just like the metaphysis, most entities can occur in the diaphysis (they just do it less).

Pathology - For Trivia

Fibrous Dysplasia:

Fibrous dysplasia is a skeletal developmental anomaly of osteoblasts – failure of normal maturation and differentiation which results in replacement of the normal medullary space.

Famously "can look like anything", with phases like Pagets (lytic, mixed, blastic) - although the most classic appearance is a *"long lesion, in a long bone, with ground glass matrix."* Sometimes the vocabulary "lytic lesion with a hazy matrix" is used instead of the word "ground glass" - for the purpose of fucking with you. The discriminator used by Helms is "**no periosteal reaction or pain.**"

Shepherd Crook
-Coxa Varus Angulation
-Classic for FD (but can be seen in Paget and OI)

Likes the ribs and long bones. If it occurs in the pelvis, it also hits the ipsilateral femur (**Shepherd Crook deformity**). If it's multiple it likes the skull and face (Lion-like faces).

The disorder can occur at any age - but the multiple lesion variety "polyostotic" - tends to occur earlier.

You could think monostotic (20's & 30's) or polyostotic (< 10 year old). When you see the polyostotic form (often with a mangled horrible horrible face… a face that only a mother could love) - you should think syndromes.

THIS vs THAT	
McCune Albright	**Mazabraud**
Polyostotic Fibrous Dysplasia	Polyostotic Fibrous Dysplasia
Girl	Woman (*middle aged*)
Café au lait spots	Soft Tissue Myxomas
Precocious Puberty	Increased Risk Osseous Malignant Transformation

Adamantinoma:
A total zebra (*probably a unicorn*). A tibial lesion that **resembles fibrous dysplasia** (mixed lytic and sclerotic). It is potentially malignant.

Nonossifying Fibroma (NOF):

These are very common. They are seen in children, and will spontaneously regress (becoming more sclerotic before disappearing). They are *rare in children not yet walking.* Just like GCTs they like to occur around the knee. They are classically described as eccentric with a thin sclerotic border (remember GCTs don't have a sclerotic border). They are called fibrous cortical defects when smaller than 2 cm.

Vocab: NOFs are the larger version (> 3cm) of a fibrous cortical defect (FCD). A wastebasket term for the both of them is simply "fibroxanthoma."

Jaffe-Campanacci Syndrome: Syndrome of multiple NOFs, café-au-lait spots, mental retardation, hypogonadism, and cardiac malformations.

Enchondroma:

This guy is a tumor of the medullary cavity composed of hyaline cartilage. They become progressively more common with age - peaking around 10-30 years old.

The sneaky thing about this lesion is that it looks different depending on the body part it is in.

- Humerus or Femur = Arcs and Rings
- Fingers or Toes = Lytic

The **ARCS AND RINGS** is the more classic textbook look with the irregularly speckled calcification of chondroid matrix. Just don't forget that this classic matrix is **not found in the fingers or toes.**

The enchondroma is actually the most common cystic lesion in the hands and feet. Just like fibrous dysplasia, this lesion does not have periostitis.

 Differentiating Enchondroma vs Low Grade Chondrosarcoma
Strategies to Deal with the Chondroid Matrix Lesion in a Long Bone

Primary Tactic: History of pain — Enchondroma vs a Low Grade Chondrosarcoma
Not Painful   *PAINful*

Secondary Tactic: Size — Enchondroma vs a Low Grade Chondrosarcoma
1-2 cm   *> 4-5 cm*

Tertiary Tactic: Glitch in the Matrix — Enchondroma vs a Low Grade Chondrosarcoma
Arcs & Rings   *Arcs & Rings Pattern*
Pattern does   *Changes - moves*
NOT Change   *around grows etc...*

When multiple — especially when in the hands you should think syndromes:

THIS vs **THAT**	
Ollier Disease	**Maffucci Syndrome** *"Marffucci Has More"* *More Cancer Risk and More Vascular Malformations*
Multiple Enchondromas (3 or more)	Multiple Enchondromas
	Hemangiomas (bunch lucent centered calcifications)
Slight increase risk in Chondrosarcoma	Increase risk in Chondrosarcoma *(probably more than Ollier)*

Eosinophilic Granuloma (EG):

This is typically included in every differential for people less than 30 (peak age is 5-10).
It can be solitary (usually) or multiple.

There are 3 classic appearances - for the purpose of multiple choice:
(1) Vertebra plana in a kid
(2) Skull with lucent "beveled edge" lesions (also in a kid).
(3) "Floating Tooth" with lytic lesion in alveolar ridge --- this would be a differential case

The appearance is highly variable and can be lytic or blastic, with or without a sclerotic border, and with or without a periosteal response. Can even have an osseous sequestrum.

Classic DDx for Vertebra Plana (MELT)	Classic DDx for Osseous Sequestrum:
• Mets / Myeloma • EG • Lymphoma • Trauma / TB	• Osteomyelitis • Lymphoma • Fibrosarcoma • EG *Osteoid Osteoma can mimic a sequestrum*

Giant Cell Tumor (GCT):

This guy has some key criteria (which lend themselves well to multiple choice tests).
They include:

- Physis MUST be closed
- Non Sclerotic Border
- Abuts the articular surface

Another trick is to show you a pulmonary met, and ask if it could be a GCT? The answer is yes (although this is rare) GCT is considered "quasi-malignant" because it can be locally invasive and about 5% will have pulmonary mets (which are still curable by resection). As a result of this, it should be resected with wide margins.

Things to know about GCTs:

- Most common in the knee - abutting the articular surface
- Most common at age 20-30 * physis must be closed
- There is an association with ABCs (they can turn into them)
- They are "quasi-malignant" - 5% have lung mets
- Fluid levels on MRI

Osteoid Osteoma *"Pain at night, relieved by aspirin."*

- *Most Classic Age:* "Adolescent" —- 10-25 ish.

- *Most Classic Look:* Oval lytic lesion ("lucent nidus") surrounded by dense sclerotic cortical bone ("periosteal reaction").

- *Most Classic Locations:* (1) Meta/diaphysis of long bones (femoral neck = most common) and (2) Posterior elements of the spine (lumbar > cervical > thoracic). Technically the fingers are more common than the spine, but that's rarely show on multiple choice.

Associations of Osteoid Osteoma
Painful Scoliosis
Growth Deformity: Increased length and girth of long bones
Synovitis: Can be seen if intra-articular, joint effusions
Arthritis: Can occur from primary synovitis, or secondarily from altered joint mechanics.

Modality Trivia:

- MRI: "Lots of edema." I'll say that again ***"large amount of edema for the size of the lesion."*** Adjacent soft tissue edema is also common - don't let that fool you.

- Nuke Bone Scan: "Double Density Sign" - very intense central activity at nidus, surrounded by less intensity of reactive bone. A common distractor is a stress fracture. Stress fractures are linear. O.O. should be round.

Scoliosis Trivia: When you have them in the spine (most common in the posterior elements of the lumbar spine), you frequently have an associated **painful scoliosis** with the **convexity pointed away from the lesion.**

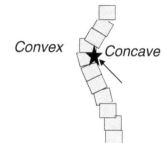
Convex   *Concave*

Treatment:

These can be treated with percutaneous radiofrequency ablation (as long as it's not within 1 cm of a nerve or other vital structure – *typically avoided in hands, spine, and pregnant patients*).

Osteoblastoma:

Basically it's an osteoid osteoma that is larger than 2 cm. It's seen in patients < 30 years old. They are most likely to show this in the posterior elements. It also occurs in the long bones (35%) and when it does it is usually diaphyseal (75%).

Aneurysmal Bone Cyst (ABC):

Classic DDx for Lucent Lesion in Posterior Elements:

Osteoblastoma
ABC
TB

Aneurysmal bone cysts are aneurysmal lesions of bone with thin-walled, blood-filled spaces (fluid-fluid level on MRI). Patients are usually < 30. They may develop following trauma.

Location: Tibia > Vert > Femur > Humerus

They can be described as primary ABC, presumably arising denovo or secondary ABC, associated with another tumor (classic GCT). They are commonly associated with other benign lesions.

Things to know about ABC:
- Up to 40% of secondary ABC's are associated with giant cell tumor of bone.
- It's on the DDx for Fluid - Fluid Level on MRI
- Patient < 30
- Tibia is the most common site

Solitary (Unicameral) Bone Cyst:

It would be unusual to see one of these in a patient older than 30. Most common in the tubular bones (90-95 %) usually humerus or femur. Unique feature: "Always located centrally."

It's going to be shown one of two ways: (1) With a fracture through it in the humerus (probably with a fallen fragment sign) or (2) As a lucent lesion in the calcaneus (probably with a fallen fragment sign).

The *fallen fragment sign* (bone fragment in the dependent portion of a lucent bone lesion) is pathognomonic of solitary bone cyst.

Brown Tumor (Hyperparathyroidism):

The "brown tumor" represents localized accumulations of giant cells and fibrous tissue (in case someone asks). They appear as lytic or sclerotic lesions with other findings of hyperparathyroidism (subperiosteal bone resorption). In other words, they need to tell you he/she has hyperparathyroidism first. They may just straight up tell you, or they will show you some bone resorption first (classically on the side of a finger, edge of a clavicle, or under a rib).

These things have different stages of healing / sclerosis. They resorb and can become totally sclerotic / healed, when the Hyper PTH is treated.

More on this in the arthritis section — later in the chapter

Chondroblastoma:

This is seen in kids (90% age 5-25). They classically show it in two ways
(1) in the epiphysis of the tibia on a 15 year old, or (2) in an epiphyseal equivalent.

So what are the epiphyseal equivalents???
- *Patella*
- *Calcaneus*
- *Carpal Bones*
- *And all the Apophyses (greater and less trochanter, tuberosities, etc...)*

Features of the tumor include; A thin sclerotic rim, extension across the physeal plate (25-50%), periostitis (30%). Actual location: femur > humerus > tibia . This may show bone marrow edema, and soft tissue edema on MRI (MRI can mislead you into thinking it's a bad thing). This is one of the only bone lesions that is often **NOT T2 bright**. They tend to reoccur after resection (like 30% of the time).

 Gamesmanship Hip: When you have a chondroblastoma in the hip, it tends to *favor the greater trochanter (more than the femoral epiphysis).*

Chondromyxoid Fibroma:

This is the least common benign lesion of cartilage. It is usually in patients younger than 30. The typical appearance is an osteolytic, elongated in shape, eccentrically located, metaphyseal lesion, with cortical expansion and a "bite" like configuration. Sorta looks like an NOF - with the classic location in the proximal metaphyseal region of the tibia.

The Hip

Greater Trochanter - Remember this is an *epiphyseal equivalent* and the chrondroblastomas prefer it to the femoral epiphysis. You can get all the other DDxs (ABC, Infection, GCT, etc... here as well). Plus, you can have avulsions of the gluteus medius and minimus.

Lesser Trochanter - An avulsion here without significant clinical history should make you think pathologic fracture.

The Intertrochanteric Region: Classic DDx here: Lipoma, Solitary Bone Cyst, and Monostotic Fibrous Dysplasia.

Classic (& sneaky non-classic) Lesions that can be shown in the calcaneus.

The suggested Promethean method is to first use location within the bone, and then use characteristic appearance as a secondary discriminator.

First let us take a closer look at the calcaneus. Remember this thing is an epiphyseal equivalent, but only in certain locations. It's probably better to think about the bone like a hybrid long bone - complete with a diaphysis, two metaphysis, and three epiphysis.

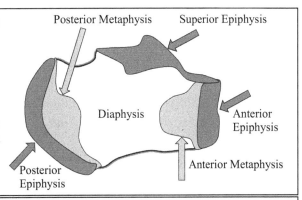

Chondroblastoma:

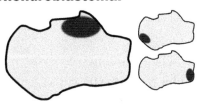

- Most classic epiphysis lesion - with a preference for the superior epiphysis near the talocalcaneal articulation (although they can be at any of the 3 epiphysis).
- Lucent lesion, that can have some internal calcifications.

Giant Cell Tumor: Can also involve the epiphysis (although it typically starts out metaphyseal and grows into the epiphysis). Remember these things required a closed physis. The Posterior Metaphysis / Epiphysis is favored.

Osteoid Osteoma:

- Talus > Calcaneus
- Similar to Chondroblastoma in favoring the superior epiphysis near the talocalcaneal articulation.
- Distinction is the sclerotic thickening of the adjacent bone and the radiolucent nidus.

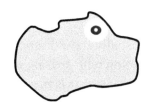

Geode: Older Patient + Subtalar degenerative change / Obvious Arthritis

Osteomyelitis & Mets:

The calcaneal apophysis (equivalent to the metaphyseal region of long bones) will have a similar predilection for collection hematogenous spread of both infection or cancer (GU or Colon).

In both cases the involvement favors the posterior meta-epiphyseal region (which has the richest blood supply), with lesions potentially growing large enough to involve the entire calcaneus.

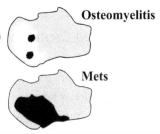

Osteomyelitis

Mets

Solitary Bone Cyst: The typical location for this lesion is the diaphysis (anterior 1/3 laterally). This will have sharp edges. A thick sclerotic edge with a multiloculated appearance is helpful. The "fallen fragment" will be more in the bottom if shown – although fractures in the calcaneus are much less common than in the arm.

Intraosseous Lipoma: This is also typically located in the diaphysis (anterior 1/3 laterally). If they show you this, it will either have (a) fat density on CT or MRI, or (b) a **central fragment** – stuck within the middle of the fat. This calcification / fat necrosis occurs about 50% of the time in the real world (nearly 100% on pictures shown on tests), and is secondary to fat necrosis.

Pseudo-cyst: This is a variation on the normal trabecular pattern, which creates a central triangular radiolucent area. This area is sometimes called the "pseudo-cyst triangle" and is obnoxiously located in the same anterior 1/3 as the SBC and Lipoma. Supposedly the persistence of thin trabeculae, visible nutrient foramen, and the classic location are helpful in telling it from the other benign entities.

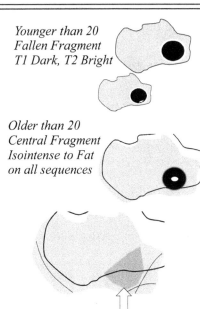

Younger than 20
Fallen Fragment
T1 Dark, T2 Bright

Older than 20
Central Fragment
Isointense to Fat
on all sequences

Metastatic Disease: Should be on the differential for any patient over 40 with a lytic lesion. As a piece of trivia renal cancer is ALWAYS lytic (usually).

- *Classic Blastic Lesions:* Prostate, Carcinoid, Medulloblastoma
- *Classic Lytic Lesions:* Renal and Thyroid

Next Step - Prostate Met vs Bone Island??? - <u>Get a Bone Scan</u>
- Bone Island should be mild (or not active)
- Prostate Met should be HOT

Multiple Myeloma (MM): Plasma cell proliferation increases surrounding osteolytic activity (in case someone asks you the mechanism). Usually in older patient (40's-80's). Plasmacytomas can precede clinical or hematologic evidence of myeloma by 3 years.

They usually have discrete margins, and can be solitary or multiple. Vertebral body destruction with sparing of the posterior elements is classic. Bone Scan is often negative, *skeletal survey is better* (but horribly painful to read), and MRI is the most sensitive.

Additional classic (testable) scenario: *MM manifesting as Diffuse Osteopenia*

Myeloma Related Conditions:

Plasmacytoma *(usually under 40):* This is a discrete, solitary mass of neoplastic monoclonal plasma cells in either bone or soft tissue (*extramedullary subtype*). It is associated with latent systemic disease in the majority of affected patients. It can be considered as a singular counterpart multiple myeloma. The lesions look like a geographic lytic area, sometimes with **expansile** remodeling.

"Mini Brain Appearance" – Plasmacytoma in vertebral body

POEMS: This is basically "<u>*Myeloma with Sclerotic Mets*</u>." It's a rare medical syndrome with plasma cell proliferation (typically myeloma) , neuropathy, and organomegaly.

Lucent Lesion Classic Looks and Locations

Long Lesion in a Long Bone	Fibrous Dysplasia
Ground Glass	Fibrous Dysplasia
Lytic lesion with a hazy matrix	Fibrous Dysplasia
Chondroid Matrix in the Proximal Humerus or Distal Femur	Enchondroma
Lucent Lesion in the Finger or Toe	Enchondroma
Epiphyseal Tibial Lesion in a Teenager	Chondroblastoma
Epiphyseal Equivalent Lesion	Chondroblastoma or Giant Cell Tumor **technically GCTs grow into the Epiphysis*
Lucent Lesion in the Greater Trochanter	Chondroblastoma
Lucent Lesion with a Fracture (Fallen Fragment) in the Humerus	Solitary Bone Cyst
Calcaneal Lesion with Central Calcification	Lipoma
Lucent Lesion in the Skull	EG
Vertebra Plana in a Kid	EG
Vertebra Plana in an Adult	Mets
Sequestrum / Nidus in the Tibia / Femur	Osteoid Osteoma
"Painful Scoliosis"	Osteoid Osteoma
Calcified Lesion in the Posterior Element of the C-Spine	Osteoblastoma

Solitary vs Multiple (Generalization for Multiple Choice Trivia)

Multiple Sclerotic Lesions	Mets
Multiple Sclerotic Lesions Centered Around a Joint	Osteopoikolosis
Multiple Lucent Lesions (older than 40)	Mets, Myeloma, Metastatic Non-Hodgkin Lymphoma

Size Matters

Nidus < 2.0 cm	Osteoid Osteoma
Nidus > 2.0 cm	Osteoblastoma
Well-defined lytic lesion in the cortex of a long bone with a sclerotic rim < 3 cm	Fibrous cortical defect
Well-defined lytic lesion in the cortex of a long bone with a sclerotic rim > 3 cm	Nonossifying fibroma
Chondral lesion in a long bone 1-2 cm	Probably an Enchondroma
Chondral lesion in a long bone > 4-5 cm	Increased risk of low-grade chondrosarcoma

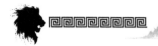
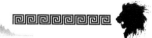

Liposclerosing Myxofibroma:

Very characteristic location – at the intertrochanteric region of the femur. Looks like a geographic lytic lesion with a sclerotic margin. Despite non-aggressive appearance, 10% undergo malignant degeneration so they need to be followed.

Osteochondroma:

Some people think of this as more of a developmental anomaly (although they still always make the tumor chapter). Actually, it's usually listed as the most common benign tumor ("exostosis"). They can be radiation induced, making them the *only benign skeletal tumor associated with radiation.*

They have a very small risk of malignant transformation (which supposedly can be estimated based on size of cartilage cap).
Supposedly a cap > 1.5 cm is concerning.

Key Points:
- They point away from the joint
- The bone marrow flows freely into the lesion

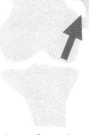

Away from Joint

Multiple Hereditary Exostosis:

AD condition with multiple osteochondromas.
They have an **increased risk of malignant transformation**.

Trevor Disease (Dysplasia Epiphysealis Hemimelica - DEH):

This is a disease characterized by the development of osteochondromas develop at the epiphysis which result in significant joint deformity (**most common in ankle** and knee) — making you terrible at tennis and soccer. Instead of pointing away from the joint (like a normal osteochondroma) these assholes point into the joint — this is why you have so many joint issues. You see this is young children. The osteochondroma looks more like an irregular mass. They tend to be treated with surgical excision.

Supracondylar Spur (Avian Spur):

This is an Aunt Minnie, and normal variant. This is an osseous process, that usually does nothing, but can compress the median nerve if the **Ligament of Struthers** smashes it.

Notice this thing points towards the joint, that is how you know it is not an osteochondroma. Also - it is not a Trevor Disease thing - because
(1) of the characteristic location and
(2) it is not originated from the epiphysis.

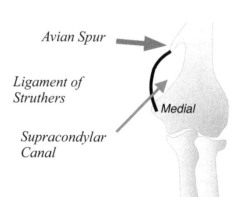

Avian Spur

Ligament of Struthers

Medial

Supracondylar Canal

Periosteal Chondroma (Juxta-Cortical Chondroma): When you see a lesion in the finger of a kid think this. It's a rare entity, of cartilaginous origin. "Saucerization" of the adjacent cortex with sclerotic periosteal reaction can be seen.

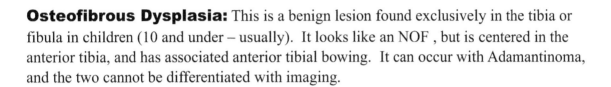

Osteofibrous Dysplasia: This is a benign lesion found exclusively in the tibia or fibula in children (10 and under – usually). It looks like an NOF , but is centered in the anterior tibia, and has associated anterior tibial bowing. It can occur with Adamantinoma, and the two cannot be differentiated with imaging.

When I say looks like NOF in the anterior tibia with anterior bowing, you say Osteofibrous Dysplasia.

Distal Femoral Metaphyseal Irregularity (Cortical Desmoid):

This is a lucency seen along the back of the posteriomedial aspect of the distal femoral metaphysis. If they show you a lateral knee x-ray, and there is an irregularity or lucency on the back of the femur this is it. It's often bilateral.

Buzzwords include "Scoop like defect" with an "irregular but intact cortex."

This is a total incidental finding and is a don't touch lesion. **Don't biopsy it, Don't MRI it.**

Just leave it alone. If you really want to know, it's probably a chronic tug lesion from the adductor magnus.

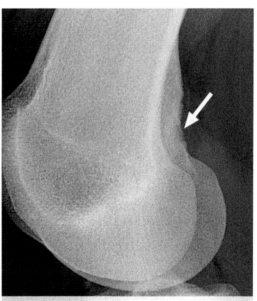

Cortical Desmoid - Scoop Like Defect

Calcium Hydroxyapatite: Most pathologic calcification in the body is calcium hydroxyapatite, which is also the most abundant form of calcium in bone.

Calcium hydroxyapatite deposition disease = ***calcific tendinitis.***

The calcium is deposited in tendons around the joint. The most common location for hydroxyapatite deposition is the shoulder. Specifically, the **supraspinatus tendon is the most frequent site of calcification**, usually at its insertion near the greater tuberosity. *The longus colli muscle (the muscle anterior to atlas -> T3) is also a favorite location for multiple choice test writers.* It may be primary (idiopathic) or secondary. Secondary causes worth knowing are: chronic renal disease, collagen-vascular disease, **tumoral calcinosis** and hypervitaminosis D.

Osteopoikilosis: It's just a bunch of bone islands. Usually in epiphyses (different from blastic mets or osteosarcoma mets). It can be inherited or sporadic but if you are forced to pick a pattern - I'd go with *autosomal dominant.*

Mets vs Osteopoikilosis - Osteopoikilosis tends to be joint centered (clustered around centered). Sclerotic mets will be all over the place. Sclerotic mets believe in nothing Lebowski.

Trivia - Osteopoikilosis patients tend to be keloid formers.

Osteopathia Striata: Linear, parallel, and longitudinal lines in metaphysis of long bones. Doesn't mean shit (usually - but can in some situations cause pain).

 Engelmann's Disease: This is also known as progressive diaphyseal dysplasia or PDD. What you see is *fusiform bony enlargement* with sclerosis of the long bones. This is a total zebra that begins in childhood.

Things to know:

- *It's Bilateral and Symmetric*
- *It likes the long bones - usually shown in the tibia*
- *It's hot on bone scan*
- *It can involve the skull – and can cause optic nerve compression*

Thalassemia: This is a defect in the hemoglobin chain (can be alpha or beta – major or minor). From the MSK Radiologist prospective, we are talking about "hair-on-end" skulls, expansion of the facial bones, "rodent faces," expanded ribs "jail-bars". It is frequently associated with extramedullary hematopoiesis.

	Thalassemia	Sickle Cell
	Will Obliterate Sinuses	Will Not Obliterate Sinuses
Lytic	Usually Asymptomatic	
Mixed *(reparative)*	Elevated Alkaline Phosphate. Fractures	
Sclerotic *(latent inactive)*	Elevated Hydroxyproline. More fractures. Sarcomas may develop.	

AVN of the Hip:

Variety of causes including Perthes in kids, sickle cell, Gaucher's, steroid use etc…. It can also be traumatic with <u>femoral neck fractures</u> (*degree of risk is related to degree of displacement* / disruption of the retinacular vessels). AVN of the hip typically involves the superior articular surface, beginning more anteriorly.

Double Line Sign:	**Rim Sign:**	**Crescent Sign:**
Best seen on T2; inner bright line (granulation tissue), with outer dark line (sclerotic bone).	Best seen on T2; high T2 signal line sandwiched between two low signal lines. This represents *fluid between sclerotic borders of an osteochondral fragment*, and **implies instability**. (Stage III).	Seen on X-ray (optimally frog leg); Refers to a subchondral lucency seen most frequently in the anterolateral aspect of the proximal femoral head. It indicates imminent collapse.
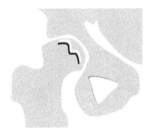	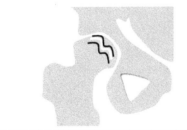	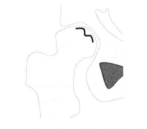

Plain Film Stages of Osteonecrosis
(there are MR stages also - presumed to be beyond the scope of this exam):

o   Zero = Normal

o   One = Normal x-ray, edema on MR

o   Two = Mixed Lytic / Sclerotic

o   Three = Crescent Sign, Articular Collapse, Joint Space Preserved

o   Four = Secondary Osteoarthritis

Paget Disease (Osteitis Deformans):

A relatively common condition that affects 4% of people at 40, and 8% at 80 *(actually 10%, but easier to remember 8%)*. M > F. Most people are asymptomatic. The pathophysiology of Paget is not well understood.

The bones **go through three phases which progress from lytic to mixed to sclerotic** *(the latent inactive phase)*. The phrase **"Wide Bones with Thick Trabecula"** make you immediately say Pagets (nothing else really does that).

Comes in two flavors: (1) Monostotic and (2) Polyostotic – with the poly subtype being much more common (80-90%).

 Buzzwords / Signs:

- *Blade of Grass Sign:* Lucent leading edge in a long bone
- *Osteoporosis Circumscripta:* Blade of Grass in the Skull
- *Picture Frame Vertebra:* Cortex is thickened on all sides (Rugger Jersey is only superior and inferior endplates)
- *Cotton Wool Bone:* Thick disorganized trabeculae
- *Banana Fracture:* Insufficiency fracture of a bowed soft bone (femur or tibia).
- *Tam O'Shanter Sign:* Thick Skull - with the frontal aspect "falling over the facial bones"
- *Saber Shin:* Bowing of the tibia
- *Ivory Vertebra:* This is a differential finding, including mets. Pagets tends to be expansile.

Complications: **Deafness is the most common complication**. Spinal stenosis from cortical thickening is very characteristic. Additional complications include cortical stress fracture, cranial nerves paresis, CHF (high output), secondary hyperparathyroidism (10%), **Secondary development of osteosarcoma (1%) – which is often highly resistant to treatment.** *As a piece of ridiculous trivia - giant cell tumor can arise from Paget.*

Trivia: Of all the tumors to which Paget may devolve to, Osteosarcoma is the Most Common.

Total Trivia: Paget bone is hypervascular and may be 5 degrees hotter than other bone (get your thermometer ready). Alk Phos will be elevated (up to 20x) in the reparative phase.

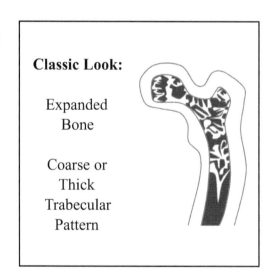

Classic Look:

Expanded Bone

Coarse or Thick Trabecular Pattern

Skull:

Large Areas of Osteolysis in the Frontal and Occipital Bones "Osteoporosis Circumscripta", in the lytic phase.

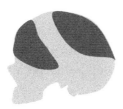

The skull will look "cotton wool" in the mixed phase.

Thickened sclerotic appearance is a good chronic look. Involves BOTH inner and outer table *(Fibrous Dysplasia favors the outer table)*

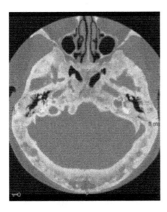

Tam O'Shanter Sign: Skull sorta looks like one of those stupid hats with the frontal aspect "falling over the facial bones"

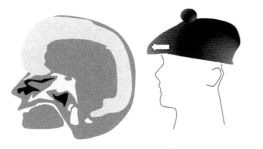

Long Bones

Advancing margin of lucency from one end to the other is the so-called "blade of grass" or "flame." Will often spare the fibula, even in diffuse disease.

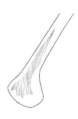

Tibia Bowing "saber shin" is also classic.

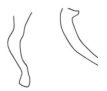

Pelvis:

Most common bone involved. "Always" involves the iliopectineal line on the pelvic brim.

Can cause advanced arthritis and acetabular protrusio.

Has a classic look on bone scan.

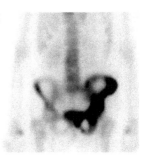

Spine:

Cortical Thickening can cause a "picture frame sign" (same as osteopetrosis). Also can give you an ivory vertebral body.

Discussed more on the next page

THIS vs THAT Pagets Spine vs Other Spine Changes

Pagets – This is discussed in detail in the MSK chapter, but is such a high yield topic that it's worth touching on again. The incidence increases with age (around 8% at age 80). It's at increased risk for fracture, and has a 1% risk of sarcoma degeneration (usually high grade).

It's shown two ways in the spine:
  (1) An enlarged "ivory vertebrae",
  (2) Picture frame vertebrae (sclerotic border)
   —- with central lysis (*mixed phase*)

Ivory

Picture Frame

Renal Osteodystrophy – Another high yield topic covered in depth in the MSK chapter. The way it's shown in the spine is the "Rugger Jersey Spine" – with sclerotic bands at the top and bottom of the vertebral body. You could also have paraspinal soft tissue calcifications

This vs That: Rugger Jersey vs "Paget" Picture Frame:

- Rugger Jersey = Top and Bottom Only
- Paget Picture Frame = All 4 margins of the vertebral body

Osteopetrosis - Another high yield topic covered in depth in the MSK chapter. This is a genetic disease with impaired osteoclastic resorption. You have thick cortical bone, with diminished marrow. On plain film or CT it can look like a Rugger Jersey Spine or Sandwich vertebra. On MR you are going to have loss of the normal T1 bright marrow signal, so it will be T1 and T2 dark.

"H-Shaped Vertebra" – This is usually a **buzzword for sickle cell**, although it's only seen in about 10% of cases. It results from microvascular endplate infarct. If you see "H-Shaped vertebra," the answer is sickle cell. If sickle cell isn't a choice the answer is Gauchers. Another tricky way to ask this is to say which of the following causes **"widening of the disc space."** Widened disc space is another way of describing a "H Shape" without saying that.

Paget on Other Imaging Modalities:

MRI: There are three marrow patterns that closely (but not exactly) follow the phases on x-ray.

Lytic / Early Mixed	Heterogenous T2; T1 is isointense to muscle, with a "speckled appearance"
Late Mixed	Maintained fatty high T1 and T2 signals
Sclerotic	Low signal on T1 and T2

This vs That: Malignant Transformation vs Active Disease:
- Both are T2 Bright and Will Enhance
- Malignant Transformation will lose the Normal T1 signal (just like a cancer would)
- *Best Sequence for Distinguishing the two?* T1 Pre Con

Nuclear Medicine: The primary utility of a bone scan is in defining the extent of disease and to help assess response to treatment. The characteristic look for Paget is "Whole Bone Involvement."

For example, the **entire vertebral body including the posterior elements,** or the entire pelvis. The classic teaching is that Paget is hot on all three phases (although often decreased or normal in the sclerotic phase).

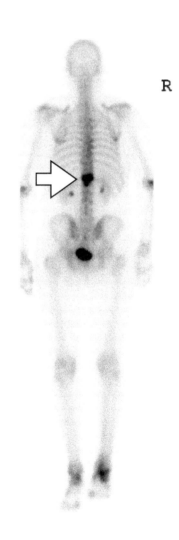

R

Tibial Bowing

Most likely shown as an Aunt Minnie: NF-1 anterior with a fibular pseudoarthrosis, Rickets with wide growth plates, or Blounts tibia vara. Pagets can also cause this.

The most likely pure trivia question is that physiologic bowing is smooth, lateral, and occurs from 18 months - 2 years.

NF-1	**Anterior Lateral** - Unilateral	May be unilateral. May have hypoplastic fibula with pseudarthrosis.
Foot Deformities	Posterior	
Physiologic Bowing	Lateral – Bilateral Symmetric	Self limiting **between 18 months and 2 years**.
Hypophosphatasia	Lateral	"Rickets in a newborn"
Rickets	Lateral	Fraying of the metaphyses and widening of the growth plates. Seen best in "fast growing bones" - knee, wrist
Blount	Tibial Vara – Often asymmetric	Early walking, Fat, black kid. Proximal tibia posteromedial physeal growth disturbance resulting in deformity
Osteogenesis Imperfecta	Involves all long bones	
Dwarfs	Short Limbs	

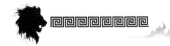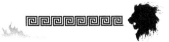
Studying / learning MSK soft tissues masses / tumors tends to create tons of anxiety. This is because Academic Radiology tends to overcomplicate the issue.

Here is the simple part - only about 20-30% of them can be accurately diagnosed on MRI. That's because they are almost all T2 bright and enhance. This is actually good news for the purpose of multiple choice, because you only need to learn the ones that don't behave like that - or are overwhelming likely due to epidemiological stats (which has to be provided for you - either directly "the patient is 65" or with clues - "arthritis = old" , "no arthritis = not old").

Here is the list I would know:

- MFH — Malignant Fibrous Histiocytoma aka - Pleomorphic Undifferentiated Sarcoma
- Synovial Sarcoma
- Lipoma, Atypical Lipoma, Liposarcoma
- Hemangioma
- Myxoma

Malignant Fibrous Histiocytoma (MFH)

Yes - they changed the name to Pleomorphic Undifferentiated Sarcoma "PUS." However, I want you to continue to think of this as MFH because it will help you remember some of the imaging features.

First, the generalizations — This is very common. It's seen in **old people**. It's seen in a **central location** (proximal arms and legs).

Features - About half the time it's **dark to intermediate on T2** (remember most soft tissue tumors are T2 bright). The way I remember this is the word "fibrous" - makes me think scar (which is dark).

Gamesmanship - These things are often associated with spontaneous hemorrhage - they outgrow their blood supply. The history is often "old lady, stood up from a chair" - has a big proximal muscular hematoma — under that hematoma is the MFH.

Trivia: Bone infarcts can turn into MFH - *"sarcomatous transformation of infarct"*
Trivia: Radiation is a risk factor.

Synovial Sarcoma:

Generalization - Seen most commonly in the **peripheral** lower extremities of patients aged 20-40.

Gamesmanship - They occur close to the joint (but **not in the joint**). To confuse the issue they may have secondary invasion into the joint (10%), however for the purpose of multiple choice tests they "never involve the joint." A common trick is to show an ultrasound of the leg with looks like a Baker's cyst - but the mother fucker is too complex - or has flow in it. *Not everything in the popliteal fossa is a Baker's cyst - especially on multiple choice.

> **Baker's Cyst Fuckery**
>
> Baker's Cyst MUST be located between the medial head of the gastrocnemius and the semimembranosus.
>
> If it's NOT - you should think Synovial Sarcoma - and "next step" MRI.

Besides the "not-a-Baker's cyst" trick - there are 3 other ways to show this. (1) as the "**triple sign**", which is high, medium, and low signal all in the same mass (probably in the knee) on T2, (2) as the "**bowl of grapes**" which is a bunch of fluid –fluid levels in a mass (probably in the knee), or (3) as a plain x-ray with a soft tissue component and calcifications – this would be the least likely way to show it.

Synovial Sarcoma Trivia:
- Most sarcomas don't attack bones; Synovial Sarcoma Can
- Most sarcomas present as painless mass; Synovial Sarcomas Hurt
- Soft tissue calcifications + Bone Erosions are highly suggestive
- They are slow growing and small in size, often leading to people thinking they are B9.
- 90% have a translocation of X-18.
- Most common malignancy in teens/young adults of the **foot**, ankle, and lower extremity

When I say "Ball-like tumor" in the extremity of a young adult, you say Synovial Sarcoma.
*When I say "Soft Tissue Tumor in the **Foot**" of a young adult, you say Synovial Sarcoma.*

MFH (PUS)	Synovial Sarcoma
OLD	YOUNG
Central (Upper Thigh, Upper Arm)	Peripheral (Foot, Knee)
T2 - Variable (Sometime Dark)	T2 - "Triple Sign"

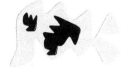

Lipoma *vs* Atypical Lipoma *vs* Liposarcoma

These exist on a spectrum, with Lipoma being totally benign, and Liposarcoma being a bad bad boy. A pearl is that, histologically, Atypical Lipoma behaves and looks just like a low grade Liposarcoma. It would be total horse-shit to ask you to tell those apart. It's more likely the distinction will be either Lipoma vs Liposarcoma.

Think about them like this:

Lipoma	Atypical Lipoma / Low Grade Liposarcoma	High Grade Liposarcoma *"The One That Fucks You Up"*
Signal Intensity parallels fat on all sequences.	May have parts that are slightly darker (or brighter) than fat on T1.	May not even have fat *(for the exam it will have some - otherwise you can't even tell for sure that it is a Liposarcoma)*
Will Fat Sat Out	May incompletely fat sat	May incompletely fat sat (or not fat sat at all)
No Sepations (or thin ones)	Thick Chunky Septations	Thick Nodular Complex Stuff
		Enhancing Components

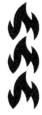

Pearls:

- Liposarcomas tend to be DEEP (retroperitoneum)
- Liposarcomas tend to be BIG
- Lipomas tend to be Superficial

Trivia: Myxoid Liposarcoma is the most common liposarcoma in patients < 20. They can be T2 Bright (expected), but T1 dark (confusing) - don't call it a cyst. Also, don't call it a comeback (I've been here for years). They'll need gad+

Hemangioma

These are common.

Here are the tricks:
- T2 bright (like most tumors)
- **Flow voids.** They have to show you flow voids (buncha dark holes).
- Hemangiomas don't respect fascial boundaries - they will infiltrate into stuff (this is a somewhat unique feature).
- Enhances Intensely - Duh - they are a vascular tumor
- They can **contain fat** - and likely will on multiple choice.

Mazabraud Syndrome

It's a totally zebra syndrome - which makes it totally appropriate for an "intermediate level exam." It has 3 main findings:

(1) Polyostotic Fibrous Dysplasia - *which makes you ugly*
(2) Multiple Soft Tissue Myxomas
(3) Difficulty finding a date to the prom — *see finding "1"

Next Step: A great next step question would be to ask for a plain film. Why a plain film? phleboliths my friend — If they show you soft tissue **phleboliths** then hemangioma is the answer.

Myxoma

If this shows up on the exam, it is almost certainly going to be shown in the setting of Mazabraud Syndrome.

What do Myxomas Look Like? They are T2 bright (like every tumor), but tend to be lower signal than muscle on T1 - which makes them sorta unique.

What does Marsellus Wallace Look Like ?   *Hint - Don't say "what?"

**CT vs MRI
for Lesion Characterization:**

CT is Good for:
-Occult Bone Destruction
-Matrix and Mineralization — Example, better look at the lucent nidus of an osteoid osteoma.

MR is Good for:
-Staging — specifically local extend and tumor spread.
-Follow up - to assess response to therapy.

Treatment High Yield Trivia:

• *Osteosarcoma:* Chemo first (to kill micro mets) , followed by wide excision

• *Ewings:* Both Chemo and Radiation, followed by wide excision.

• *Chondrosarcoma:* Usually just wide excision (they are usually low grade, and main concern is local recurrence).

• *Giant Cell Tumor:* Because it extends to the articular surface usually requires arthroplasty.

Other Soft Tissue Masses (and related conditions)

Pigmented Villonodular Synovitis (PVNS) : PVNS is an uncommon benign neoplastic process that may involve the synovium of the joint diffusely or focally. It can also affect the tendon sheath.

Intra-Articular Disease : Basically, it's **Synovial Proliferation + Hemosiderin Deposition**. The knee is by far the most common joint affected (65-80%). On plain film, features you will probably see are a joint effusion with or without marginal erosions. Osseous erosions with preservation of the joint space and normal mineralization is typical. It is not possible to distinguish PVNS from *synovial chondromatosis (see below)* on plain film. MRI will be obvious with **blooming on gradient echo**, and this is the most likely way they will show this. Treatment is with complete synovectomy, although recurrence rate is 20-50%.

Trivia: Unusual in kids, but when present is typically polyarticular.

Giant Cell Tumor of the Tendon Sheath (PVNS of the tendon): Typically found in the hand (palmar tendons). Can cause erosions on the underlying bone. Will be soft tissue density, and be T1 and T2 dark *(contrasted to a **glomus tumor** which is T1 dark, **T2 bright,** and will enhance uniformly).*

Primary Synovial Chondromatosis: There are both primary and secondary types; secondary being the result of degenerative changes in the joint. The primary type is an extremely high yield topic. It is a metaplastic / true neoplastic process (not inflammatory) that results in the formation of multiple cartilaginous nodules in the synovium of joints, tendon sheaths, and bursea. These nodules will eventually progress to loose bodies. It usually affects one joint, and that one joint is usually the knee (70%). It is usually a person in their 40's or 50's.

Joint bodies (which are usually multiple and uniform in size) may demonstrate the ring and arc calcification characteristic of chondroid calcification. Treatment involves removal of the loose bodies with or without synovectomy.

PVNS	Synovial Chondromatosis
Benign Neoplasia	Benign Neoplasia
Associated with Hemarthrosis	NOT Associated with Hemarthrosis
Never Calcifies	May Calcify

Secondary Synovial Chondromatosis: A lower yield topic than the primary type. This is secondary to degenerative change, and typically seen in an older patient. There will be extensive degenerative changes, and the fragments are usually fewer and larger when compared to the primary subtype.

Diabetic Myonecrosis:

This is basically infarction of the muscle seen in poorly controlled type 1 diabetics. It **almost always involves the thigh (80%)**, or calf (20%). MRI will show marked edema with enhancement and irregular regions of muscle necrosis. You **should NOT biopsy this:** it delays recovery time and has a high complication rate.

Lipoma Arborescens:

 This is a zebra that affects the synovial lining of the joints and bursa.

The buzzword is "**frond-like**" deposition of fatty tissue.

It's seen in late adulthood (50's-70's), with the most common location being the suprapatellar bursa of the knee. Although it **can develop in a normal knee, it's often associated with OA, Chronic RA, or prior trauma**. It's usually unilateral. On MRI it's going to behave like fat – T1 and T2 bright with response to fat saturation.

A sneaky trick is to show this on gradient – and have you pick up the chemical shift artifact at the fat-fluid interface.

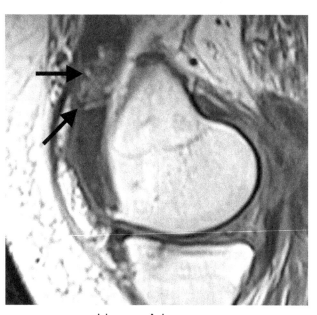

Lipoma Arborescens

This could also be shown on ultrasound with a "frond-like hyperechoic mass" and associated joint effusion.

Bone Biopsy

The route of biopsy should be discussed with the orthopedic surgeon, to avoid contaminating compartments not involved by the tumor (or not going to be used in the resection process).

Special considerations:
- Pelvis: Avoid crossing gluteal muscles (may be needed for reconstruction).
- Knee: Avoid the joint space via crossing suprapatellar bursa or other communicating bursae. Avoid crossing the quadriceps tendon unless it is involved.
- Shoulder: Avoid the posterior 2/3rd (axillary nerve courses post -> anterior, therefore a posterior resection will denervate the anterior 1/3).

"Don't Touch Lesions"
Characteristically Benign Lesions that look Aggressive but are NOT – and should NOT be biopsied because of possibly misleading pathology.

Myositis Ossificans	Circumferential calcifications with a lucent center	Can look scary on MRI if imaged early because of edema, and avid enhancement
Avulsion Injury	Typical location near the pelvis	Can have an aggressive periosteal reaction
Cortical Desmoid	Characteristic location on the posterior medial epicondyle of the distal femur. Bilateral 30% of the time.	Can be hot on bone scan. NOT a desmoid (despite the name). It's actually a tug lesion from the medial gastrocnemius and ADDuctor magnus.
Synovial Herniation Pit "Pitt's Pit"	Characteristic location in the anterosuperior femoral neck.	Lytic appearing lesion Associated with femoral acetabular syndrome (probably).

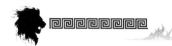 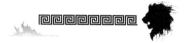

Arthritis is tricky. Anne Brower wrote a book *called Arthritis in Black and White*, which is probably the best book on the subject. The problem is that book is 415 pages. So, I'm going to try and offer the 10 page version.

Epidemiology

Although there are over 90 different rheumatic diseases recognized by the American College of Rheumatology, only a few tend to show up on multiple choice tests (and at the view box).

You can broadly categorize arthritis into 3 categories:
- Degenerative (OA, Neuropathic)
- Inflammatory (RA and Variants)
- Metabolic (Gout, CPPD)

Degenerative:

Osteoarthritis is the most common cause. The pathogenesis is that you have mechanical breakdown (hard work) which leads to cartilage degeneration (fissures, micro-fractures) and fragmentation of subchondral bone (sclerosis and subchondral cysts). You get all the classic stuff, joint space narrowing (<u>NOT symmetric</u>), subchondral cysts, endplate changes, vacuum phenomenon, etc... The poster boy is the osteophyte.

Neuropathic Joint. The way the case is classically shown is a bad joint followed by the reason for a bad joint (syringomyelia, spinal cord injury, etc...). A way to think about this is *"osteoarthritis with a vengeance."* The buzzword is "Surgical Like Margins." Basically nothing else causes this kind of destruction. I like to describe the joints as a **d**eformity, with **d**ebris, and **d**islocation, having **d**ense subchondral bone, and **d**estruction of the articular cortex. The classic scenario is a shoulder that looks like it's been amputated, and then they show you a syrinx.

Charcot Foot - The classic example of a <u>**d**iabetic</u> neuropathic foot with the **d**eformity, with **d**ebris, and **d**islocation, having **d**ense subchondral bone, and **d**estruction of the articular cortex - favoring the midfoot eventually causing a *"rocker-bottom deformity"* of the foot resulting from the collapse of the longitudinal arch.

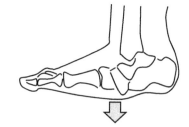

This vs That - Charot vs Infection: Diabetics get neuropathic feet and infections - so there can be overlap. To tell them apart you can <u>look for the presence of an ulcer or sinus tract</u> (that infers infection). Location is helpful - charcot prefers the midfoot (osteomyelitis prefers the pressure points of the forefoot - metatarsal heads, IP joints - and the posterior plantar aspect of the calcaneus).

Inflammatory:

Erosive Osteoarthritis *(Inflammatory Osteoarthritis).* The buzzword is "gull wing", which describes the central erosions. It is seen in postmenopausal women and favors the DIP joints.

Rheumatoid Arthritis: There is a ton of trivia

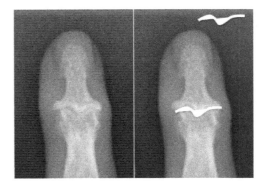

Erosive OA - Gullwing

related to this disease. It's not a disease of bone production. Instead it is characterized by osteoporosis, soft tissue swelling, marginal erosions and <u>uniform joint space narrowing</u>. It's often bilateral and symmetric. Classically spares the DIP joints (opposite of erosive OA).

Trivia: The 5th Metatarsal head is the first spot in the foot

RA in the Hand Pearls - Expect the PIP joints to be involved AFTER the MCP joints. The First CMC is classically spared (or is the last carpal to be involved). The first CMC should NOT be first. Obviously OA loves the first CMC so this is helpful in separating them. Psoriasis, on the other hand, also tends to make the first CMC go last.

- **Felty Syndrome:** RA > 10 years + Splenomegaly + Neutropenia

- **Caplan Syndrome:** RA + Pneumoconiosis

The distribution of RA vs OA in the hip is a classic teaching point:

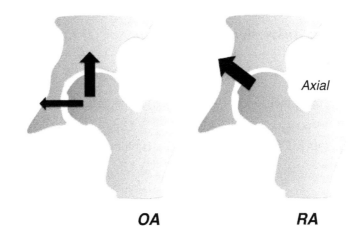

Axial

OA   RA

Rheumatoid Variants:

- Psoriatic Arthritis
- Reiter's syndrome *(Reactive arthritis)*
- Ankylosing Spondylitis
- Inflammatory Bowel Disease

Psoriatic Arthritis: This is seen in 30% of patients with psoriasis. In almost all cases (90%) the skin findings come first, then you get the arthritis. As a point of trivia, there is a strong correlation between involvement of the nail and involvement of the DIP joint. The classic description is "erosive change with bone proliferation (IP joints > MCP joints). The erosions start in the margins of the joint and progress to involve the central portions (can lead to a "pencil sharpening" effect). The hands are the most commonly affected (second most common is the feet). Up to 40% of cases will have SI joint involvement (asymmetric).

Additional Buzzwords
- "Fuzzy Appearance" to the bone around the joint (bone proliferation)
- Sausage Digit – whole digit has soft tissue swelling
- Ivory Phalanx – sclerosis and/or bone proliferation (most commonly the great toe)
- Pencil in Cup Deformities
- Ankylosis in Finger
- "Mouse Ears"
- Acro-osteolysis

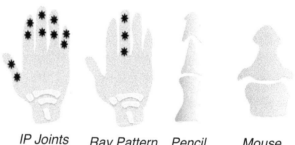

IP Joints   Ray Pattern   Pencil in Cup   Mouse Ears

When I say Ankylosis in the Hand, You Say (1) Erosive OA or (2) Psoriasis

RA	Psoriasis	*Mutilans*
Symmetric	Asymmetric	Severe bone resorption leading to soft tissue "telescoping" collapse.
Proximal (favors MCP, carpals)	Distal (favors IP joints)	*Trivia:* If you pulled on the patient's fingers they would lengthen - but who would want to touch a patient ? Yuck!
Osteoporosis	No Osteoporosis	
No Bone Proliferation	Bone Proliferation - the form of periostitis	
Can Cause "Mutilans" When Severe	Can Cause "Mutilans" When Severe	

Reiter's (Reactive Arthritis):

Apparently Reiter was a Nazi (killed a bunch of people with typhus vaccine experiments). So, people try not to give him any credit for things (hence the name change to Reactive arthritis). Regardless of what you call it, it's **a very similar situation to Psoriatic arthritis** – both have bone proliferation, erosions, and asymmetric SI joint involvement.

The difference is that **Reiter's is rare in the hands** (tends to affect the feet more). Just remember Reiter's favors things below the waist (like the penis = urethritis, and the foot).

Reiter's Triad:
Urethritis *Conjunctivitis* *Arthritis* *(Can't See or Climb a Tree to Pee on a Nazi named Reiter).*

You Know Who Else Was A Nazi? **Henry Ford** - Google It.

Ankylosing Spondylitis: This disease favors the spine and SI joints. The classic buzzword is **"bamboo spine"** from the syndesmophytes flowing from adjacent vertebral bodies. Shiny corners is a buzzword, for early involvement. As you might imagine, these spines are susceptible to fracture in trauma. **SI joint involvement is usually the first site (symmetric).** The joint actually widens a little before it narrows. As a point of trivia, these guys can have an upper lobe predominant interstitial lung disease, with small cystic spaces.

Next Step - Any significant Ank Spon / DISH + Even Minor Trauma = Whole Spine CT

Random High Yield Topic: Ankylosing Spondylitis in the Hip
When the peripheral skeleton is involved in patient's with Ank Spond, think about the shoulders and hips (hips more common). Hip involvement can be very disabling.
Heterotopic Ossification tends to occur post hip replacement or revision. It occurs so much that they often get postoperative low dose radiation and NSAIDs to try as prophylactic therapy.
If they show you normal SI joints - then show you anything in the spine it's not AS. It has to hit the SI joints first (especially on multiple choice).

Inflammatory Bowel Disease (Enteropathic) – Allegedly 20% of patient's with Crohns & UC have a chronic inflammatory arthritis. The imaging findings occurs in two distinct flavors.

(A): Axial Arthritis (favors SI joints and spine) – often unrelated to bowel disease
(B): Peripheral Arthritis – this one varies depending on the severity of the bowel disease.

SI Joint Involvement Patterns (Rheumatoid Variants)

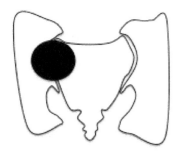

Unilateral = Infection

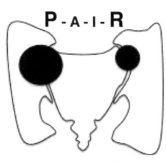

P - A - I - **R**

**Asymmetric =
Psoriasis, Reiters**

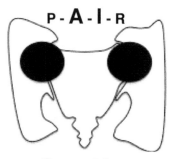

P - **A** - I - R

**Symmetric =
Inflammatory Bowel, AS**

Psoriatic Arthritis	Reiters (Reactive)	Ankylosing Spondylitis
M = F	M > F	M>F
Asymmetric SI Joint	Asymmetric SI Joint	Symmetric SI Joint
Hands, Feet, Thoracolumbar Spine	Feet, Lumbar Spine, SI joint	SI joint, Spine (whole thing)

——

Metabolic:

Gout: This is a crystal arthropathy from the deposition of uric acid crystals in and around the joints. It's almost always in a man over 40. The big toe is the classic location.

Buzzwords / Things to Know:
- Earliest Sign = Joint Effusion
- Spares the Joint Space (until late in the disease); Juxta-articular Erosions - away from the joint.
- "Punched out lytic lesions"
- "Overhanging Edges"
- Soft tissue tophi

Gout on MR

- Juxta-articular soft tissue mass (LOW ON T2).
- The tophus will typically enhance.

Gout Mimickers:

There are 5 entities that can give a similar appearance to a gouty arthritis, although they are much less common. This is the mnemonic I was taught in training:

"**A**merican **R**oentgen **R**ay **S**ociety **H**ooray"
- *Amyloid*
- *RA (cystic)*
- *Reticular Histocytosis (the most rare)*
- *Sarcoid*
- *Hyperlipidemia*

CPPD: Calcium Pyrophosphate Dihydrate Disease is super common in old people. It often causes chondocalcinosis (although there are other causes). Synovitis + CPPD = "Pseudogout." CPPD loves the triangular fibrocartilage of the wrist, the peri-odontoid tissue, and intervertebral disks. Another important phrase is **"degenerative change in an uncommon joint"** – shoulder, elbow, patellofemoral joint, radiocarpal joint. Having said that, **pyrophosphate arthropathy is most common at the knee**.

- *If you see isolated disease in the patellofemoral, radiocarpal, or talonavicular joint, think CPPD.*
- *Hooked MCP Osteophytes with chondrocalcinosis in the TFCC is a classic look (although hemochromatosis can also look that way).*

CPPD can (and does commonly) cause SLAC wrist by degenerating the SL Ligament.

THIS vs THAT — *OA vs CPPD ?*

There are many overlapping features including joint space narrowing, subchondral sclerosis, subchondral cyst, and osteophyte formation. However, CPPD has some unique features, such as an "atypical joint distribution" – favoring compartments like the patellofemoral or radiocarpal. Subchondral cyst formation can be bigger than expected.

Hemochromatosis:

This iron overload disease also is known for calcium pyrophosphate deposition and resulting chondrocalcinosis. It has a similar distribution to CPPD (MCP joints). Both CPPD and Hemochromatosis will have "hooked osteophytes" at the MCP joint.

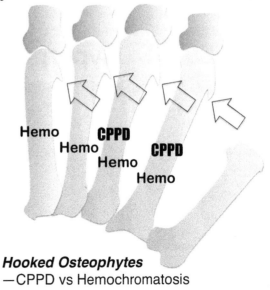

THIS *vs* **THAT**- *CPPD and Hemochromatosis:* Hemochromatosis has uniform joint space loss at ALL the MCP joints. CPPD favors the index and middle finger MCPs.

Trivia: As a point of trivia, therapy for the systemic disease does NOT affect the arthritis.

Hooked Osteophytes
—CPPD vs Hemochromatosis

"Milwaukee Shoulder" - This is an apocalyptic destruction of the shoulder (**almost looks neuropathic**) secondary to the demon mineral **hydroxyapatite**.

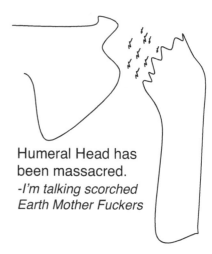

The articular surface changes will be very advanced, and you have a lot of intra-articular loose bodies.

The humeral head will look like it needed the United Nations to delivery a binding resolution to keep the hydroxyapatite from fucking destroying it.

Humeral Head has been massacred.
-I'm talking scorched Earth Mother Fuckers

Classic History: Old women with a history of trauma to that joint.

Hyperparathyroidism - As you may remember from medical school, this can be primary or secondary, and its effects on calcium metabolism typically manifest in the bones. Here are your buzzwords: "Subperiosteal bone resorption" of the radial aspect of the 2nd and 3rd fingers, rugger-jersey spine, brown tumors, and terminal tuft erosions.

The classic ways this can be shown:
- *Superior and inferior rib notching – bone resorption*
- *Resorption along the radial aspect of the fingers with brown tumors*
- *Tuft Resorption*
- *Rugger Jersey Spine*
- *Pelvis with Narrowing or "Constricting" of the femoral necks, and wide SI joints.*

Hyperparathyroidism

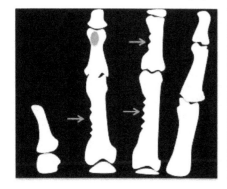 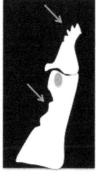 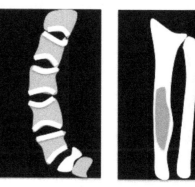

Subperiosteal Resorption, Tuft Resorption and *brown tumors*   Rugger Jersey Spine   Brown Tumor

Problem Solving:

If you are given a picture of a hand or foot and asked what the arthritis is, it will probably be obvious (they show a gull-wing for erosive OA, or bad carpals for RA, or the pencil in cup for psoriasis, or the 5th metatarsal for RA). If it's not made obvious with an "Aunt Minnie" appearance, I like to use this approach to figure it out (I also use this in the real world).

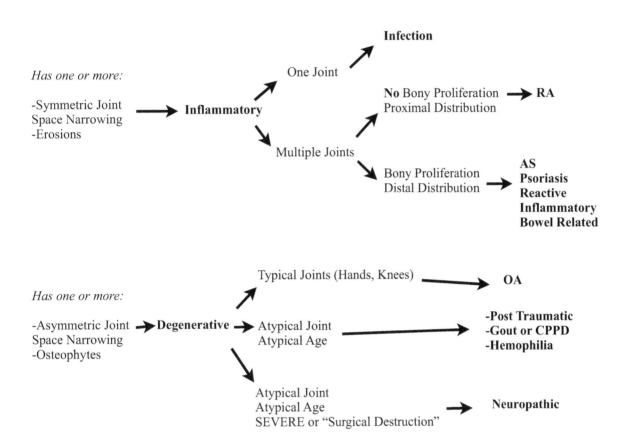

Spine Degenerative Change:

In the real world it's usually just multilevel degenerative change. But in multiple choice world you should be thinking about other things. Shiny corners with early AS, or flowing syndesmophytes with later AS. DISH with the bulky osteophytes sparing the disc space. The big bridging lateral osteophyte is classically shown for psoriatic arthritis.

Vertebral Ossifications			Cervical Spine: *Gamesmanship*
"Flowing Syndesmophytes"	Ankylosing Spondylitis	Bamboo Spine	**Fusion:** Either congenital (Klippel-Feil) or Juvenile RA.
Diffuse Paravertebral Ossifications	DISH	Ossification of ALL	**Erosions of the Dens:** CPPD and RA famously do this.
Focal Lateral Paravertebral Ossification	Psoriatic Arthritis	Ossification of Annulus Fibrosis	**Bad Kyphosis** = NF1

DISH (Diffuse Idiopathic Skeletal Hyperostosis) :

You see ossification of the anterior longitudinal ligament involving more than 4 levels with **sparing of the disc spaces**, you say DISH. The **thoracic spine is most commonly used**. These guys often have bony proliferation at pelvis, ischial tuberosities, trochanters, and iliac crests. There is **no sacroiliitis** (helps you differentiate from AS).

OPLL (Ossification of the Posterior Longitudinal Ligament):

This is an ossification of the posterior longitudinal ligament. It is associated with DISH, ossification of the ligamentum flavum, and Ankylosing Spondylitis. It favors the cervical spine of old Asian men. It can cause spinal canal stenosis, and can lead to cord injury after minor trauma. A key point is that it's bad news in the cervical spine (where it is most common); in the thoracic spine it is usually asymptomatic.

Destructive Spondyloarthropathy.:

This is associated with patients on renal dialysis (for at least 2 years), and it most commonly affects the C-spine. It looks like bad degenerative changes or CPPD. Amyloid deposition is supposedly why it happens.

Misc Stuff That's Sorta in the Arthritis Category:

Systemic Lupus Erythematosus:

The Aunt Minnie look is **reducible deformity of joints without articular erosions**. *Joint space narrowing and erosions are uncommon findings.* They can show you the hands with ulnar subluxations at the MCPs on Norgaard view, then they reduce on AP (because the hands are flat).

This ligamentous laxity also increases risk of **patellar dislocations**.

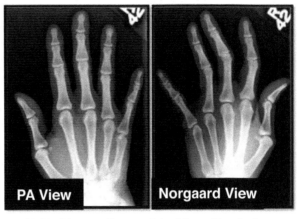

SLE: Shows Reversible Ulnar Deviation

Jaccoud's Arthropathy: This is **very similar to SLE** in the hand (people often say them together). You have non erosive arthropathy with ulnar deviation of the 2nd-5th fingers at the MCP joint. The **history is post rheumatic fever**.

Mixed Connective Tissue Disease: One unique feature is that it is positive for some antibody – Ribonucleoprotein (RNP) - and therefore *serology is essential to the diagnosis.*

Juvenile Idiopathic Arthritis: This occurs before age 16 (by definition). What you see is a washed out hand that has a proximal distribution (**carpals are jacked**), and is ankylosed (**premature fusion of growth plates**). Serology is often negative (85%). In the knees, you see enlargement of the epiphyses and <u>widened intercondylar notch</u> – similar to findings in hemophilia.

 Buzzword: "Epiphyseal Overgrowth"

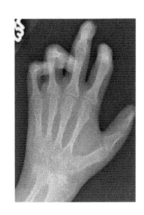

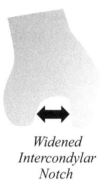

Widened Intercondylar Notch

Amyloid Arthropathy: This is seen with patients on dialysis (less commonly in patients with chronic inflammation such as RA). The pattern of destruction can be severe – similar to septic arthritis or neuropathic spondyloarthropathy. The distribution is key, with **bilateral involvement of the shoulders, hips, carpals, and knees** being typical. **Carpal tunnel syndrome is a common clinical manifestation**. The **joint space is typically preserved** until later in the disease. When associated with dialysis, it's rare before 5 years of treatment, but very common after 10 years (80%).

Pituitary Gigantism: If they happen to show you x-rays of Andre the Giant, look for "**widening of the joint space in an adult hip**" – can be a classic buzzword. Late in the game, the cartilage will actually outgrow its blood supply and collapse, leading to **early onset osteoarthritis**. The formation of endochondral bone at existing chondro-osseous junctions results in widening of osseous structure.

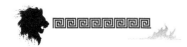 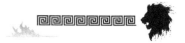
This is a confusing topic and there are entire books on the subject. I'm going to attempt to hit the main points, and simplify the subject.

Bone marrow consists of three components: (1) Trabecular Bone – the support structure, (2) Red Marrow – for making blood, and (3) Yellow Marrow –fat for a purpose unknown at this time.

Marrow Conversion: The basic rules are that yellow marrow increases with age, in a predictable and progressive way. This is usually completed by the mid 20s. You are born with all red marrow, and the conversion of red to yellow occurs from the extremities to the axial skeleton (feet and hands first). Within each long bone the progression occurs epiphyses / apophyses first -> diaphysis -> followed by the distal metaphysis , and finally the proximal metaphysis. **Red marrow can be found in the humeral heads and femoral heads as a normal variant in adults.**

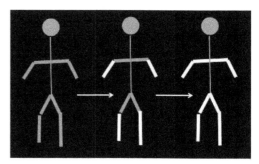

Red Marrow Coverts to Yellow Marrow from Distal to Proximal

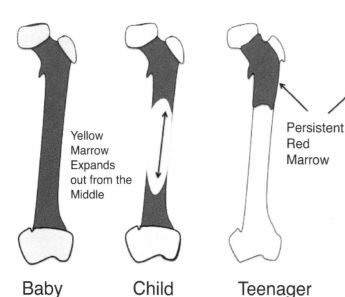

Yellow Marrow Expands out from the Middle

Persistent Red Marrow

Baby   Child   Teenager   Adult

As a child, you have diffuse red marrow except for ossified epiphyses and apophyses.

As adults, you have yellow marrow everywhere except in the axial skeleton, and proximal metaphyses of proximal long bones.

Few Pearls on Marrow:

- Yellow marrow increases with age (as trabecular bone decreases with osteoporosis, yellow marrow replaces it).
- T1 is your money sequence: Yellow is bright, Red is darker than yellow (near iso-intense to muscle).
- Red marrow should never be darker than a normal disk or muscle on T1 (think about muscle as your internal control).
- Red marrow increases if there is a need for more hematopoiesis (reconversion – occurs in exact reverse order of normal conversion)
- Marrow turns yellow with stress / degenerative change in the spine

Three most classic marrow questions:

(1 Q) What is the normal pattern of conversion ?

(A) The epiphyses convert to fatty marrow almost immediately after ossification. Distal then proceeds medial / proximal (diaphysis first, then metaphysis).

(2 Q) What is the normal pattern of REconversion ?

(A) The pattern of reconversion: This occurs in the reverse order of normal marrow conversion, beginning in the axial skeleton and heading peripheral. The last to go are the more distal long bones. Typically, the epiphyses are spared unless the hematopoietic demand is very high.

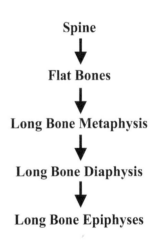

Spine
↓
Flat Bones
↓
Long Bone Metaphysis
↓
Long Bone Diaphysis
↓
Long Bone Epiphyses

(3 Q) What areas are spared / normal variants?

(A) Patchy areas of red marrow may be seen in the proximal femoral metaphysis of teenagers. **Distal femoral sparing is seen in teenagers and menstruating women.**

Leukemia:

Proliferation of leukemic cells results in replacement of red marrow. **Marrow will look darker than muscle (and normal disks) on T1**. On STIR, marrow may be brighter than muscle because of the increased water content. T2 is variable, often looking like diffuse red marrow.

 They can show leukemia in two main ways:

(1) Lucent metaphyseal bands in a kid

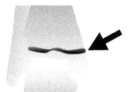

(2) T1-weighted MRI showing marrow darker than adjacent disks and muscle. Remember that Red Marrow is still 40% fat and should be brighter than muscle on T1.

Most infiltrative conditions affect the marrow diffusely. The exceptions are *multiple myeloma, which has a predilection for focal "speckled" deposits, and Waldenstrom's macroglobulinemia, which causes infarcts.*

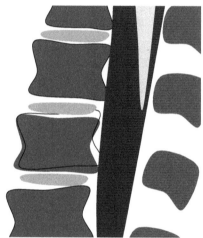

T1 Sag - Marrow is Darker than Disk —

Chloroma (Granulocytic Sarcoma)

Just say *"destructive mass in a bone of a leukemia patient."* It's some kind of colloid tumor.

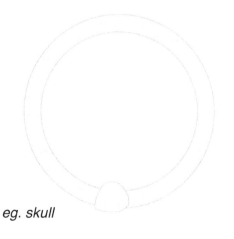

eg. skull

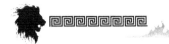
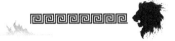
It's absolutely incredible that I even need to go over this, but dinosaur radiologists love this stuff. Plus it is popular in Europe, so logically it belongs on an intermediate exam in the US.

Anisotropy: The most common and most problematic issues with ultrasounding tendons is this thing called "anisotropy." The tendon is normally hyperechoic, but if you look at it when it's NOT perpendicular to the sound beam it can look hypoechoic (injured?).

It's the biggest pain in the ass:

• Supraspinatus tendon – as it curves along the contours of the humeral head
• Long Head of the Biceps – In the bicipital groove

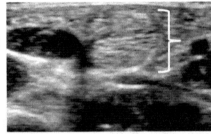

Normal Appearing Hyperechoic Tendon

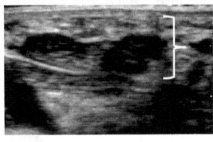

Exact same tendon - now appearing hypoechoic - when scanned non perpendicular

Tears: The tendon is usually hyperechoic. Focal hypoechoic areas are tears. It can be really tricky to tell if it's partial or complete (that's what MRI is for).

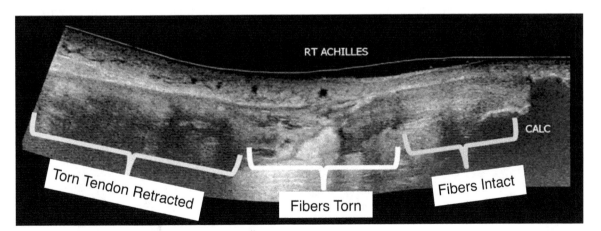

Tenosynovitis: As discussed above, there are a variety of causes. If they show it on ultrasound, you are looking for increased fluid within the tendon sheath. You could also see associated peritendinous subcutaneous hyperemia on Doppler.

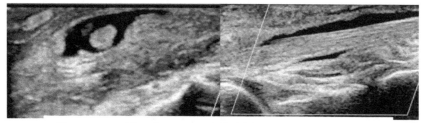

Tenosynovitis - Increased fluid in the tendon sheath

Plantar Fasciitis: This is another pathology that lends itself to a *"what is it ?"* type of ultrasound question. Hopefully, they at least tell you this is the foot (they could label the calcaneus). The finding will be thickening of the plantar fascia (greater than 4 mm), with loss of the normal fibrillar pattern. If you see calipers on the plantar fascia – this is going to be the answer.

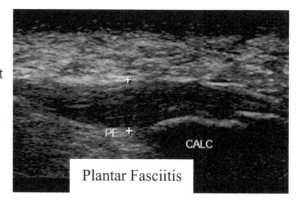

Plantar Fasciitis

Trivia - <u>Most commonly involves the central band</u> (there are 3 bands - people who don't know anatomy think there are two).

Calcific Tendonitis: As described above, this is very common and related to hydroxyapatite. The most common site is the supraspinatus tendon, near its insertion. It will shadow just like a stone in the GB.

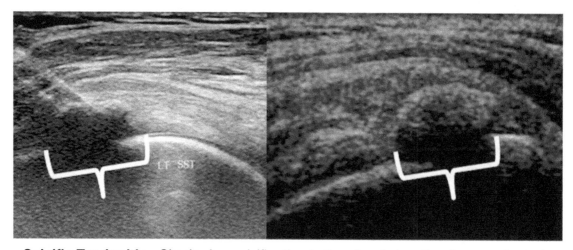

Calcific Tendonitis - Shadowing calcification in the classic location (supraspinatus)

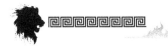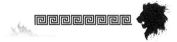
An important point to remember is that the target is not actually the joint. The target is the capsule. In other words, you just need the needle to touch a bone within the capsule. The trick is to do this without causing contamination or damaging an adjacent structure (like an artery). *General Tip* - Avoid putting air in the joint, as this will cause susceptibility artifact.

Hip: The general steps are as follows: (1) Mark the femoral artery. (2) Internally rotate the hip (slightly) to localize the femoral head-neck junction (your target). (3) Clean and numb the skin. (4) Advance a 20-22 gauge spinal needle into the joint - straight down on the superior head neck junction. (5) Inject a small amount of contrast to confirm position. Contrast should flow away from the tip. If the contrast just stays there it's not in the capsule. (6) Put the rest of the contrast in.

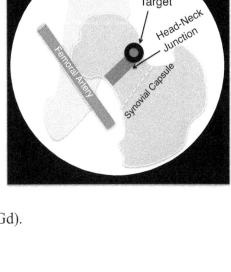

Trivia: Capsule is widest at the head-neck junction.

Trivia: The cocktail injected is around 14 cc total (4 cc Lidocaine, 10 cc Visipaque, and only about 0.1 cc Gd).

Shoulder: The general steps are as follows: (1) Supinate the hand (externally rotate the shoulder) (2) Clean and numb the skin. (3) Advance a 20-22 gauge spinal needle into the joint - straight down on the junction between the middle and inferior third of the humeral head - 2 mm inside the cortex. (4) Once you strike bone, pull back 1 mm and turn the bevel towards the humeral head - this should drop into the joint (5) Inject a small amount of contrast to confirm position. Contrast should flow away from the tip. If the contrast just stays there it's not in a space. (6) Put the rest of the contrast in.

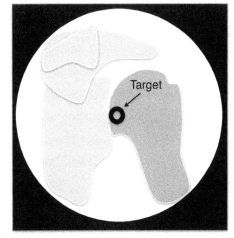

Trivia: The cocktail injected is around 12cc total (4cc Lidocaine, 8cc Visipaque, and only about 0.1 cc Gd).

Special Situations - Problem Solving

So there are three main reasons that you might get asked to put a needle in a joint

1 - Needs Arthrogram to Evaluate the Labrum

2 - Needs Steroid / Lidocaine Injection for Pain Management

3 - Possible Joint Infection - Needs Aspiration

Only one of these is going to end up getting imaged (the arthrogram), the other two just need the needle in the correct spot - and it doesn't matter what you had to do to get it there.

Scenario 1 - Patient is allergic to (has a phobia of) Gd, but needs an arthrogram?

You could try a CT Arthrogram. So - not Gad, just Visipaque and Lidocaine.

Scenario 2 - Patient is allergic to (has a phobia of) CT Contrast (Visi or Omni), but needs a steroid joint injection?

You can inject air into the joint (instead of visi) to confirm placement - then put the steroid in.

Scenario 3 - Patient is allergic to (has a phobia of) CT Contrast (Visi or Omni), but needs an arthrogram ?

This situation is different. You can't inject air because you will end up with a big blooming mess on MR. CT isn't an option either - because obviously you need the CT Contrast or it's not an arthrogram. Your only choices would be to either (1) pre-medicate them, or (2) use the force (trust your feelings...) and hope you can get in the joint without confirming positioning with fluoro.

Blank for Scribbles

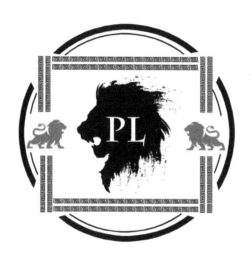

12

VASCULAR

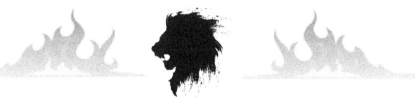

PROMETHEUS LIONHART, M.D.

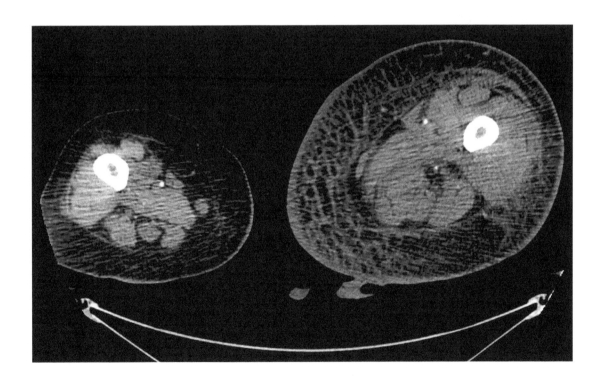

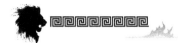 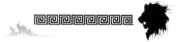

Aorta: The thoracic aorta is divided anatomically into four regions; the root, the ascending aorta, the transverse aorta (arch), and the descending aorta. The "root" is defined as the portion of the aorta extending from the aortic valve annulus to the sino-tubular junction. The diameter of the thoracic aorta is largest at the aortic root and gradually decreases *(average size is 3.6 cm at the root, 2.4 cm in the distal descending).*

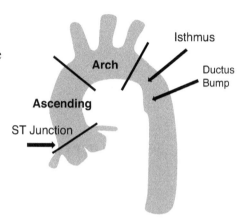

- *Sinuses of Valsalva:* There are 3 outpouchings (right, left, posterior) above the annulus that terminate at the ST Junction. The right and left coronaries come off the right and left sinuses. The posterior cusp is sometimes called the "non-coronary cusp."

- *Isthmus:* The segment of the aorta between the origin of the left Subclavian and the ligamentum arteriosum.

- *Ductus bump:* Just distal to the isthmus is a contour bulge along the lesser curvature, which is a normal structure (not a pseudoaneurysm).

Aortic Arch Variants: There are 4 common variations:

Normal (75%), Bovine Arch (15%) – common origin of brachiocephalic artery and left common carotid artery, left common carotid coming off the brachiocephalic proper (10%), and in 5% of people the left vertebral artery originates separately from the arch. Branching with regards to right arch, left arch and double arch was discussed in more detail in the cardiac chapter.

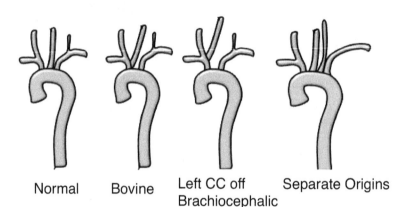

Normal   Bovine   Left CC off   Separate Origins
                    Brachiocephalic

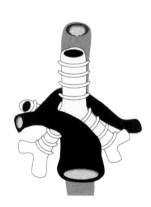

Pulmonary Sling: Aberrant Left pulmonary artery coming off the right pulmonary artery.

-Unique as the only anomaly to create indentations in the posterior trachea and anterior esophagus.

-Unique as the only anomaly that can cause stridor in a patient with a normal left sided arch.

Adamkiewicz:

The thoracic aorta puts off multiple important feeders including the great anterior medullary artery (Artery of Adamkiewicz) which serves as a dominate feeder of the spinal cord.

This thing usually comes off on the **left side (70%) between T9-T12.**

"Beware of the Hairpin Turn"
-The classic angiographic appearance of the artery is the "hairpin turn" as its anastomosis with the anterior spinal artery.

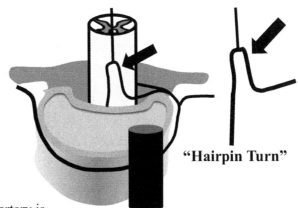

"Hairpin Turn"

Mesenteric Branches:

The anatomy of the SMA and IMA is high yield, and can be shown on a MIP coronal CT, or Angiogram. I think that knowing the inferior pancreaticoduodenal comes off the SMA first, and that the left colic (from IMA) to the middle colic (from SMA) make up the Arc of Riolan are probably the highest yield facts.

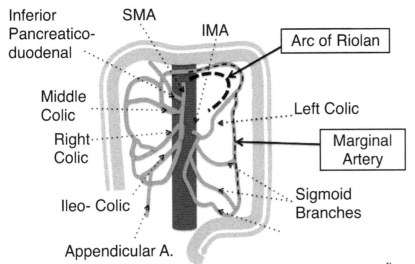

Inferior Pancreatico-duodenal

SMA

IMA

Arc of Riolan

Middle Colic

Left Colic

Right Colic

Marginal Artery

Ileo- Colic

Sigmoid Branches

Appendicular A.

Celiac Branches:

The classic branches of the celiac axis are the common hepatic, left gastric, and the splenic arteries.

The "common" hepatic artery becomes the "proper" hepatic artery after the GDA.

This "traditional anatomy" is actually only seen in 55% of people.

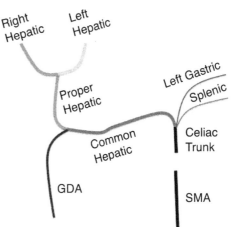

Right Hepatic

Left Hepatic

Proper Hepatic

Left Gastric

Splenic

Common Hepatic

Celiac Trunk

GDA

SMA

Celiac Anatomy - Remember this can be shown with an angiogram, CTA, or MRA.

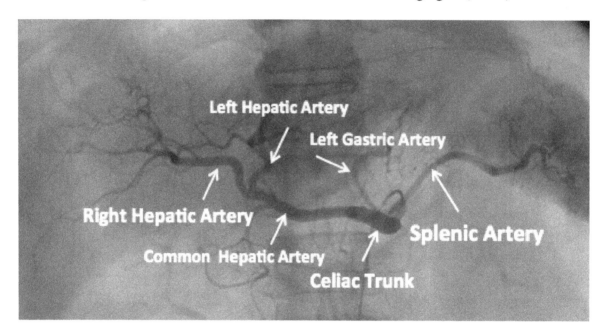

Variant Hepatic Artery Anatomy – The right hepatic artery and left hepatic arteries may be "replaced" (originate from a vessel other than the proper hepatic) or duplicated - which anatomist called "accessory." This distinction of "replaced" vs "accessory" would make a great multiple choice question.

Trivia to know:

• Replaced = Different Origin, usually off the left gastric or SMA

• Accessory = Duplication of the Vessel, with the spare coming off the left gastric or SMA

• If you see a **vessel in the fissure of the ligamentum venosum** (where there is not normally a vessel), it's probably an accessory or **replaced left hepatic artery arising from the left gastric artery**.

• **The proper right hepatic artery is anterior to the right portal vein, whereas the replaced right hepatic artery is posterior to the main portal vein.** This positioning of the replaced right increases the risk of injury in pancreatic surgeries.

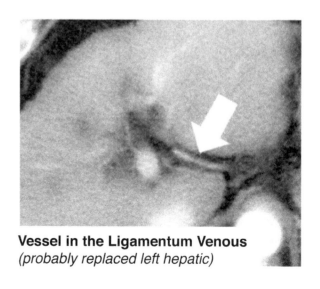

Vessel in the Ligamentum Venous
(probably replaced left hepatic)

Iliac Anatomy: The branches of the internal iliac are high yield, with the most likely question being "which branches are from the posterior or anterior divisions?" A *useful mnemonic is "I Love Sex," Illiolumbar, Lateral Sacral, Superior Gluteal, for the posterior division.*

My trick for remembering that the mnemonic is for posterior and not anterior is to think of that super religious girl I knew in college — *I Like Sex in the butt / posterior.*

I don't think they will actually show a picture, it's way more likely to be a written question.

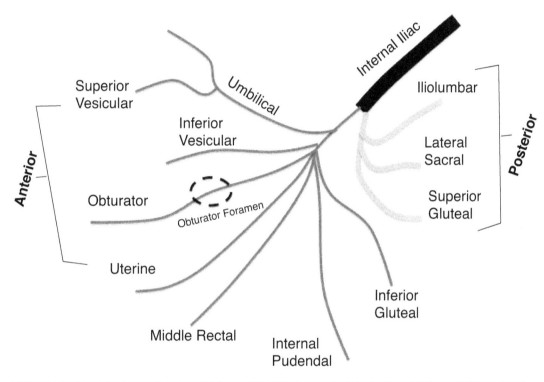

Anterior Division	Posterior Division
Umbilical	Iliolumbar
Superior Vesicular (off umbilical)	Lateral Sacral
Inferior Vesicular	Superior Gluteal
Uterine (if you have a uterus)	*Inferior Gluteal *** sometimes*
Middle Rectal	
Internal Pudendal	
Inferior Gluteal	
Obturator	

Trivia: The ovarian arteries arise from the anterior-medial aorta 80-90% of time.

Persistent Sciatic Artery – An anatomic variant, which is a **continuation of the internal iliac**. It passes posterior to the femur in the thigh and then will anastomose with the distal vasculature. Complications worth knowing include aneurysm formation and early atherosclerosis in the vessel. The classic vascular surgery boards question is "external iliac is acutely occluded, but there is still a strong pulse in the foot", the answer is the patient has a persistent sciatic.

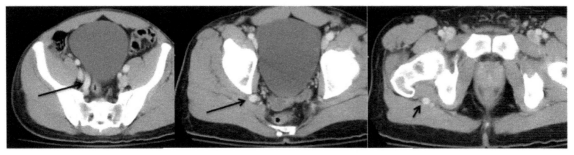

Persistent Sciatic Artery

Mesenteric Arterial Collateral Pathways:

Celiac to SMA: The conventional collateral pathway is Celiac -> Common Hepatic -> GDA -> Superior Pancreatic Duodenal -> Inferior Pancreatic Duodenal -> SMA.

Arc of Buhler: This is a variant anatomy (seen in like 4% of people), that represents a collateral pathway from the celiac to the SMA. The arch is independent of the GDA and inferior pancreatic arteries. This rare collateral can have an even more rare aneurysm, which occurs in association with stenosis of the celiac axis.

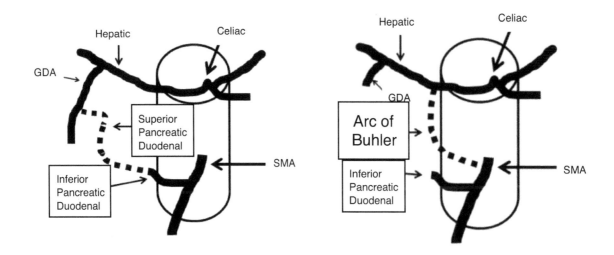

SMA to IMA: The conventional collateral pathway is SMA -> Middle Colic -> Left Branch of the Middle Colic -> Arc of Riolan (as below) -> Left Colic - > IMA.

Arc of Riolan – Also referred to as the meandering mesenteric artery. Classically a **connection between the middle colic of the SMA and the left colic of the IMA.**

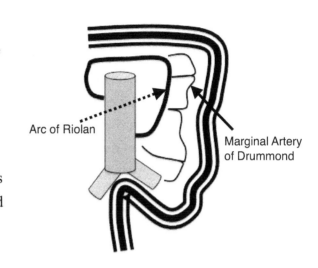

Marginal Artery of Drummond – This is another **SMA to IMA connection**. The anastomosis of the terminal branches of the ileocolic, right colic and middle colic arteries of the SMA, and of the left colic and sigmoid branches of the IMA, form a **continuous arterial circle or arcade along the inner border of the colon.**

IMA to Iliacs: The conventional collateral pathway is IMA -> Superior Rectal -> Inferior Rectal -> Internal Pudendal -> Anterior branch of internal iliac.

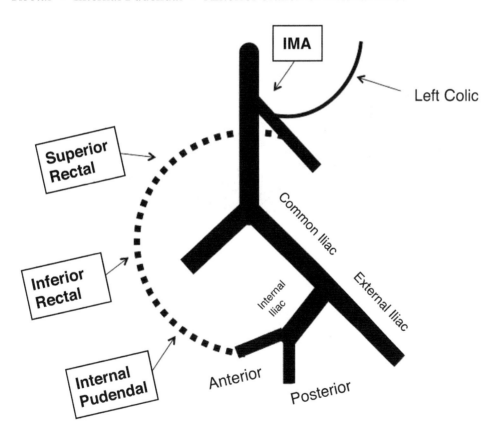

Winslow Pathway – This is a collateral pathway that is seen in the setting of aorto-iliac occlusive disease. The pathway apparently can be inadvertently cut during transverse abdominal surgery. The pathway runs from subclavian arteries -> internal thoracic (mammary) arteries -> superior epigastric arteries -> inferior epigastric arteries -> external iliac arteries.

Corona Mortis – Classically described as a vascular connection between the **obturator and external iliac.** Some authors describe additional anastomotic pathways, but you should basically think of it as any vessel **coursing over the superior pubic rim**, regardless of the anastomotic connection. The "crown of death" is significant because it can (a) be **injured in pelvic trauma** or (b) be **injured during surgery – and is notoriously difficult to ligate.** Some authors report that it causes 6-8% of deaths in pelvic trauma. The last piece of trivia is that it could hypothetically cause a type 2 endoleak.

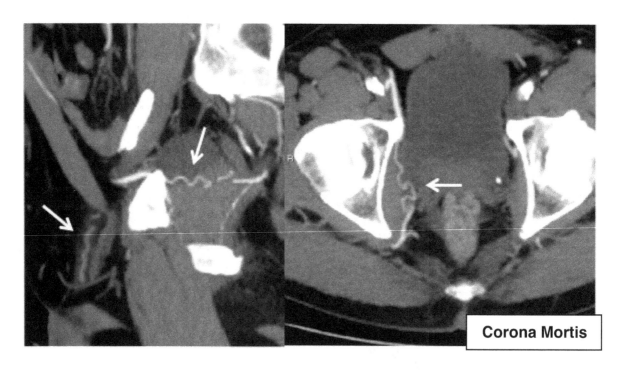

Corona Mortis

Upper Extremity Anatomy:

The scalene muscles make a triangle in the neck. If you have ever had the pleasure of reading a brachial plexus MRI finding this anatomy in a sagittal plane is the best place to start (in my opinion). The relationship to notice (because it's testable) is that the subclavian vein runs anterior to the triangle, and the subclavian artery runs in the triangle (with the brachial plexus).

Trivia to Remember: The subclavian artery runs posterior to the subclavian vein.

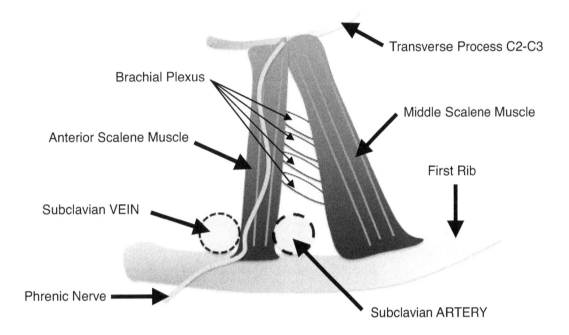

The subclavian artery has several major branches: the vertebral, the internal thoracic, the thyrocervical trunk, the costocervical trunk, and the dorsal scapular.

As the subclavian artery progresses down the arm, anatomists decided to change it's name a few times. This name changing makes for great multiple choice fodder.

The highest yield thing you can know with regard to upper extremity vascular anatomy is when stuff becomes stuff:

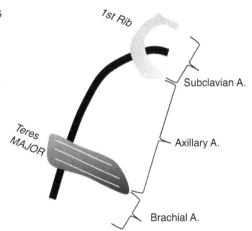

- **Axillary Artery:** Begins at the first rib
- **Brachial Artery:** Begins at the lower border of the teres <u>major</u> (major NOT minor!)
- **Brachial Artery:** Bifurcates to the ulnar and radial

Upper Extremity Normal Variants:

* Anterior Interosseous Branch (Median Artery) persists and supplies the deep palmar arch of the hand.

* **"High Origin of the Radial Artery"** – Radial artery comes off either the axillary or high brachial artery (remember it normally comes off at the level of the radial head).

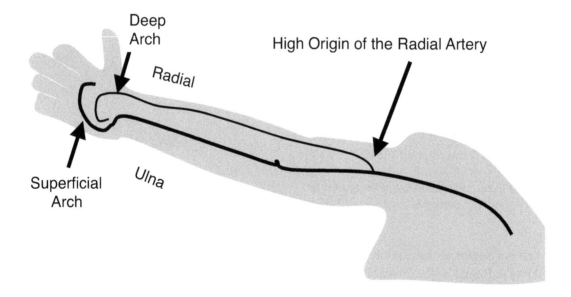

Lower Extremity Anatomy:

Every medical student knows the aorta bifurcates into the right and left common iliac arteries, which subsequently bifurcate into the external and internal iliac arteries. The nomenclature pearl for **the external iliac is that it becomes the common femoral once it gives off the inferior epigastric** *(at the inguinal ligament).*

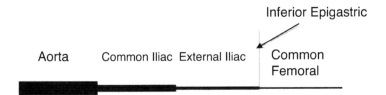

Once the inferior epigastric comes off (level of the inguinal ligament) you are dealing with the common femoral artery(CFA). The CFA divides into the deep femoral (profunda) and superficial femoral. The deep femoral courses lateral and posterior. The superficial femoral passes anterior and medial into the flexor muscle compartment (ADDuctor / Hunter's Canal). At the point the vessel emerges from the canal it is then the popliteal artery. At the level of the distal border of the popliteus muscle the popliteal artery divides into the **anterior tibialis (the first branch)** and the tibioperoneal trunk. The anterior tibialis courses anterior and lateral, then it <u>transverses the interosseous membrane</u>, running down the front of the anterior tibia and terminating as the dorsalis pedis. The tibioperoneal trunk bifurcates into the posterior tibialis and fibular (peroneal) arteries. A common quiz is "what is the most medial artery in the leg?" , with the answer being the posterior tibial (felt at the medial malleolus). Notice how lateral the AT is - you can imagine it running across the interosseous membrane, just like it's suppose to.

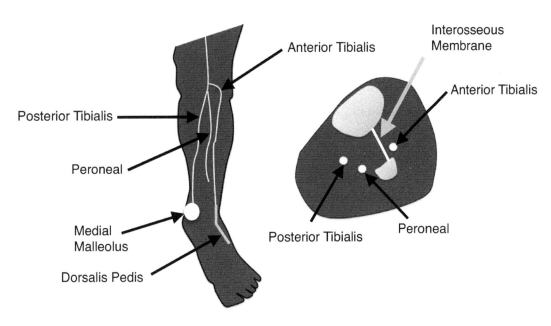

Mesenteric Venous Collaterals:

Gastric Varices: As described in more detail in the GI chapter, portal hypertension shunts blood away from the liver and into the systemic venous system. Spontaneous portal-systemic collaterals develop to decompress the system. The thing to know is that **most gastric varices are formed by the left gastric (coronary vein)** . That is the one they always show big and dilated on an angiogram. Isolated gastric varices are secondary to splenic vein thrombosis. Gastric Varices (80-85%) drain into the inferior phrenic and then into the left renal vein, forming a gastro-renal shunt.

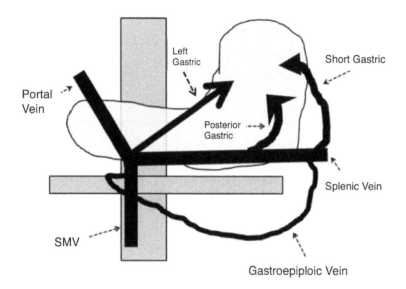

- Left Gastric (Coronary) = Cardia
- Posterior and Short Gastric = Fundus

Splenorenal Shunt: Another feature of portal hypertension, this is an abnormal collateral between the splenic vein and renal vein. This is actually a desirable shunt because it is **not associated with GI bleeding.** However, **enlarged shunts are associated with hepatic encephalopathy** (discussed in greater detail in the BRTO section of the IR chapter). A common way to show this is an enlarged left renal vein and dilatation of the inferior vena cava at the level of the left renal vein.

Caval Variants

Left Sided SVC – The most common congenital venous anomaly in the chest. In a few rare cases these can actually result in a right to left shunt. They are only seen in isolation in 10% of cases (the other 90% it's "duplicated"). The location and appearance is a total **Aunt Minnie**.

Trivia to know:

• Most commonly associated CHD is the ASD

• Associated with an unroofed coronary sinus

• Nearly always (92% of the time) it drains into the coronary sinus

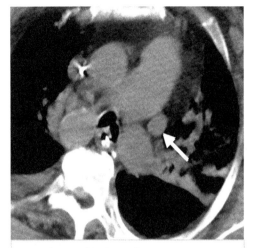

Left Sided SVC - *When you see that son of a bitch right there, that thing can only be one of two things - a lymph node or a duplicated SVC.*

Duplicated SVC – The above discussed "Left Sided SVC" almost never occurs in isolation. Instead, there is almost always a "normal" right sided SVC, in addition to the left sided SVC. It is in this case (which is the majority of cases of left sided SVC) that the terminology "duplicated SVC" is used. It is so common that people will use the terms duplicated and left sided interchangeably. But, technically to be duplicated you need a right sided and left sided SVC (even if the right one is a little small - which is often the case in the setting of a left SVC).

Duplicated IVC - There are two main points worth knowing about this: (1) that the appearance is an **Aunt Minnie**, and (2) it's **associated with Renal stuff**. Renal associations include horseshoe and crossed fused ectopic kidneys.

Also these dudes often have circumaortic renal collars (see below).

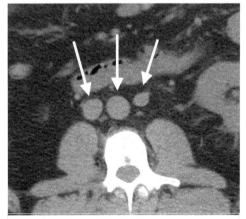

Duplicated IVC *(IVCs are the bread, Aorta is the cheese or peanut butter… or bacon)*

Circumaortic Venous Collar – Very common variant with an additional left renal vein that passes posterior to the aorta. It only matters in two situations (a) renal transplant, (b) IVC filter placement. The classic question is that the **anterior limb is superior**, and the posterior limb is inferior.

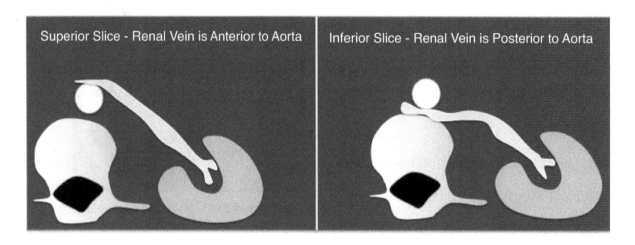

Azygos Continuation – This is also known as absence of the hepatic segment of the IVC. In this case, the hepatic veins drain directly into the right atrium. Often the IVC is duplicated in these patients, with the left IVC terminating in the left renal vein , which then crosses over to join the right IVC.

The first thing you should think when I say azygous continuation is **polysplenia** (reversed IVC/Aorta is more commonly associated with asplenia).

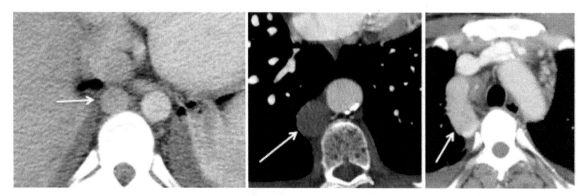

Azygos Continuation - *No IVC in the Liver, Dilated Azygos in the Chest*

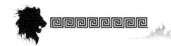 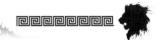

There are 3 "acute aortic syndromes", aortic dissection, intramural hematoma, and penetrating ulcer. Lets take these one at a time and talk about the trivia.

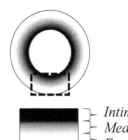

Intima
Media
Externa

Anatomy Review:

Remember vessels have 3 layers: Intima, Media, and that other one no one gives a shit about.

Penetrating Ulcer:

This is an ulceration of an atheromatous plaque that has eroded the inner elastic layer of the aortic wall. When it reaches the media it produces a hematoma within the media.

- **#1 Risk Factor = Atherosclerosis**
  (Delicious Burger King and Tasty Cigarettes)

- **Classic Scenario:** Elderly patient with hypertension and atherosclerosis usually involving the descending thoracic aorta

- **Genesis:** Eating like a pig and smoking results in atherosclerosis. Nasty atherosclerotic plaque erodes through the intima. Hematoma forms in the media (intramural hematoma). With severe disease can eventually progress to a pseudo aneurysm (and maybe even rupture)

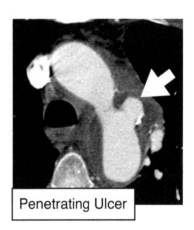
Penetrating Ulcer

- **Pearl:** Look for a gap in the intimal calcifications (that's how you know it's truly penetrated through the intima, and not just some funky contour abnormality).

- **Classification:** All 3 AASs can be classified as type A or B Stanford, based on their locations before (type A) or after the takeoff the of the left subclavian (type B).

- **These things often result in a saccular morphology around the arch.** In general, sac like aneurysm above the diaphragm is related to penetrating ulcer. Sac like aneurysm below the diaphragm is gonna be septic ("mycotic").

Relationship between Penetrating Ulcer and Dissection:
—*Controversial (which usually means it won't be tested)* – famous last words

If forced to answer questions on this relationship, I would go with the following:
- Penetrating Ulcers are caused by atherosclerosis (this is a fact)
- Penetrating Ulcer can lead to Dissection (this is probably true in some cases)
- Atherosclerosis does NOT cause Dissection (which is confusing, may or may not be true, and is unlikely to be tested). What is true is that the presence of dense calcified plaque can stop extension of a dissection tear.
- Dissections often occur in the aortic root – where you have the highest flow pressures
- Penetrating Ulcers nearly never occur in the root – as these flow pressures prevent atherosclerosis (wash those cheeseburger crumbs away).

Treatment of Penetrating Ulcer ?

- "Medical" = Similar to Type B Dissections. If they do get treated (grafted etc…) they tend to do WORSE than dissections (on average)

- Q: When are they Surgical ?
- A: Hemodynamic instability, Pain, Rupture, Distal Emboli, Rapid Enlargement

Dissection

- The most common cause of acute aortic syndrome (70%)
- **Hypertension** is the main factor – leads to an intimal tear resulting in two lumens
- Marfans, Turners, and other Connective Tissue Diseases increase risk

Classic Testable Scenarios:
- Pregnancy — known to increase risk
- Cocaine Use in a young otherwise healthy person
- Patient with "Hypertension" and a sub-sternal "Tearing Sensation."

Chicken vs Egg: Some people say that hypertensive pressures kill the vasa vasorum (the little vessels inside the vessel walls) leading to development of intramural hematoma which then ruptures into the intima. This is the "inside out" thinking. Other people think the hypertensive forces tear the inner layer directly ("outside in" thinking).
Honestly… who gives a shit? Not even sure why I mentioned that.

Dissection Continued...

There are two general ways to classify these things:

(1) Time: Acute (< 2 weeks), or Chronic
(2) Location:
- **Stanford A:** Account for 75% of dissections and involves the ascending aorta and arch <u>proximal to the take-off of the left subclavian</u>. These guys need to be <u>treated surgically.</u>

- **Stanford B:** Occur <u>distal to the take-off of the left subclavian</u> and are <u>treated medically</u> unless there are complications (organ ischemia etc...)

THIS vs THAT:		Floating Viscera Sign:
True Lumen	**False Lumen**	This is a classic angiographic sign of abdominal aortic dissection.
Continuity with undissected portion of aorta	"CobWeb Sign" – slender linear areas of low attenuation	It is shown as opacification of abdominal aortic branch vessels during aortography (catheter placed in the aortic true lumen), with the branch vessels— (celiac axis, superior mesenteric artery, and right renal artery) arising out of nowhere.
Smaller cross sectional areas (with higher velocity blood)	**Larger** cross section area (slower more turbulent flow)	
Surrounded by calcifications (if present) 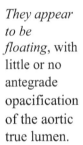	**Beak Sign** - acute angle at edge of lumen - seen on axial plane	*They appear to be floating*, with little or no antegrade opacification of the aortic true lumen. 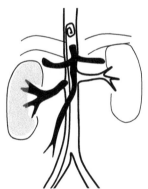
Usually contains the origin of celiac trunk, SMA, and **RIGHT** renal artery	Usually contains the origin of **LEFT** renal artery	
	Surrounds true lumen in Type A Dissection	

***just remember false is left (like left handed people are evil, or false) – then everything else is true.*

Dissection Flap in the Abdomen - Vocab Trivia:

- **Static** = dissection flap in the feeding artery (usually treated by stenting)
- **Dynamic** = dissection flap dangling in front of ostium (usually treated with fenestration).

It can be hard to tell these apart. If asked I'd expect them to just use the vocab words.

THIS vs THAT: Aneurysm with Mural Thrombus VS Thrombosed Dissection

- The dissection should spiral, the thrombus tends to drop straight down
- Intimal Calcs – the dissection will displace them.

Intramural Hematoma

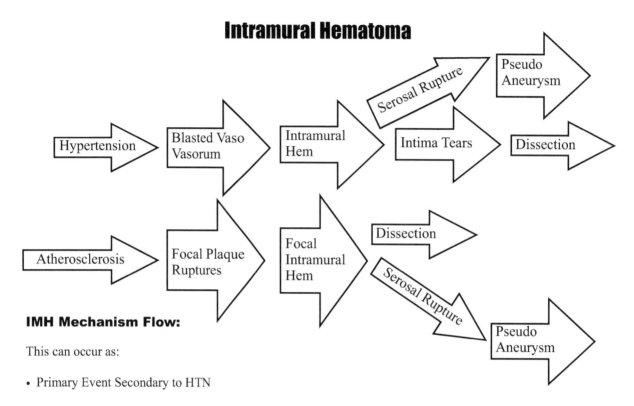

IMH Mechanism Flow:

This can occur as:

- Primary Event Secondary to HTN

- Secondary Event usually From Atherosclerosis, but also as a Focal Hematoma on the road to dissection

For the purpose of multiple choice – the cause is HTN

Ways this can be shown:

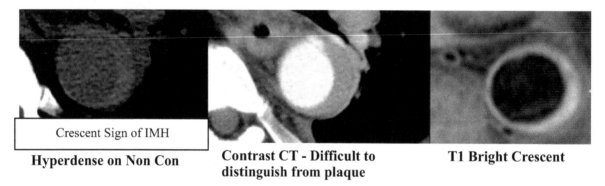

Crescent Sign of IMH

Hyperdense on Non Con | **Contrast CT - Difficult to distinguish from plaque** | **T1 Bright Crescent**

Treatment:
- Also uses the Stanford A vs B idea
- Some people will say Type A = Surgery, Type B medical
- This is controversial and unlikely to be tested

Predictors of Shitty Outcome:
- Most of these will spontaneously regress. These are the things that make that less likely:
  - Hematoma Thickness Greater than 2 cm
  - Association with aneurysmal dilation of the aorta – 5 cm or more
  - Progression to dissection or penetrating ulcer
  - IMH + Penetrating Ulcer has a worse outcome compared to IMH + Dissection

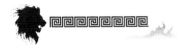 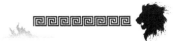
THIS vs THAT: Aneurysm vs Pseudo-aneurysm – The distinction between a true and false aneurysm lends itself well to multiple choice testing. A true aneurysm is an enlargement of the lumen of the vessel to 1.5 times its normal diameter. True = 3 layers are intact. In a false (pseudo) aneurysm all 3 layers are NOT intact, and it is essentially a contained rupture. The risk of actual rupture is obviously higher with false aneurysm. It can sometimes be difficult to tell, but as a general rule fusiform aneurysms are true, and saccular aneurysms might be false. Classic causes of pseudoaneurysm include trauma, cardiologists (groin sticks), infection (mycotic), pancreatitis, and some vasculitides. On ultrasound they could show you the classic yin/yang sign, with "to and fro" flow on pulsed Doppler. The yin/yang sign can be seen in saccular true aneurysms, so you shouldn't call it on that alone (unless that's all they give you). To and Fro flow within the aneurysm neck + clinical history is the best way to tell them apart.

SVC Syndrome - Occurs secondary to complete or near complete obstruction of flow in the SVC from external compression (lymphoma, lung cancer) or intravascular obstruction (Central venous catheter, or pacemaker wire with thrombus). A less common but testable cause is fibrosing mediastinitis (just think histoplasmosis). The dude is gonna have face, neck, and bilateral arm swelling.

Traumatic Pseudoaneurysm –

Again a pseudoaneurysm is basically a contained rupture. The most common place to see this (in a living patient) is the **aortic isthmus (90%)**. This is supposedly the result of tethering from the ligamentum arteriosum. The second and third most common sites are the ascending aorta and diaphragmatic hiatus - respectively. Ascending aortic injury is actually probably number one, it just kills them in the field so you don't see it. They could show you a CXR with a wide mediastinum, deviation of the NG Tube to the right, depressed left main bronchus, or left apical cap and want you to suspect acute injury.

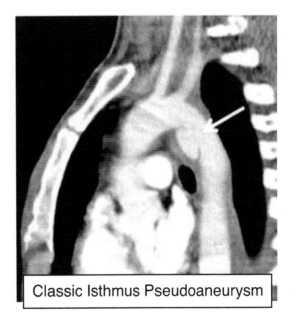
Classic Isthmus Pseudoaneurysm

Ascending Aortic Calcifications - There are only a few causes of ascending aortic calcifications, as atherosclerosis typically spares the ascending aorta. **Takayasu and Syphilis** should come to mind. The real-life significance is the clamping of the aorta may be difficult during CABG.

Aneurysm - Defined as enlargement of the artery to 1.5 times its expected diameter (> 4 cm Ascending and Transverse, > 3.5 cm Descending, > 3.0 cm Abdominal). Atherosclerosis is the most common overall cause. Medial degeneration is the most common cause in the ascending aorta. Patients with connective tissue (Marfans, Ehlers Danlos) diseases tend to involve the aortic root. *When I say cystic medial necrosis you should think Marfans.* Aneurysms may develop in any segment of the aorta, but most involve the infra-renal abdominal aorta. This varies based on risk factors, rate of growth, etc... but a general rule is surgical repair for aneurysms at 6cm in the chest (5.5 cm with collagen vascular disease) and 5 cm in the abdomen.

Sinus of Valsalva Aneurysm – Aneurysms of the valsalva sinus (aortic sinus) are rare in real life, but have been known to show up on multiple choice tests. Factoids worth knowing are that they are more common in Asian Men, and **typically involve the right sinus**. They can be congenital or acquired (infectious). VSD is the most common associated cardiac anomaly. Rupture can lead to cardiac tamponade. Surgical repair with Bentall procedure.

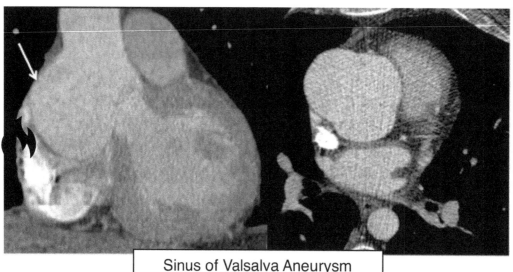

Sinus of Valsalva Aneurysm

Endoleaks - There are 5 types, and type 2 is the most common. These are discussed in detail in the IR chapter.

Rupture / Impending Rupture- Peri-aortic stranding, rapid enlargement (10 mm or more per year), or pain are warning signs of impending rupture. A retroperitoneal hematoma adjacent to an AAA is the most common imaging finding of actual rupture. The most common indicator for elective repair is the maximum diameter of the aneurysm , "Sac Size Matters," with treatment usually around 6 cm (5.5 cm in patients with collagen vascular disease). A thick, circumferential mural thrombus is thought to be protective against rupture. Enlargement of the patent lumen can indicate lysis of thrombus and predispose to rupture.

Findings of Impending Rupture	
Draped Aorta Sign	Posterior wall of the aorta drapes over the vertebral column.
Increased Aneurysm Size	10 mm or more increased per year
Focal Discontinuity in Circumferential Wall Calcifications	
Hyperdense Crescent Sign	Well-defined peripheral crescent of increased attenuation. One of the most specific manifestations of impending rupture.

Mycotic Aneurysm – These are most often **saccular** and most often **pseudoaneurysms**. They are prone to rupture. They most often occur via hematogenous seeding in the setting of septicemia (**endocarditis**). They can occur from direct seeding via a psoas abscess or vertebral osteomyelitis (but this is less common). **Most occur in the thoracic or supra-renal aorta** (most atherosclerotic aortic aneurysms are infra-renal). Typical findings include saccular shape, lobular contours, peri-aortic inflammation, abscess, and peri-aortic gas. They tend to expand faster than atherosclerotic aneurysms. In general small, asymptomatic, and unruptured.

 Gamesmanship - If you see a saccular aneurysm of the aorta (especially the abdominal aorta) you have to lead with infection.

NF 1 – One of the more common neurological genetic disorders, which you usually think about causing all the skin stuff (Café au lait spots and freckling), and bilateral optic gliomas. Although uncommon, vascular findings also occur in this disorder. **Aneurysms and stenoses are sometimes seen in the aorta and larger arteries**, while dysplastic features are found in smaller vessels. **Renal artery stenosis can occur, leading to renovascular hypertension** (found in 5% of children with NF). **The classic look is orificial renal artery stenosis presenting with hypertension in a teenager or child.** The mechanism is actually Dysplasia of the arterial wall itself (less common from peri-arterial neurofibroma).

Marfan Syndrome – Genetic disorder caused by mutations of the fibrillin gene (step 1 question). There are lots of systemic manifestations including ectopic lens, being tall, pectus deformity, scoliosis, long fingers etc… Vascular findings can be grouped into aneurysm, dissection, and pulmonary artery dilation:

- *Aneurysm:* Dilation with Marfans is classically described as **"Annuloaortic ectasia"**, with dilatation of the aortic root. The dilation usually begins with the aortic sinuses, and then progresses into the sinotubular junction, ultimately involving the aortic annulus. **Dilatation of the aortic root leads to aortic valve insufficiency**. Severe aortic regurgitation occurs that may progress to aortic root dissection or rupture. The mechanism for all this nonsense is that disruption of the media elastic fibers causes aortic stiffening, and predisposes to aneurysm and dissection. The buzzword for the Marfans ascending aneurysm is **"tulip bulb."** They are usually repaired earlier than normal aneurysm (typically around 5.5 cm).

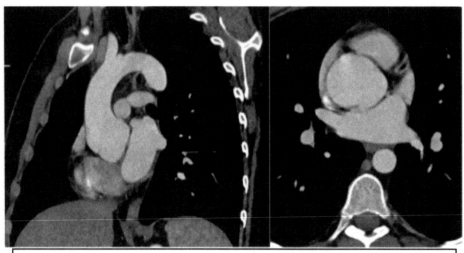

Marfan's - *Annuloaortic Ectasia*, with dilation of the aortic root

- *Dissection:* Recurrent dissections are common, and even "triple barreled dissection" can be seen (dissections on both sides of a true channel).

- *Pulmonary Artery Enlargement:* Just like dilation of the aorta, pulmonary artery enlargement favors the root.

Loeys Dietz Syndrome - Despite the name, this is actually not a Puerto Rican DJ. Instead think of this as the really shitty version of Marfans. They have a terrible prognosis, and rupture their aortas all the time. **Vessels are very tortuous** (twisty). They also have crazy wide eyes (hypertelorism).

Loeys Dietz Classic Triad:
1. Hypertelorism (frog eyes),
2. Bifid uvula or cleft palate
3. Aortic aneurysm with tortuosity

Classic Look: Crazy twisty vertebral arteries

Ehlers-Danlos - This one is a disorder in collagen, with lots of different subtypes. They have the stretchy skin, hypermobile joints, blood vessel fragility with bleeding diatheses. Invasive diagnostic studies such as conventional angiography and **other percutaneous procedures should be avoided** because of the excessive risk of arterial dissection. Imaging characteristics of aortic aneurysms in Ehlers-Danlos syndrome **resemble those in Marfan syndrome, often involving the aortic root.** Aneurysms of the abdominal visceral arteries are common as well.

Syphilitic (Luetic) Aneurysm – This is super rare and only seen in patients with untreated tertiary syphilis. There is classically a saccular appearance and it involves the ascending aorta as well as the aortic arch. Classic description **"saccular asymmetric aortic aneurysm with involvement of the aortic root branches. "** Often heavily calcified **"tree bark" intimal calcifications**. Coronary artery narrowing (at the ostium) is seen 30% of the time. Aortic valve insufficiency is also common.

Aortoenteric Fistula - These come in two flavors: (a) Primary, and (b) Secondary.

* **Primary:** Very, very, very rare. Refers to an A-E fistula without history of instrumentation. They are only seen in the setting of aneurysm and atherosclerosis.

* **Secondary:** Much more common. They are **seen after surgery** with or without stent graft placement.

The question is usually what part of the bowel is involved, and the answer is **3rd and 4th portions of the duodenum**. The second most likely question is A-E fistula vs perigraft infection (without fistula)? The answer to that is unless you see contrast from the aorta into the bowel lumen (usually duodenum), you can't tell. Both of them have ectopic perigraft gas > 4 weeks post repair, both have perigraft fluid and edema, both lose the fat place between the bowel and aorta (tethering of the duodenum to the anterior wall of the aorta), both can have pseudoaneurysm formation.

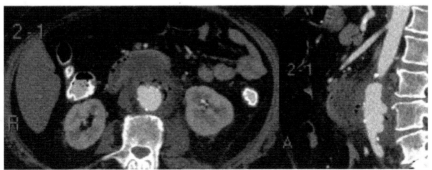

Aortoenteric Fistula - *Primary Type*

Inflammatory Aneurysms - Most are **symptomatic**, more common in **young men**, and associated with increased risk of rupture regardless of their size. Unlike patients with atherosclerotic AAA, most with the inflammatory variant have an **elevated ESR**. Their etiology is not well understood but may be related to periaortic retroperitoneal fibrosis or other autoimmune disorders (SLE, Giant Cell, RA). **Smoking is apparently a strong risk factor**, and smoking cessation is the first step in medical therapy. **In 1/3 of cases hydronephrosis or renal failure** is present at the time of diagnosis because the inflammatory process usually involves the ureters. Imaging findings include a thickened wall and inflammatory or fibrotic changes in the periaortic regions. Often there is asymmetrical thickening of the aorta with sparing of the posterior wall (helps differentiate it from vasculitis).

Leriche Syndrome - Refers to complete occlusion of the aorta distal to the renal arteries (most often at the aortic bifurcation). It is often secondary to bad atherosclerosis. There can be large collaterals.

Clinical Triad:

- Limp Dick (impotence)
- Ass claudication
- Absence femoral pulses

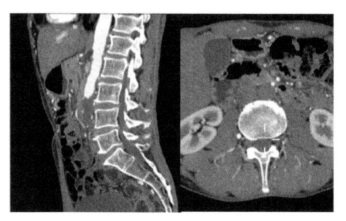

Leriche Syndrome - *Complete occlusion of the aortal distal to the renal arteries*

Mid Aortic Syndrome (Coarctation of the Abdominal Aorta) - Refers to progressive narrowing of the abdominal aorta and its major branches. Compared to Leriche, this is higher, and longer in segment. It's also a total freaking zebra. It tends to affect children / young adults. This thing is characterized by progressive narrowing of the aorta. It is **NOT secondary to arteritis or atherosclerosis** but instead the result of some intrauterine insult (maybe) with fragmentation of the elastic media.

This also has a clinical triad:

- **HTN (most common presenting symptom)** - *this is the most common cause of death if not treated*
- Weak or Absent Femoral Pulses
- Claudication
- Renal failure

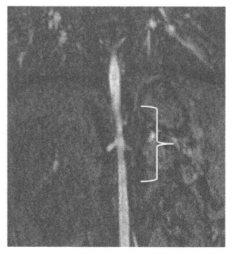

Mid Aortic Syndrome - *Narrow aorta without arteritis or atherosclerosis*

Aortic Coarctation -

- There are two subtypes (as shown in the chart)

- Strong Association with **Turners Syndrome** (15-20%).

- **Bicuspid Aortic valve** is the most common associated defect (80%).

- They have more **berry aneurysms**.

- **Figure 3 sign** (appearance of CXR).

- **Rib Notching**: most often involves 4th - 8th ribs. It does NOT involve the 1st and 2nd because those are fed by the costocervical trunk.

THIS vs THAT: Coarctation of the Aortic (Narrowing the of the Aortic Lumen)	
Infantile	**Adult**
Presents with heart failure within the first week of life.	Leg Claudication BP differences between arms and legs.
Pre-Ductal (Before the left Subclavian A.)	Post-Ductal (Distal to left Subclavian A.)
Aortic Arch = Hypoplastic	Aortic Arch = Normal Diameter
	Collateral Formation is More Likely

Pseudocoarctation - This is a favorite of multiple choice writers. You will have elongation with narrowing and kinking of the aorta. It really looks like a coarctation, BUT there is **NO pressure gradient, collateral formation, or rib notching** - that is the most likely question. The second most likely question is the area of aneurysmal dilation may occur distal to the areas of narrowing in pseudocoarctation, and they may become progressively dilated and should therefore be followed.

Thoracic Outlet Syndrome – Congenital or acquired compression of the Subclavian vessels (artery and vein), and brachial plexus nerves as they pass through the thoracic inlet. *It is a spectrum: Nerve (95%) >>>>>> Subclavian Vein >> Subclavian Artery*. With symptoms varying depending on what is compressed. **Compression by the anterior scalene muscle is the most common cause**. However, cervical rib, muscular hypertrophy, fibrous bands, Pagets, tumor etc… can all cause symptoms. Treatment is usually surgical removal of the rib / muscle. The classic way to show this is arms up and arms down angiography (occlusion occurs with arms up).

Paget Schroetter – This is **essentially thoracic outlet syndrome, with development of a venous thrombus in the Subclavian vein**. It's sometimes called "effort thrombosis" because it's associated with athletes (pitchers, weightlifters) who are raising their arms a lot. They will use catheter directed lysis on these dudes, and surgical release of the offending agent as above. Stenting isn't usually done (and can only be done after surgery to avoid getting the stent crushed).

Pulmonary Artery Aneurysm/Pseudoaneurysm – Think about three things for multiple choice; (1) **Iatrogenic from Swan Ganz catheter *most common** (2) Behcets,   (3) Chronic PE. When they want to lead Swan Ganz they may say something like "patient in the ICU." The buzzwords for Behcets are: "Turkish descent", and "mouth and genital ulcers."

- **Hughes-Stovin Syndrome:** This is a zebra cause of pulmonary artery aneurysm that is similar (and maybe the same thing) as Behcets. It is characterized by recurrent thrombophlebitis and pulmonary artery aneurysm formation and rupture.

- **Rasmussen Aneurysm:** This has a cool name, which instantly makes it high yield for testing. This is a pulmonary artery **pseudoaneurysm secondary to pulmonary TB**. It usually involves the upper lobes in the setting of reactivation TB.

- **Tetralogy of Fallot Repair Gone South:** So another possible testable scenario is the patch aneurysm, from the RVOT repair.

Splenic Artery Aneurysm: The most common visceral arterial aneurysm (3rd most common abdominal - behind aorta and iliac).

Etiology of these things depends on who you ask. Some source will say arteriosclerosis is the most important cause. However, it seems that most sources will say that arteriosclerosis less important and things like *portal hypertension* and a *history of multiple pregnancy* are more important. **More common in pregnancy, and more likely to rupture in pregnancy.**

> **- High Risk For Rupture -**
> - Liver Transplantation
> - Portal Hypertension
> - Pregnancy
> - Connective Tissue Disorders
> - Alpha 1 Antitrypsin Def

Most are located in the distal artery. False aneurysms are associated with pancreatitis.

An important mimic is the islet cell pancreatic tumor (which is hypervascular). Don't be a dumb ass and try to biopsy the aneurysm. If you are forced to choose *which ones to treat* I guess I'd go with: anything over 2 cm, any pseudoaneurysm, and any in a women planning on getting pregnant.

SMA Aneurysm: All SMA aneurysms should be treated - as there is a high rate of rupture and association with mesenteric ischemia.

Hepatic Artery Aneurysm: Treated if the patient is symptomatic or size exceeds 2cm (just like the spleen). In patients with FMD or polyarteritis nodosa - typically they are treated regardless of size.

Median Arcuate Ligament Syndrome (Dunbar Syndrome) : This is compression of the celiac artery by the median arcuate ligament (fibrous band that connects the diaphragm). Most people actually have some degree of compression, but it's not a syndrome until there are symptoms (abdominal pain, weight loss). Typical age is 20-40 years old. The buzzword is **"hooked appearance."** It's classically shown on angiography and they will want you to know that it gets **worse with expiration**. It can actually lead to the development of pancreaticoduodenal collaterals and aneurysm formation. It's treated surgically.

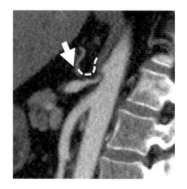

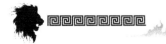 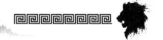
This can be broadly classified as acute or chronic.

Chronic: Significant Stenosis of 2 out of 3 main mesenteric vessels + symptoms ("food fear") , LUQ pain after eating, pain out of proportion to exam). Some practical pearls are that you can have bad disease and no symptoms if you have good collaterals. Alternatively if you have bad one-vessel disease you can have symptoms if you have crappy collaterals. Remember that the *splenic flexure ("Griffith's Point") is the most common* because it's the watershed of the SMA and IMA.

Acute: This comes from 4 main causes. Arterial, Venous, Non-occlussive, and Strangulation.

- **Arterial:** Occlusive emboli (usually more distal, at branch points), or Thrombus (usually closer to the ostium). Vasculitis can also cause it. The SMA is most commonly affected. Bowel typically has a **thinner wall** (no arterial inflow), and is **NOT typically dilated**. After reperfusion the bowel wall will become thick, with a target appearance.

- **Venous: Dilation with wall thickening** *(8-9mm, with < 5mm being normal)* is more common. Fat stranding and ascites are especially common findings in venous occlusion.

- **Non-Occlusive**: Seen in patients in shock or on pressors. This is the most difficult to diagnose on CT. The involved bowel segments are often thickened. Enhancement is variable. *Look for delayed filling of the portal vein at 70 seconds.*

- **Strangulation:** This is almost always secondary to a closed loop obstruction. This is basically a mixed arterial and venous picture, with **congested dilated bowel**. Hemorrhage may be seen in the bowel wall. The lumen is often fluid-filled.

Trivia: Mesenteric Ischemia has a described association with SMA Aneurysm.

Mesenteric Ischemia			
Arterial	**Venous**	**Strangulation**	**Non-Occlusive**
Thin Bowel Wall (thick after reperfusion)	Thick Bowel Wall	Thick Bowel Wall	Thick Bowel Wall
Diminished Enhancement	Variable	Variable	Variable
Bowel *Not Dilated*	Moderate Dilation	Severe Dilation (and fluid filled)	Bowel *Not Dilated*
Mesentery *Not Hazy* (until it infarcts)	<u>Hazy</u> with Ascites	<u>Hazy</u> with Ascites, and "whirl sign" with closed loop.	Mesentery *Not Hazy* (until it infarcts)

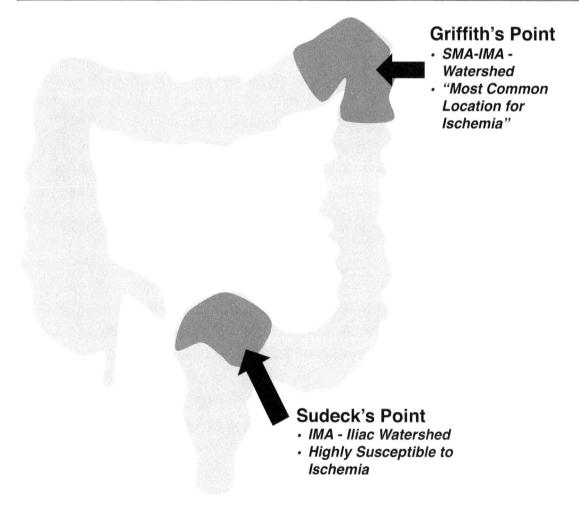

Griffith's Point
- *SMA-IMA - Watershed*
- *"Most Common Location for Ischemia"*

Sudeck's Point
- *IMA - Iliac Watershed*
- *Highly Susceptible to Ischemia*

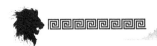
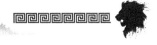
This is my general algorithm if I see angry (thick walled) bowel

—

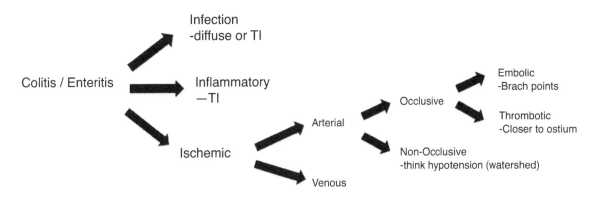

Colonic Angiodysplasia – This is the second most common cause of colonic arterial bleeding (diverticulosis being number one). This is primarily **right sided** with angiography demonstrating a cluster of small arteries during the arterial phase (along the antimesenteric border of the colon), with *early opacification of dilated draining veins* that persists late into the venous phase. There is an **association with aortic stenosis which carries the eponym Heyde Syndrome** (which instantly makes it high yield for multiple choice).

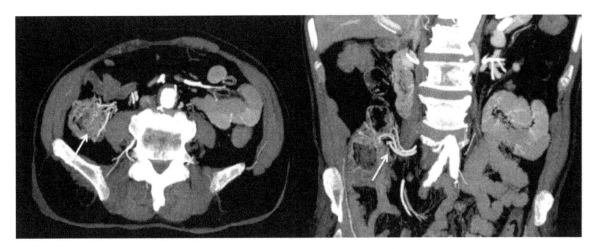

Colonic Angiodysplasia

Osler Weber Rendu (Hereditary Hemorrhagic Telangiectasia) – This is an AD multi-system disorder characterized by multiple AVMs. On step 1 they used to show you the tongue / mouth with the telangiectasis and a history of recurrent bloody nose. Now, they will likely show multiple hepatic AVMs or multiple pulmonary AVMs. Extensive shunting in the liver can actually cause biliary necrosis and bile leak. They can have high output cardiac failure. ***Most die from stroke or brain abscess.***

 Gamesmanship "Next Step" - If the syndrome is suspected, these guys need CT of the Lung & Liver (with contrast), plus a Brain MR / MRA

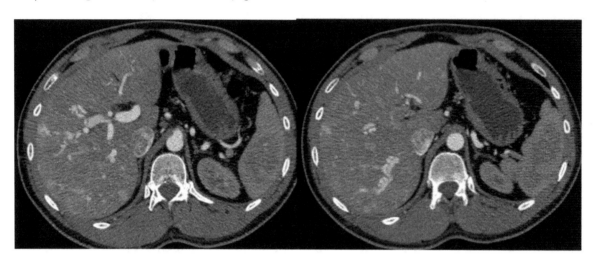

Renal Artery Stenosis – Narrowing of the renal artery most commonly occurs secondary to atherosclerosis (75%). This type of narrowing is usually near the ostium, and can be stented. FMD is the second most common cause and typically has a beaded appearance sparing the ostium (should not be stented). Additional more rare causes include PAN, Takayasu, NF-1, and Radiation.

FMD (Fibromuscular Dysplasia) – A non-atherosclerotic vascular disease, primarily affecting the renal arteries of young white women.

Things to know:

- Renovascular HTN in Young Women = FMD

- Renal arteries are the most commonly involved (carotid #2, iliac #3)

- There are 3 types, but just remember medial is the most common (95%)

- They are predisposed to spontaneous dissection

 - Buzzword = String of Beads

- Treatment = Angioplasty WITHOUT stenting. Eating walnuts helps (seriously, there is a paper on it). Eating cashews does not help (same paper), which is too bad because cashews are delicious... and walnuts taste like shit.

Nutcracker Syndrome – Usually a healthy female 30s-40s. The left renal vein gets smashed as it slides under the SMA, with resulting abdominal pain (left flank) and hematuria. The left renal vein gets smashed a lot, but it's not a syndrome without symptoms. Since the left gonadal vein drains into the left renal vein, it can also cause left testicle pain in men, and LLQ pain in women.

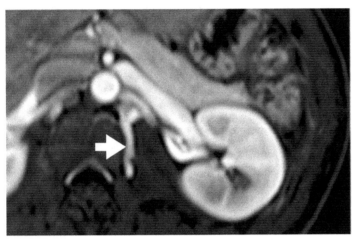

Nutcracker: Renal Vein, Smashed by SMA. Note the prominent venous collateral (arrow)

Nutcracker Diagnostic Gold Standard: Retrograde venography with renal / caval pressure measurements

SAM (Segmental Arterial Mediolysis) – Targets the splanchnic arteries in the elderly, and the coronaries in young adults. Not a true vasculitis, with no significant inflammation. It's complicated but essentially the media of the vessel turns to crap, and you get a bunch of aneurysms. The aneurysms are often multiple. The way this is shown is **multiple abdominal splanchnic artery saccular aneurysms, dissections, and occlusion** – *this is the disease hallmark. Can also be shown as spontaneous intra-abdominal hemorrhage.*

> WTF is a *"Splanchnic"* Artery ?
>
> Typically the splanchnic circulation of the GI tract refers to the Celiac, SMA, and IMA.

Pelvic Congestion Syndrome – This is a controversial entity, sometimes grouped in the fibromyalgia spectrum. Patients often have "chronic abdominal pain." They also often wear a lot of rings and drink orange soda. The classic demographic is a depressed, multiparous, pre-menopausal women with chronic pelvic pain. Venous obstruction at the left renal vein (nutcracker compression) or incompetent ovarian vein valves leads to **multiple dilated parauterine veins**. This very "real" diagnosis can be treated by your local Interventional Radiologist via ovarian vein embolization.

Testicular Varicocele – Abnormal dilation of veins in the pampiniform plexus. Most cases are idiopathic and **most (98%) are found on the left side** *(left vein is longer, and drains into renal vein at right angle)*. They can also occur on the left, secondary to the above mentioned "nutcracker syndrome." They **can cause infertility**. "Non-decompressible" is a buzzword for badness. Some sources state that neoplasm is actually the most likely cause of **non-decompressible varicocele** in men over 40 years of age; (left renal malignancy invading the renal vein). Right-sided varicocele can be a sign of malignancy as well. When it's new, and on the right side (in an adult), you should raise concern for a pelvic or abdominal malignancy. New right-sided varicocele in an adult should make you think renal cell carcinoma, retroperitoneal fibrosis, or adhesions.

Non-Decompressible = Bad

Right = Bad

Left = Ok

Bilateral = Ok (probably)

 Gamesmanship - This diagnosis is the classic next step question of all next step questions because you need to recognize when this common diagnosis is associated with something bad.

• Isolated Right Varicocele = Get an ABD CT (or MR, or US)

• Non-decompressible Varicocele = Get an ABD CT (or MR, or US)

• Bilateral Decompressible Varicoceles = Might need treatment if infertile etc.., but doesn't need additional cancer hunting imaging.

• Isolated Left Varicocele = Might need treatment if infertile etc.., but doesn't need additional cancer hunting imaging.

Uterine AVM – This can present with life threatening massive genital bleeding. Rarely they can present with CHF. They come in two flavors (a) Congenital, and (b) Acquired. **Acquired occurs after D&C**, abortion, or multiple pregnancies. They are most likely to show this on color Doppler with serpiginous structures in the myometrium with low resistance high velocity patterns. This one needs embolization. Could look similar to retained products of conception (clinical history will be different, and *RPOC is usually centered in the endometrium rather than the myometrium*).

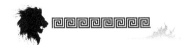 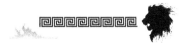

May Thurner – A syndrome resulting in DVT of the left common iliac vein. The pathology is **compression of the left common iliac vein by the right common iliac artery**. Treatment is thrombolysis and stenting. *If they show you a swollen left leg, this is probably the answer.* PE and acute limb ischemia from severe venous obstruction (Phlegmasia cerulea dolens) are two described complications.

Popliteal Aneurysm – This is the most common peripheral arterial aneurysm (2nd most common overall, to the aorta). The main issue with these things is distal thromboembolism, which can be limb threatening. There is a strong and frequently tested association with AAA.

- *30-50% of patients with popliteal aneurysms have a AAA*

- *10% of patients with AAA have popliteal aneurysms*

- *50-70% of popliteal aneurysms are bilateral*

The **most dreaded complication of a popliteal artery aneurysm is an acute limb** from thrombosis and distal embolization of thrombus pooling in the aneurysm.

Popliteal Entrapment – Symptomatic compression or occlusion of the popliteal artery due to the developmental relationship with the **medial head of the gastrocnemius** (less commonly the popliteus). Medial deviation of the popliteal artery is supposedly diagnostic. This usually occurs in young men (<30). These patients may have *normal pulses that decrease with plantar flexion or dorsiflexion of the foot.* They will show you either a MRA or conventional angiogram in rest and then stress (dorsi / plantar flexion) to show the artery occluding.

Hypothenar Hammer – Caused by blunt trauma (history of working with a jack-hammer) to the ulnar artery and superficial palmar arch. The impact occurs against the hook of the hamate. Arterial wall damage leads to aneurysm formation with or without thrombosis of the vessel. Emboli may form, causing distal obstruction of digits (this can cause confusion with the main DDx Buergers). Look for **corkscrew configuration of the superficial palmar arch, occlusion of the ulnar artery, or pseudoaneurysm of the ulnar artery**.

Venous Thromboembolism (VTE) - Blanket term used to refer to PE and DVT (PE and DVT are both forms of VTE).

Trivia: You are <u>more likely to develop VTE if you are paraplegic</u> vs tetraplegic.

Having said that, VTE is more likely in "motor complete" AIS A patients (those that have lost motor and sensory) vs motor incomplete AIS B,C,D (those with some residual sensory or motor function) -- which is more intuitive. Quad being worse than tetra for VTE risk makes zero sense (and therefore makes a good trivia question).

Peripheral Vascular Malformations - About 40% of vascular malformations involve the extremities (the other 40% are head and neck, and 20% is thorax). Different than hemangiomas, vascular malformations generally increase proportionally as the child grows. This dude Jackson classified vascular malformation as either low flow or high flow. Low flow would include venous, lymphatic, capillary, and mixes of the like. **High flow has an arterial component.** Treatment is basically determined by high or low flow.

Klippel-Trenaunay Syndrome (KTS) - This is often combined with **Parkes-Weber which is a true high flow AV malformation.** KTS has a triad of port wine nevi, bony or soft tissue hypertrophy (localized gigantism), and a venous malformation. A persistent sciatic vein is often associated. The marginal vein of Servelle (some superficial vein in the lateral calf and thigh) is pathognomonic (it's basically a great saphenous on the wrong side).

Additional trivia: 20% have GI involvement and can bleed, if the system is big enough it can eat your platelets (**Kasabach Merritt**). Basically, **if you see a MRA/MRV of the leg with a bunch of superficial vessels (and no deep drainage) you should think about this thing**.

- *KTS* = Low Flow (venous)

- *Parkes Weber* = High Flow (arterial)

- *"Klippel Trenaunay Weber"* = Something people say when they (a) don't know what they are talking about, or (b) don't know what kind of malformation it is and want to use a blanket term.

ABIs – So basic familiarity with the so called "Ankle to Brachial Index" can occasionally come in handy, with regard to peripheral arterial disease. This is basically a ratio of systolic pressure in the leg over systolic blood pressure in the arm. Diabetics can sometimes have unreliable numbers (usually high), because dense vascular calcifications won't let the vessels compress.

Opinions vary on what the various cut off numbers mean. Most people will agree that you can safely deploy the phrase "peripheral arterial disease" if the resting ABI is less than 0.90

You can also deploy the following generalizations: 0.5-0.3 = claudication, < 0.3 = rest pain

**More on this in the IR chapter

Intimal Hyperplasia – "The bane of endovascular intervention." This is not a true disease but a response to blood vessel wall damage. Basically this is an exuberant healing response that leads to intimal thickening which can lead to stenosis. You hear it talked about the most in IR after they have revascularized a limb. Re-Stenosis that occurs 3-12 months after angioplasty is probably from intimal hyperplasia. It's sneaky to treat and often resists balloon dilation and/ or reoccurs. If you put a bare stent in place it may grow through the cracks and happen anyway. If you put a covered stent in, it may still occur at the edges of the stent. The take home point is that it's a pain in the ass, and if they show an angiogram with a stent in place, that now appears to be losing flow, this is probably the answer.

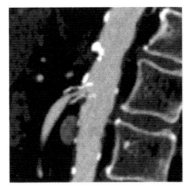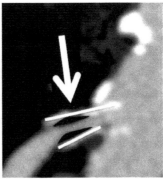

Intimal Hyperplasia
-dark stuff growing along the inside of the stent walls

Cystic Adventitial Disease – This uncommon disorder classically **affects the popliteal artery, of young men**. Basically you have one or **multiple mucoid-filled cysts** developing in the outer media and adventitia. As the cysts grow, they compress the artery.

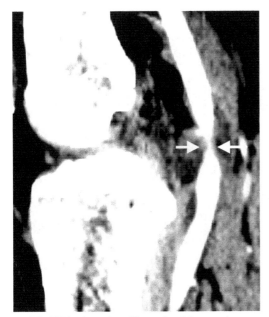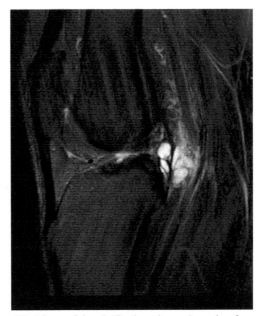

MIP CTA showing Vascular Narrowing

Fluid sensitive MR showing a bunch of cysts around the vessel, extrinsically narrowing it

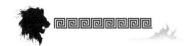 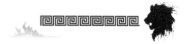

Basically all vasculitis looks the same, with wall thickening, occlusions, dilations, and aneurysm formation. The trick to telling them apart is the age of the patient, the gender / race, and the vessels affected. Classically, they are broken up into large vessel, medium vessel, small vessel ANCA +, and small vessel ANCA negative.

Large:

Takayasu - "The pulseless disease." This vasculitis loves **young Asian girls** (usually 15-30 years old). If they mention the word "Asian," this is likely to be the answer. Also, if they show you a **vasculitis involving the aorta** this is likely the answer. In the acute phase there will be both **wall thickening and wall enhancement**. There can be occlusion of the major aortic branches, or dilation of the aorta and its branches. The aortic valve is often involved (can cause stenosis or AI). In the late phase there is classically diffuse narrowing distally. The pulmonary arteries are commonly involved, with the typical appearance of peripheral pruning.

If anyone was a big enough jerk to ask, there are 5 types with variable involvement of the aorta and its branches. Which type is which is beyond the scope of the exam, just know type 3 is most common - involves arch and abdominal aorta.

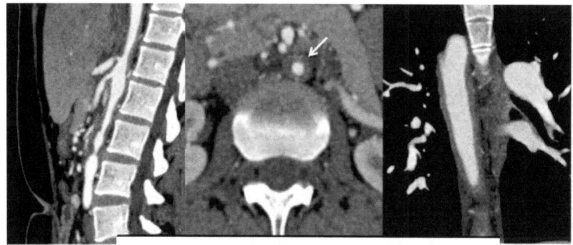

Takayasu - Wall Thickening Involving the Aorta

Giant Cell (GCA) – The most common primary system vasculitis. This vasculitis loves **old men** (usually 70-80)** *although there are a few papers that will say this is slightly more common in women.* This vasculitis involves the aorta and its major branches particularly those of the external carotid (**temporal artery**). This can be shown in two ways: (1) an ultrasound of the temporal artery, demonstrating wall thickening, or (2) CTA / MRA or even angiogram of the armpit area (Subclavian/ Axillary/ Brachial), demonstrating wall thickening, occlusions, dilations, and aneurysm. Think about it as the **part of the body that would be compressed by crutches** (old men need crutches).

Trivia worth knowing:

• ESR and CRP are markedly elevated,

• Disease responds to steroids.

• "Gold Standard" for diagnosis is temporal artery biopsy (although it's often negative).

• Clinical connection between GCA and <u>polymyalgia rheumatica</u>, (they might be different phases of the same disease). History might be "morning stillness in shoulders and hips."

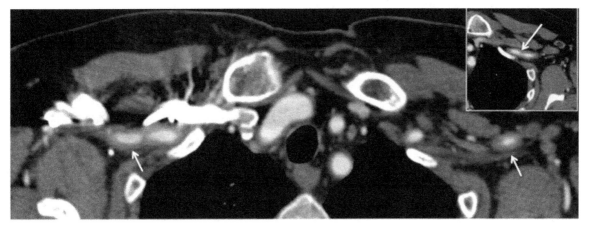

Giant Cell - *"Armpit"* Vessel Thickening

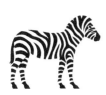
Cogan Syndrome – Total Zebra probably not even worth mentioning. It is a large vessel vasculitis that targets children and young adults. It likes the eyes and ears causing optic neuritis, uveitis, and audiovestibular symptoms resembling Menieres. They can also get aortitis, and those that do have a worse prognosis.

Basically, **kid with eye and ear symptoms + or – aortitis.**

Medium

PAN (Polyarteritis Nodosa) – This is one of two vasculitides (*the other being Buergers*) that is more common in men. **PAN is more common in a MAN**. This can effect a lot of places with the big 3 being Renal (90%), Cardiac (70%), and GI (50-70%). Typically we are talking about **microaneurysm formation**, primarily at branch points, followed by infarction. I would expect this to be shown either as a CTA or angiogram of the **kidneys with microaneurysms**, or a kidney with areas of infarct (multiple wedge shaped areas).

Trivia to know is the **association with Hep B.**

Also, as a point of trivia the micro-aneurysm formation in the kidney can also be seen in patients who abuse Crystal Meth (sometimes called a "speed kidney").

Kawasaki Disease – Probably the most common vasculitis in children (HSP also common). Think about this as a cause of coronary vessel aneurysm. A **calcified coronary artery aneurysm shown on CXR is a very rare aunt Minnie**.

-Coronary Artery Aneurysms > 8mm are "Giant" and prone to badness including MI

-Coronary Artery Aneurysms < 8mm may regress

Clinical Trivia:
"Fever for 5 Days"
• Strawberry Tongue • Neck Lymph Nodes • Rash of Palms of Hands / Soles of Feet • Sore Throat Diarrhea
• "Etiology Unknown"

Small Vessel Disease (ANCA +)

Wegeners - I think about upper respiratory tract (sinuses), lower respiratory tract (lungs), and kidneys. cANCA is (+) 90% of the time. Ways this is shown are the **nasal perforation** (like a cocaine addict) and the **cavitary lung lesions**.

Churg Strauss – This is a necrotizing pulmonary vasculitis which is in the spectrum of Eosinophilic lung disease. They always have asthma and eosinophilia. **Transient peripheral lung consolidation** or ground glass regions is the most frequent feature. Cavitation is rare (this should make you think Wegeners instead). They are pANCA (+) 75% if the time.

Microscopic Polyangiitis – Affects the kidneys and lungs. Diffuse pulmonary hemorrhage is seen in about 1/3 of the cases. It is pANCA (+) 80% of the time.

As I've previously mentioned, you aren't supposed to say "Wegener" - because apparently he ate his boogers, and was a Nazi. He also could not (more likely deliberately chose not to) correctly pronounce the word "Gyro." No matter how many times people corrected him. Dude- it is "YEE-roh."

Wegener was truly one of histories greatest assholes.

So we don't say his name. Instead say "Granulomatosis with polyangiitis."

You know who else was a Nazi?? Henry Ford. No one ever talks about that… Google it - he wrote a book called *"The International Jew, the World's Foremost Problem,"* and got an award from Hitler.

Small Vessel Disease (ANCA -)

HSP (Henoch-Schonlein Purpura) – The most common vasculitis in children (usually age 4-11). Although it is a systemic disease, GI symptoms are most common (painful bloody diarrhea). It is a common lead point for intussusception. They could show this two classic ways: (1) ultrasound with a **doughnut sign for intussusception**, or (2) as a ultrasound of the **scrotum showing massive skin edema**. A less likely (but also possible) way to show this case would be multi-focal bowel wall thickening, or a plain film with thumbprinting.

Behcets – Classic history is mouth ulcers and genital ulcers in someone with Turkish descent. It can cause thickening of the aorta, but for the purpose of multiple choice test I expect the question will be **pulmonary artery aneurysm**.

Buergers – This vasculitis is strongly associated with **smokers**. It affects both small and medium vessels in the arms and legs (more common in legs). Although it is more commonly seen in the legs, it is more commonly tested with a hand angiogram. The characteristic features are extensive arterial occlusive disease with the development of corkscrew collateral vessels. It usually affects more than one limb. **Buzzword = Auto-amputation**.

Gamesmanship Hand Angiograms:

If they are showing you a hand angiogram, it's going to be either Buergers of Hypothenar Hammer Syndrome (HHS).

My strategy centers around the ulnar artery.

(1) Ulnar artery involved = HHS. The most helpful finding is a pseudo-aneurysm off the ulnar artery - this is a slam dunk for HHS.

(2) Ulnar artery looks ok - then look at the fingers - if they are out, go with Buergers. It sure would be nice to see some "corkscrew collaterals" - to make it a sure thing.

Be careful, because the fingers can be out with HHS as well (distal emboli), but the ulnar artery should be fucked. Look at that ulnar artery first.

Location - Location

Central =
Think Takayasu

Mid-Clavicle =
Think Thoracic
Syndrome

Armpit =
Think Giant Cell

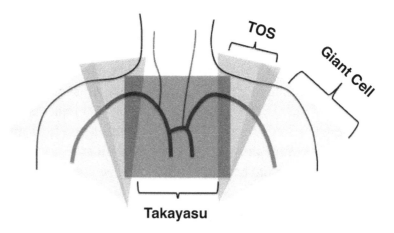

Large Vessel	
Takayasu	Young Asian Female – thickened aneurysmal aorta
Giant Cell	Old Person with involvement of the "crutches" / armpit region (Subclavian, axillary, brachial).
Cogan Syndrome	Kid with eye and ear symptoms + Aortitis
Medium Vessel	
PAN	PAN is more common in a MAN (M > F). Renal Microaneurysm (similar to speed kidney). Associated with Hep B.
Kawasaki	Coronary Artery Aneurysm
Small Vessel (ANCA +)	
Wegeners	Nasal Septum Erosions, Cavitary Lung Lesions
Churg Strauss	Transient peripheral lung consolidations.
Microscopic Polyangiitis	Diffuse pulmonary hemorrhage
Small Vessel (ANCA -)	
HSP	Kids. Intussusception. Massive scrotal edema.
Behcets	Pulmonary artery aneurysm
Buergers	Male smoker. Hand angiogram shows finger occlusions.

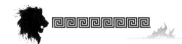 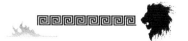

General Vascular Ultrasound Concepts — Stenosis:

The waveform will go through changes before entering a stenosis, within the stenosis, and after exiting the stenosis.

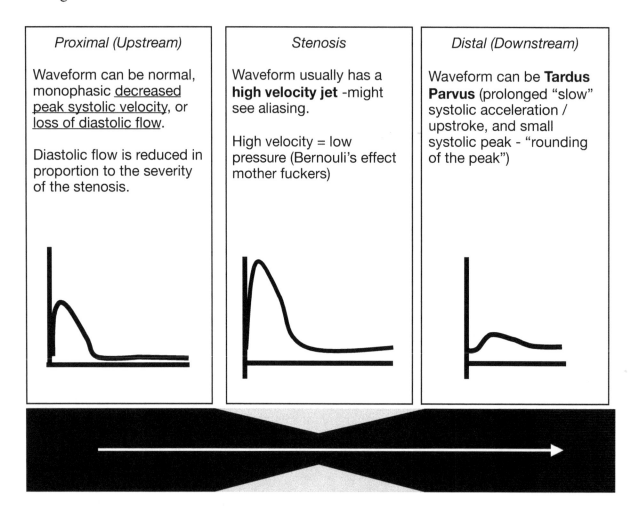

Proximal (Upstream)	*Stenosis*	*Distal (Downstream)*
Waveform can be normal, monophasic <u>decreased peak systolic velocity</u>, or <u>loss of diastolic flow</u>. Diastolic flow is reduced in proportion to the severity of the stenosis.	Waveform usually has a **high velocity jet** -might see aliasing. High velocity = low pressure (Bernouli's effect mother fuckers)	Waveform can be **Tardus Parvus** (prolonged "slow" systolic acceleration / upstroke, and small systolic peak - "rounding of the peak")

Fuckery with words: It would be correct to say that Tardus Parvus is found downstream from a stenosis. It would also be correct to say that Tardus Parvus is the result of upstream stenosis. See what I did right there? I'm not the only one who can pull some shit like that...

High Yield Topics of Carotid Doppler

Stenosis: They will show you an elevated velocity (normal is < 125cm/s). They may also show you the ICA/CCA ratio (normal is < 2), or the ICA end diastolic velocity (< 40 cm/s is normal).

Here are the rules:

• Less that 50% stenosis will not alter the peak systolic velocity

• 50-69% Stenosis: ICA PSV 125-230 cm/s , ICA/CCA PSV ratio: 2.0-4.0 , ICA EDV 40-100

• >70 % Stenosis: ICA PSV > 230 cm/s, ICA/CCA PSV ratio: > 4.0 , ICA EDV >100

Proximal Stenosis: OK here is the trick; they will show a tardus parvus waveform. **If they show it unilateral, it is stenosis of the innominate. If it's bilateral then it's aortic stenosis.**

Subclavian Steal: This is discussed in greater detail in the cardiac chapter, but this time lets show it on ultrasound. As a refresher, we are talking about stenosis and/or occlusion of the proximal subclavian artery with retrograde flow in the ipsilateral vertebral artery.

How will they show it? They are going to show two things: (1) Retrograde flow in the left vertebral, and (2) a stenosis of the subclavian artery with a high velocity.

How they can get really sneaky? They can show this thing called "early steal." Steal is apparently a spectrum, which starts with mid-systolic deceleration with antegrade late-systolic velocities. Some people think the "early steal" waveform looks like a rabbit.

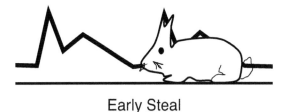

Early Steal

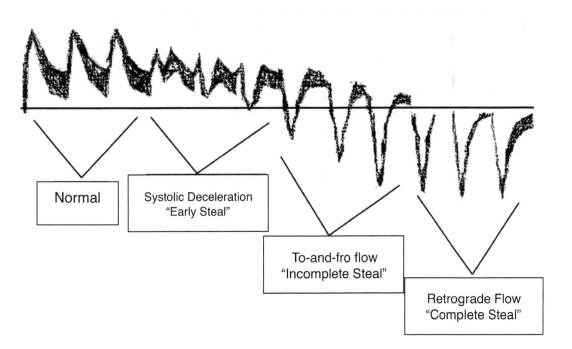

| Normal | Systolic Deceleration "Early Steal" | To-and-fro flow "Incomplete Steal" | Retrograde Flow "Complete Steal" |

THIS vs THAT: Gamesmanship Internal Carotid vs External Carotid

This really lends itself well to multiple choice test questions. The big point to understand is that the brain is always on. You need blood flow to the brain all the time, which means diastolic flow needs to be present all the time, and thus continuous color flow throughout the cardiac cycle. The external carotid feeds face muscles... they only need to be on when you eat and talk.

Internal Carotid	External Carotid
Low Resistance	High Resistance
Low Systolic Velocity	High Systolic Velocity
Diastolic velocity does not return to baseline	Diastolic velocity approaches zero baseline
Continuous color flow is seen throughout the cardiac cycle	Color flow is intermittent during the cardiac cycle

Temporal Tap – It is a technique Sonographers use to tell the external carotid from the internal carotid. You tap the temporal artery on the forehead and look for ripples in the spectrum. The tech will usually write "TT" on the strip - when they do this.

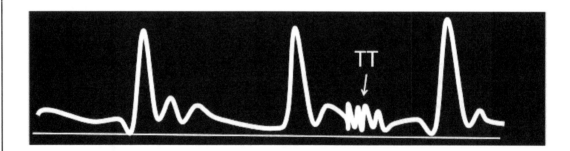

*You can also **look for branches** to tell the external carotid vs the internal.*

Aortic Regurgitation: - Just like aortic stenosis they are going to show you bilateral CCAs. In this case you are going to get **reversal of diastolic flow**.

Brain Death – Apparently in the ever-feuding monarchies of Europe, ultrasound can be used for brain death studies. **A loss of diastolic flow suggests cessation of cerebral blood flow.**

Aneurysms - In case someone asks you, distal formation of an aneurysm (such as one in the skull) cannot be detected by ultrasound, because proximal flow remains normal.

Intra-Aortic Balloon Pump - Remember these guys are positioned so that the superior balloon is 2 cm distal to the take off of the left subclavian artery, and the inferior aspect of the balloon is just above the renals (you don't want it occluding importing stuff when it inflates). When the balloon does inflate it will displace the blood in this segment of the aorta - smashing it superior and inferior to the balloon. The balloon will inflate during early diastole (right after the aortic valve closes) because this is when the maximum amount of blood is available for displacement.

What does this do to the internal carotid (ICA) waveform? You are going to see an extra bump or "augmentation" as the balloon inflates and displaces blood superior.

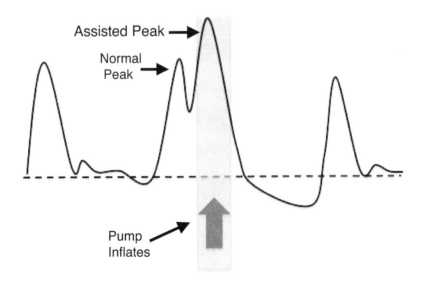

Which wave would you measure to evaluate the velocity?
The first one (the one that is not assisted).

Doppler Evaluation in the LVAD

Bro... WTF is a "LVAD" ?

The Left Ventricular Assist Device is a surgically implanted device that helps pump blood from the left ventricle to the aorta. It's done in the setting of severe heart failure, typically as a bridge to cardiac transplantation, or in those who are simply too evil to die of natural causes (Dick Cheney) and require an intermediate step while the Darth Vader suit is prepped.

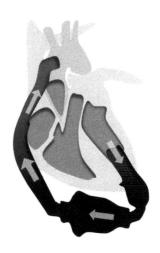

Testable Doppler Changes:

LVAD Waveforms will lose the normal high resistance spiked look of the ICA, CCA, Vertebral Arteries. Instead they are mostly flat, with a **tardus parvus** look. The flow is continuous through systole and diastole. The little spikes you see during systole are from the small amount of residual LV function.

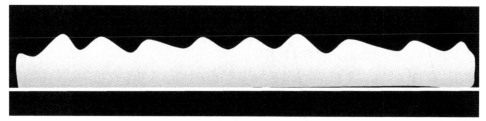

ICA - LVAD Patient

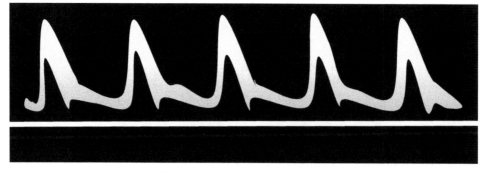

ICA - Normal Patient

Classic Carotid Doppler Cases

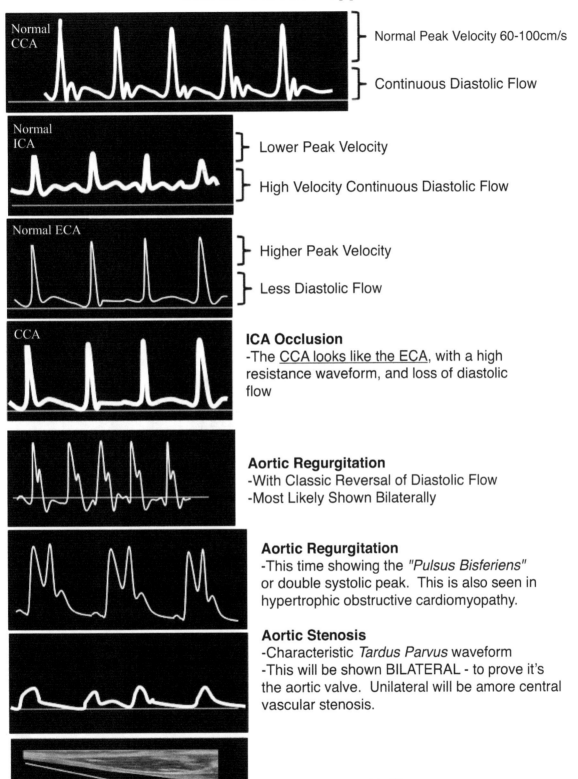

Normal CCA — Normal Peak Velocity 60-100cm/s — Continuous Diastolic Flow

Normal ICA — Lower Peak Velocity — High Velocity Continuous Diastolic Flow

Normal ECA — Higher Peak Velocity — Less Diastolic Flow

CCA

ICA Occlusion
-The <u>CCA looks like the ECA</u>, with a high resistance waveform, and loss of diastolic flow

Aortic Regurgitation
-With Classic Reversal of Diastolic Flow
-Most Likely Shown Bilaterally

Aortic Regurgitation
-This time showing the *"Pulsus Bisferiens"* or double systolic peak. This is also seen in hypertrophic obstructive cardiomyopathy.

Aortic Stenosis
-Characteristic *Tardus Parvus* waveform
-This will be shown BILATERAL - to prove it's the aortic valve. Unilateral will be amore central vascular stenosis.

Dissection - with Flap

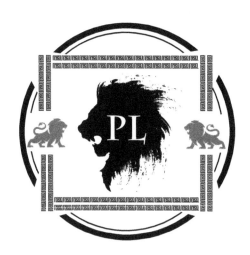

13

INTERVENTIONAL

PROMETHEUS LIONHART, M.D.

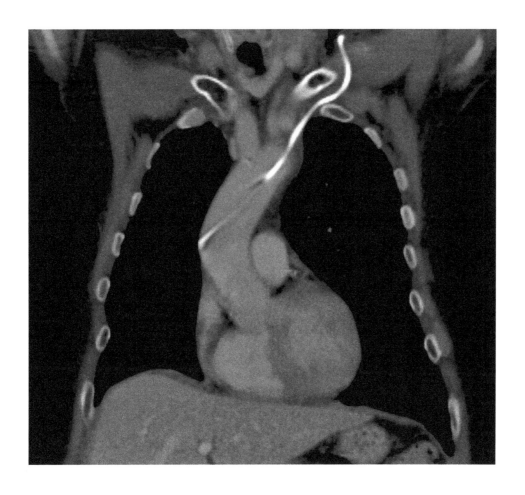

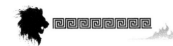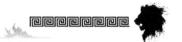
Puncture Needles:

- The smaller the "gauge" number, the bigger the needle. It's totally counterintuitive. For example, an 8G Needle is much bigger than a 16G Needle. *This is the opposite of a "French," which is used to describe the size of a catheter or dilator. The larger the French, the larger the catheter.*

- The Gauge "**G**" refers to the OUTER diameter of the needle.

Wires:

Just some general terminology:

- 0.039 inch = 1mm
- 0.035 inch is the usual size for general purposes
- 0.018 and 0.014 are considered microwires
- "Glide Wires" are hydrophilic coated wires that allow for easier passage of occlusions, stenosis, small or tortuous vessels.

Puncture Needle sizes are designated by the **OUTER** diameter

Catheter and Dilator sizes are designated by the **OUTER** diameter

Sheaths are designated by their **INNER** lumen size, (the maximum capacity of a diameter they can accommodate)

Catheters – General

- 3 French = 1 mm (6 French = 2 mm, 9 French = 3 mm) **Diameter in mm = Fr / 3**
- Important trivia to understand is that the French size is the external diameter of a catheter (not the caliber of the internal lumen).
- *The standard 0.035 wire will fit through a 4F catheter (or larger)*

Sheaths

- Sheaths are used during cases that require exchange of multiple catheters. The sheath allows you to change your catheters / wires without losing access.
- They are sized according to the largest catheter they will accommodate.
- The outer diameter of a vascular sheath is usually 1.5F to 2F larger than the inner lumen.

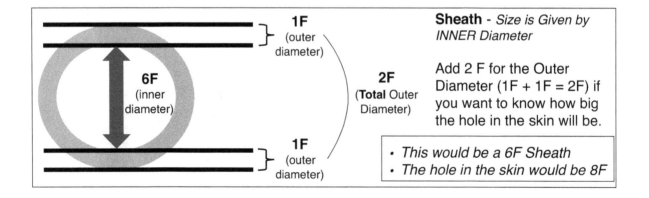

Gamesmanship — *Various Forms of Fuckery That Can Be Performed ~*

There are a few classic ways this can be asked. You can get all these questions right if you understand the following trivia:

- 3 French = 1 mm, so 1 French = 0.3 mm
- Puncture Needles, Guide Wires, and Dilators are designated with sizes that describe their OUTER diameters.
- Sheaths are designated with sizes that describe their INNER diameter
- The rubber part of the sheath is about 2F (0.6 mm) thick, so the hole in the skin is about 0.6mm bigger than the size of the sheath.
- Wire DIAMETERs are given in INCHES (example "0.035 wire" is 0.035 inches thick)
- Wire LENGTHS is typically given in CENTIMETERS (example "180 wire" is 180 cm long)

Example Quiz 1: *What is the size of a puncture hole in mm of a 6 French sheath?*

Diameter in mm = Fr / 3
2.7 mm = (6 + 2) / 3

- 6 French Describes the Inner Diameter
- Add 2 French for the thickness of the rubber
- Total is 8 French

Answer = 2.7 mm

Example Quiz 2: *What is the size of a puncture hole in mm of a 6 French sheath, placed coaxially into a short access sheath ?*

**This is some second level fuckery.

6 French sheath is being placed inside of another sheath
6 French sheath is actually 8 French Big (remember you add 2F for the rubber wall).
So you need a sheath that can accommodate an 8 French Diameter. Remember that sheaths are named for what they can accommodate, so you need an 8 French Sheath.
8 French sheath is actually 10 French Big (remember you add 2F for the rubber wall).

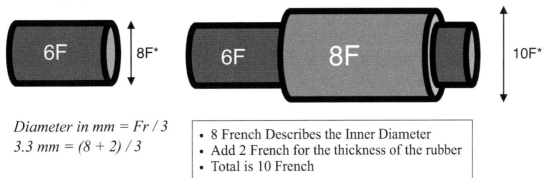

Diameter in mm = Fr / 3
3.3 mm = (8 + 2) / 3

- 8 French Describes the Inner Diameter
- Add 2 French for the thickness of the rubber
- Total is 10 French

Answer = 3.3 mm

Puncture Needles - The Legend Continues:

Some Conversions:

- 16G needle has an outer diameter of 1.65 mm, = 5 F catheter;

- 20G needle has an outer diameter of 0.97 mm, = 3 F catheter.

Some Needle Wire Rules:

Old School Seldinger Technique:

- 18G needle will accept a 0.038 inch guidewire

- 19G needle will allow a 0.035 inch guidewire

> **Remember 0.035 is probably the most common wire used. Thus the 19G is the standard needle in many IR suites.*

Micro Puncture Style:

- Initial puncture is performed with a 21G (rather than a typical 18G or 19G) needle.

- 21G needle will allow a 0.018 inch guidewire

- After you have that tiny wire in, you can exchange a few dilators up to a standard 4F-5F system with the popular 0.035 wire.

Micro Puncture is Good when….	*Micro Puncture is Bad when….*
- *Access is tough (example = a fucking antegrade femoral puncture)* - *You suck ("lack experience")* - *Anatomically sensitive areas (internal jugular, dialysis access)*	- *Scarred Up Groins* - *Big Fat People* - *When you try and upsize, sometimes that flimsy 0.018 won't give enough support for antegrade passage of a dilator.*

Guidewires - The Legend Continues to Continue:

There are two main flavors of guidewires:

(1) Non-Steerable - These are used as supportive rails for catheters. These are NOT for negotiating stenosis or selecting branches

(2) Steerable - These have different shaped tips that can be turned or flipped into tight spots. Within this category is the "hydrophilic" coated which are used to fit into the tightest spots.

Hydrophilic Guidewires - *"Slippery when wet"*. They are sticky when dry, and super slippery when wet. At most academic institutions dropping one of these slippery strings on the floor will result in "not meeting the milestone" and "additional training" (weekend PICC workups).

- *Next Step Questions:* Could revolve around the need to "wipe the wire with a wet sponge each time it is used."

- *Next Step Questions:* Pretty much any situation where you can't get into a tight spot. This could be a stenotic vessel, or even an abscess cavity.

Length - Here is the testable trivia regarding wire length.

- Remember *Diameter* is in *INCHES*, Length is in CENTIMETERS

- 180 cm is the standard length

- 260 cm is the long one. These are used if you are working in the upper extremity (from a groin access), working in the visceral circulation and need to exchange catheters, using a guide cath that is longer than 90 cm, through-and-through situation ("body flossing").

- Minimal guidewire length = length of catheter + length of the guidewire in the patient.

Floppy Tips - A lot of wires have pointy ends and soft floppy ends. The floppy ends are usually available in different sizes. The testable point is that **the shorter the floppy part the greater the chance of vessel dissection.** For example, a 1 cm floppy tip has a greater risk of dissection compared to a 6 cm floppy tip. The practical tip is to choose a wire with a long floppy tip (unless you are trying to squeeze into a really tight spot).

Guidewires - The Legend Continues to Continue to Continue

Stiffness: I feel like there are two primary ways to ask questions about stiffness:

(1) Your classic *"right tool for the right job"* questions.
Unfortunately, these are often *"read my mind, and understand my prejudices"* questions.
The following are probably the clearest scenarios:

- Bentson (floppy tip) = Classic guidewire test for acute thrombus lysability

- Lunderquist (super stiff) = "The coat hanger." This thing is pretty much only for aortic stent grafting.

- Hydrophilic = Trying to get into a tight spot. Yes a Bentson is also an option, but this is more likely the "read my mind" choice.

(2) *Which is "Stiffer ?"* or *Which is "Less Stiff ?"* types of question. Basically just have a general idea of the progression. A second-order style question would be *"Which is more or less likely to cause dissection?"* Remember the rule is "more stiff = more dissection."

Less ➡ **More Stiff**

"Noodle Like"	Normal	Supportive	Stiff	Hulk Smash !!
Bentson	Hydrophilic	Stiff Hydrophilic	Flexfinder	Lunderquist
	Standard 0.035 J or Straight	"Heavy Duty" J or Straight	Amplatzer Stiff or Extra Stiff	Backup Meier
			0.018 Platinum Plus	
			V18 - *shapeable tip*	

Trivia: Stiff guidewires should NEVER be steered through even the mildest of curves. You should always introduce them through a catheter (that was originally placed over a conventional guidewire).

J Tip Terminology: A "J Shaped" Tip supposedly has the advantages of not digging up plaque and of missing branch vessels. Often you will see a number associated with the J (example 3 mm, 5 mm, 10 mm, 15 mm etc…). *This number refers to the radius of the curve.* Small curves miss small branch vessels, larger curves miss larger branch vessels. The classic example is the 15mm curve that can be used to avoid the profunda femoris during the dreaded arterial antegrade stick.

Catheters - The Legend Continues
— Fuckery with Numbers

If you look at a "buyers guide" or the packaging of an angiographic catheter you may (if you look hard enough) find 3 different numbers. I think it would be easy to write a question asking you to ID the numbers, or asking what size sheath or wire you can use with the catheter.

The three numbers that you are going to see on the package are: the outer diameter size (in French), the inner diameter size (in INCHES), and the length (in CENTIMETERS).

Example Question 1: *What size is this catheter?*

VANDELAY INDUSTRIES	
FINE ANGIOGRAPHIC CATHETERS	**Answer = 4F**
4, 110, 0.035	

Remember that the outer diameter of a catheter defines it's size (unlike the sheath which is defined by the inner diameter), and that these sizes are given in French. 4F catheters are very commonly used. 110 and 0.035 are not catheter sizes available for humans existing outside of middle earth.

Remember that length of the catheter is given in centimeters. The standard lengths vary from about 45 cm to 125 centimeters.

Lastly the inner diameter of a catheter is given in inches and will pair up with the size wire. For example, the largest wire a 0.035 catheter will accommodate is a 0.035.

Example Question 2: *What size sheath and guidewire can you use with this catheter?*

VANDELAY INDUSTRIES	Answer =
FINE ANGIOGRAPHIC CATHETERS	• **4F Sheath or Larger**
4, 110, 0.035	• **0.035 wire or Smaller**
	a 0.038 wire would NOT fit

It's a 4F sheath because sheaths are defined by their INNER diameter. So a 4F snake can crawl through a 4F tube. Obviously a bigger tube (5F, 6F, etc...) will also have enough room for a 4F snake.

It's a 0.035 wire because the inner diameter measurements are given in inches, just like the guidewires. In this case the tube is the catheter and the wire is the snake. So a bigger snake (any wire thicker than 0.035) wouldn't fit.

Catheters - Selective vs Non-Selective

Just like Guidewires can be grouped into "steerable" or "non-steerable" , catheters can be grouped into "non-selective (flush) catheters" and "selective catheters".

- *Non-Selective Catheters:* These things are used to inject contrast into medium and large shaped vessels. This is why you"ll hear them called "flush catheters."

- *Selective Catheters:* These things come in a bunch of different shapes/angles with the goal of "selecting" a branch vessel (as the name would imply).

Non-Selective Catheters

Pigtail: For larger vessels this is the main workhorse. It's called a "pigtail" because the distal end curls up as you retract the wire. This curled morphology keeps it out of small branch vessels. The catheter has both side and end holes.

Q: What might happen if you consistently inject through the pigtail like a pussy?

A: All the contrast will go out the proximal side holes and not the tip. Eventually, if you keep flushing like a pansy you will end up with a clot on the tip.

Q: What should you do prior to giving it the full on alpha male injection ?

A: Give a small test injection to make sure you aren't in or up against a small branch vessel. Pigtails are for use in medium to large vessels.

Q: What if the pigtail fails to form as you retract the wire?

A: Push the catheter forward while twisting.

Straight Catheter: This one doesn't curl up as you retract the wire. Otherwise, it's the same as a pigtail with side holes and an end hole. The utility of this catheter is for smaller vessels (with the caveat that they still need decent flow).

The *classic location is the iliac.*

Catheters - Selective vs Non-Selective cont...

Selective Catheters

Selective catheters come in two main flavors: (1) end hole only, or (2) side + end holes (*that's what she said*).

End Hole Only	Side + End Holes *"Girl who went to catholic school"*
Hand Injection Only *high flow injection can displace the catheter, or cause dissection*	Works fine with Pump Injected runs *(can handle a rapid bolus without displacing)*
Utility = Diagnostic Angiograms and Embolization Procedures	Utility = Classic would be a SMA Angiogram
	NEVER use with Embolotherapy. The fucking coils can get trapped in the sideholes or the particulate matter/mush may go out a side hole and go crush the wrong vessel. *"Non-targeted"* they call it.

I think the above chart is probably good enough to get most reasonable selective catheter questions correct. Unfortunately, it's also possible that you could be asked a *"read my mind, understand my prejudices"* type of question in the form of *"which catheter would you use?"*

This is how I would guess - if forced.

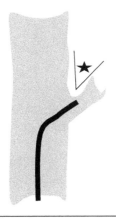 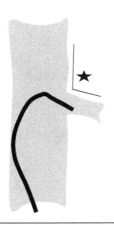 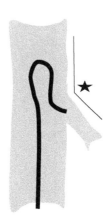

Acute Angle (< 60)	Angle of 60-120	Obtuse Angle (> 120)
Example = Aortic Arch Vessels	Example = Renals, *Maybe SMA and Celiac*	Example = Celiac, SMA, IMA
"Angled Tip Catheter"	"Curved Catheter"	"Recurved"
-*Berenstein* or *Headhunter*	*"RDC" Renal Double Curve, or a "Cobra"*	*Sidewinder* (also called a *Simmons*), or a *"Sos Omni"*

WTF is a "Recurve" ?

For whatever reason Academic Angio guys tend to spaz if residents don't understand why a *"recurve"* is different than a regular curved catheter.

Basically any curved catheter has a "**p**rimary" curve and a "**s**econdary" curve. On a regular curved cath both are in the same direction. However, on a recurved cath the primary goes one way, and the secondary goes the other.

These catheters are good for vessels with an obtuse angle. You pull the catheter back to drop into them.

I trained under a guy who was always very impressed with himself when he could perform a basic catheter maneuver like this. After dropping into the IMA he would sometimes slowly turn to one of the female techs and say *"that's why I'm the king."*

I was really afraid he was going to break his own arm, jerking himself off that hard.

That guy (or someone like him) is probably writing questions for the IR section (guessing / not confirmed - but makes me smile to think so).

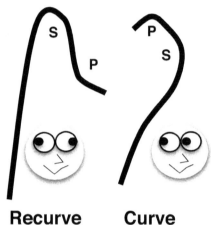

Recurve   **Curve**

Vocab

"Co-Axial Systems" - Basically one catheter inside another catheter/sheath. The most basic example would be a catheter inside the lumen of an arterial sheath.

"Guide Catheters" - These are large catheters meant to guide up to the desired vessel. Then you can swap them for something more conventional for distal catheterization.

"Introducer Guide" - This is another name for a *long sheath*. The assholes are trying to trick you.

"Microcatheter" - These are little (2-3 French). They are the weapon of choice for tiny vessels (example "super-selection" of peripheral or hepatic branches).

"Vascular Sheath" - It's a sheath (plastic tube) + hemostatic valve + side-arm for flushing

Flow Rate

"Give me 20 for 30" — typical angio lingo for a run at 20cc/sec for a total of 30cc.

How do you decide what the correct flow rate is ? For the purpose of multiple choice, I'll just say memorize the chart below. In real life you have to consider a bunch of factors: catheter size, catheter pressure tolerance, flow dynamics, vessel size, volume of the distal arterial bed (hand arteries can tolerate less blood displacement compared to something like the spleen), and interest in the venous system (a common concern in mesenteric angiography - hence the relatively increased volumes in the SMA, IMA, and Celiac on the chart).

Bigger Artery = Higher Rate. You want to try and displace 1/3 of the blood per second to get an adequate picture.

Typical Rates / Volumes			
Rate 1-2mL/sec Volume 4-10 mL	**Rate 4-8mL/sec Volume 8-15 mL**	**Rate 5-7mL/sec Volume 30-40 mL**	**Rate 20-30mL/sec Volume 30-40 mL**
Bronchial Artery Intercostal Artery	Carotid Subclavian <u>Renal</u> Femoral IMA	Celiac SMA	Aorta, Aortic Arch, IVC, Pulmonary Artery
	IMA are typically given a higher volume (15-30 mL)		*Abdominal Aorta has a slightly lower rate (15-20 mL/sec) as it is smaller than the Thoracic Aorta*

Maximum Flow Rates:

These are determined by the INTERNAL diameter, length, and number of size holes. In general, *each French size gives you about 8ml/s*.

These are the numbers I would guess if forced to on multiple choice. In the real world its (a) written on the package and (b) a range of numbers

3F = 8 ml/s, 4F = 16 ml/s, 5F = 24 ml/s.

Catheter Flushing

Double Flush Technique - This is used in situations where even the smallest thrombus or air bubble is going to fuck with someone's golf game (neuro IR / cerebral angiograms). The technique is to (1) aspirate the catheter until you get blood in the catheter, then (2) you attach a new clean saline filled syringe and flush.

Single Flush Technique - This is used everywhere else (below the clavicles). The technique is to (1) aspirate until you get about 1 drop of blood in a saline filled syringe, and (2) tilt the syringe 45 degrees and flush with saline only.

What if you accidentally mixed the blood in with the saline?

Discard the syringe and double flush

What if you are unable to aspirate any blood ?

Hopefully you are just jammed against a side wall. Try pulling back or manipulating the catheter. If that doesn't work then you have to assume you have a clot. In that case your options are to (1) pull out and clear the clot outside the patient, or (2) blow the clot inside the patient - you would only do this if you are embolizing that location anyway (and a few other situations that are beyond the scope of this exam).

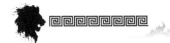 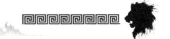
Arterial Access

General "Next Step" Scenarios:

- *You meet resistance as you thread the guidewire.* Next Step = STOP! *"Resistance"* is an angio buzzword for something bad. Pull the wire out and confirm pulsatile flow. Reposition the needle if necessary.

- *The wire will not advance beyond the top of the needle even after you pull the wire back and have normal pulsatile flow.* Next Step = Flatten the needle against the skin. You are assuming the need to negotiate by a plaque.

- *The wire stops after a short distance.* Next Step = Look under fluoro to confirm correct anatomic pathway. If it is normal then you could put a 4F sheath in and inject some contrast. After that monkeying around with a hydrophilic wire is the conventional answer.

Femoral Artery Access - This is the most common arterial access route.

Anatomy review = the external iliac becomes the CFA after it gives off the inferior epigastric.

The ideal location is over the femoral head (which gives you something to compress against), distal to the inguinal ligament / epigastric artery and proximal to the common femoral bifurcation.

- If you stick too high (above inguinal ligament): You risk retroperitoneal bleed
- If you stick too low, you risk AV Fistula
- If you stick at the bifurcation: You risk occluding branching vessels with your sheath.

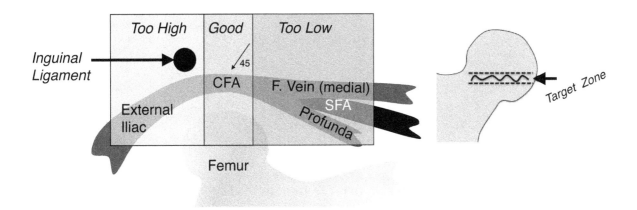

Brachial Access - Possible situations when you might want to do this:

- Femoral Artery is dead / unaccessible.

- The patient's abdominal pannus, vagina, or ball sack is really stinky.

- Upper limb angioplasty is needed

Special Testable Facts/Trivia:

- Holding pressure is often difficult. Even a small hematoma can lead to **medial brachial fascial compartment syndrome** (cold fingers, weakness) – and is a surgical emergency which may require fasciotomy.

- The **risk of stroke is higher** (relative to femoral access), if the catheter has to pass across the great vessels / arch.

- A sheath larger than a 7F may require a surgical cut down.

- The vessel is smaller and thus more prone to spasm. Some people like to give prophylactic "GTN" - glyceryl trinitrate, to prevent spasm.

Which arm ?

- Left Side if headed south (abdominal aorta or lower extremity).

- Right Side if headed north (thoracic aorta or cerebral vessels).

- All things equal = Left side (it's usually non-dominant, and avoids the most cerebral vessels).

- Blood pressure difference greater than 20 Systolic suggest a stenosis (choose the other arm).

Radial Access - This is also a thing. There are two pieces of trivia that I think are the most testable about this access type.

(1) **Bedrest is not required after compression**.

(2) You need to **perform an "Allen Test" prior to puncture.** The "Allen Test" confirms collateral flow via the ulnar artery to the hand (just in case you occlude the radial artery). The test is done by manually compressing the radial and ulnar arteries. A pulse ox placed on the middle finger should confirm desaturation. Then you release the ulnar artery and saturation should improve, proving the ulnar artery is feeding the hand.

Translumbar Aortic Puncture - This was more commonly performed in the dark ages / Cretaceous period. You still see them occasionally done during the full-on thrash that is the typical type 2 endoleak repair.

Trivia:

- The patient has to lay on his/her stomach (for hours!) during these horrible thrashes

- Hematoma of the psoas happens pretty much every case, but is rarely symptomatic.

- Known supraceliac aortic aneurysm is a contraindication

- Typically "high" access - around the endplate of T12 - is done. Although you can technically go "low" - around L3.

- The patient "Self compresses" after the procedure by rolling over onto his/her back.

- Complaining about a "mild backache" occurs with literally every one of these cases because they all get a psoas hematoma.

Pre Procedure Trivia: Prior to an arterial stick you have to know some anticoagulation trivia.

- Stop the heparin 2 hours prior to procedure (PTT 1.2x of control or less; normal 25-35 sec)
- INR of 1.5 is the number I'd pick if asked (technically this is in flux)
- Stop Coumadin at least 5-7 days prior (vitamin K 25-50 mg IM 4 hours prior, or FFP/ Cryo)
- Platelet count should be > 50K (some texts say 75)
- Stop ASA/Plavix 5 days prior (according to SIR)
- Per the ACR - diagnostic angiography, routine angioplasty, and thrombolysis are considered "clean procedures." Therefore, antibiotic prophylaxis is unnecessary.

Post Procedure Trivia: By the book, you want 15 minutes of compression. You can typically pull a sheath with an ACT of <150-180. Heparin can get turned back on 2 hours post (assuming no complications). Groin check and palpate pulses should be on the post procedure nursing orders.

Closure Devices: Never used if there is a question of infection at the access site.

Venous Access:

PICC lines: Use the non-dominant arm. The preference is basilic > brachial > cephalic. You don't place these in patients with CRF, on dialysis, or maybe going to be on dialysis.

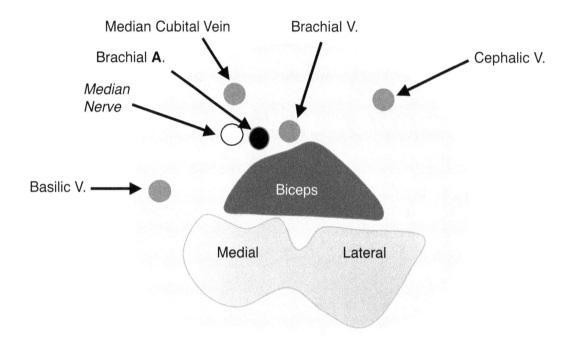

Central Lines/Port: The right IJ is preferred. External jugular veins can be used. Subclavian access is contraindicated in patients with a contraindication to PICC lines. Don't place any tunneled lines/ports in septic patients (they get temporary lines).

National Kidney Foundation-Dialysis Outcome Quality Initiative (NKF-KDOQI): Order of preference for access: RIJ > LIJ > REJ > LEJ. *"Fistula First Breakthrough Initiative"*: is the reason you don't place PICCs in dialysis patients.

What is the preferred access site for a dialysis catheter? The right IJ is the preferred access, because it is the shortest route to the preferred location (the cavoatrial junction). It will thrombose less than the subclavian (and even if it does, you don't lose drainage from the arm – like you would with a subclavian). Femoral approach is less desirable because the groin is a dirty dirty place.

Bleeding

The word *"hypotension"* in the clinical vignette after an arterial access should make you think about high sticks / retroperitoneal bleeds.

Things that won't help:

- Yelling "Mother Fucker!!" - trust me, I've tried this

Things that might help:

- Placing an angioplasty balloon across the site of the bleeding (or inflow) vessel.

> **Applying Pressure**
> *- Where dat hole be?*
>
> The hole in the skin and the hole in the artery don't typically line up.
>
> - *Antegrade Puncture* = Below the skin entry point
> - *Antegrade Puncture on a Fatty* = Well Below the skin entry point
> - *Retrograde Puncture* = Above the skin entry

Pseudoaneurysm Treatment: As described in the vascular chapter, you can get a pseudoaneurysm after a visit to the cardiology cath lab (or other rare causes). A lot of the time, small ones (< 2 cm) will undergo spontaneous thrombosis. The ones that will typically respond to interventional therapy are those with long narrow necks, and small defects. There are 3 main options for repair: (1) open surgery, (2) direct ultrasound compression, or (3) thrombin injection.

Next Step: Pain disproportionate to that expected after a percutaneous stick = Get an US to look for a pseudoaneurysm

Direct Compression	Direct compression of the neck (if possible avoid compression of the sac). Enough pressure should be applied to stop flow in the neck.	Painful for the Patient (and the Radiologist), can take 20 mins to an hour. Don't compress if it's above the inguinal ligament.
Thrombin Injection	Needle into apex of cavity *(aim towards the inflow defect)* - inject 0.5-1.0 ml (500-**1000 units**). Do NOT aspirate blood into syringe - will clot.	***Contraindications:*** Local infection , Rapid Enlargement, Distal Limb Ischemia, Large Neck (risk for propagation), Pseudoaneurysm cavity size < 1cm.
Surgery	May be needed if thrombin injection fails, there is infection, there is tissue breakdown, or the aneurysm neck is too wide.	

Pseudoaneurysm Treatment Cont:

Which option do you pick? For the purpose of multiple choice I would suggest the following:

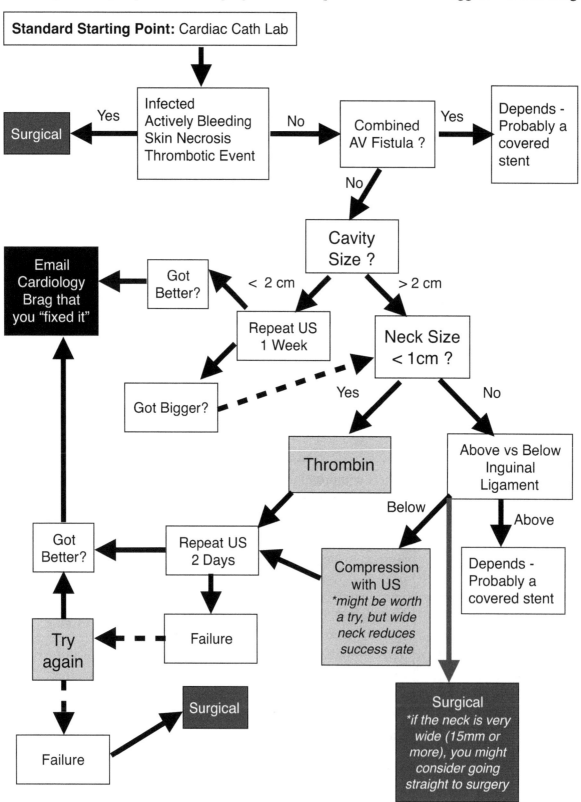

Pseudoaneurysm Treatment Cont:

*This algorithm on the prior page assumes the Test Writer agrees that **Thrombin is superior to Compression** (it hurts less, and probably has a higher success rate). Most modernly trained guys will think like this. However, some conservative strategies favor trying to compress all the ones below the Inguinal ligament first - then trying thrombin second line. Simply read the test writers mind to know his / her bias prior to answering.*

Thrombin Injection - Where do you stick the needle ?

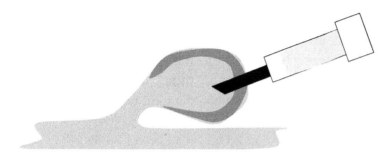

The needle should be placed in the apex of the cavity *(tip directed towards the inflow defect).*

Ultrasound Compression - Where do you compress ?

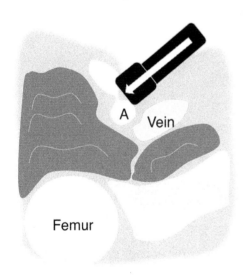

Orthogonal plane to the neck of the pseudoaneurysm. Pressure is directed to obliterate flow in the neck / sac.

Trivia - Seriously Watch the Wording Carefully:

- Anticoagulation has no effect on thrombin injection treatment - primary success**
- Anticoagulation does* increase the risk of recurrence (10%?) after thrombin injection treatment
- Anticoagulation is NOT a contraindication to attempting direct compression, although it DOES reduce success rate and most people will tell you to stop them prior to the procedure (if possible).
- Failure to respond to thrombin = Occult vascular issue (big puncture site laceration, infection)
- Untreated Pseudoaneurysm for greater than 30 days tend to resist compression and thrombin therapy to variable degrees. They do best if treated within 2 weeks.
- Attempted compression of a Pseudoaneurysm above the inguinal ligament can cause a RP bleed. It is still safe to try and thrombin inject

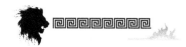 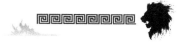

General Tips/Trivia regarding angioplasty: The balloon should be big enough to take out the stenosis and stretch the artery (slightly). The ideal balloon dilation is about 10-20% over the normal artery diameter. Most IR guys/gals will claim success if the residual stenosis is less than 30%. Obviously you want the patient anticoagulated, to avoid thrombosis after intimal injury. The typical rule is 1-3 months of anti-platelets (aspirin, clopidogrel) following a stent.

"Primary Stenting": This is angioplasty first, then stent placement. You want to optimize your result. Stenting after angioplasty usually gives a better result than just angioplasty alone (with a few exceptions – notably FMD – to which stenting adds very little). An important idea is that a stent can't do anything a balloon can't. In other words, the stent won't open it any more than the balloon will, it just prevents recoil.

Balloon Expanding vs Self Expanding: Stents come in two basic flavors, balloon expandable or self expandable. Location determines the choice.

Self Expandable stents are good for areas that might get compressed (superficial locations).

• Classic Examples = Cervical Carotid or SFA.

Balloon Expandable stents are good for more precise deployment

• Classic Example = Renal ostium

Closed vs Open Cell Stents - Vascular stent designs may be categorized as (a) closed-cell - where every stent segment is connected by a link (less flexible, with better radial force) or (b) open-cell in which some stent segment connections are deliberately absent (flexible/ conforms to tortuous vessels, less radial force).

Nitinol (magic?): Nitinol is said to have a "thermal memory." It is soft at room temperature, but can become more rigid at body temperature. This is exploited for self-expanding stents.

Drug Eluting Stents – These things have been used for CAD for a while. The purpose of the "drug" is to retard neointimal hyperplasia.

Balloon Selection - Balloons should be 10-20% larger than the adjacent normal (non-stenotic) vessel diameter. A sneaky move would be to try and get you to measure a post-stenotic dilation.

A rough guessing guide (if forced):

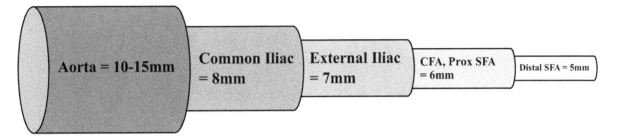

Aorta = 10-15mm

Common Iliac = 8mm

External Iliac = 7mm

CFA, Prox SFA = 6mm

Distal SFA = 5mm

**Popliteal would be 4 mm

As a general rule, larger balloons allow for more dilating force but the risk of exploding the vessel or creating a dissection is also increased.

Stent Selection - Stents should be 1-2 cm longer than the stenosis and 1-2 mm wider than the un-stenosed vessel lumen

Special Situations -

(1) **You have more than 30% residual stenosis (failed you have).** The first thing to do (if possible) is to measure a pressure gradient. If there is no gradient across the lesion, you can still stop and claim victory. If there is a gradient you might be dealing with *elastic recoil* (the lesion disappeared with inflation, but reappeared after deflation). The next step in this case is to place a stent.

(2) **You can't make the waist go away with balloon inflation.** Switch balloons to either a higher pressure rated balloon, or a "cutting balloon."

(3) **You caused a distal embolization.** First do an angiographic run. If the limb / distal vessels look fine then you don't need to intervene. If you threatened the limb, then obtain ipsilateral access and go after the clot ("aspiration").

(4) **You exploded the vessel ("Extravasation").** This is why you always leave the balloon on the wire after angioplasty. If you see extravasation get that balloon back in there quickly, and perform a low pressure insufflation proximal to the rupture to create tamponade. You may need to call vascular surgery ("the real doctors").

(5) What if you are trying to cross a tight stenosis and you see something like this ?

This is the classic *"spiral"* of a *dissecting wire.*

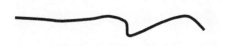

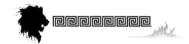 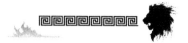

"EVAR" = EndoVascular abdominal aortic Aneurysm Repair. These include the bifurcated iliac systems and unilateral aortic + iliac systems.

"TEVAR" = Thoracic EndoVascular aortic Aneurysm Repair.

> **THIS vs THAT: Endografts vs Open Repair:**
>
> • 30 Day Mortality is LESS for Endovascular Repair (like 30% less)
> • Long Term Aneurysm Related Mortality (and total mortality) is the SAME for open vs endovascular repair
> • Graft Related Complications and Re-interventions are HIGHER with Endovascular Repair

Indications for EVAR:

(1) AAA larger than 5 cm (or more than 2x the size of the normal aorta)

(2) AAA growing "rapidly" (more than 0.5 cm in 6 months)

Anatomy Criteria for EVAR:

• Proximal landing zone must be:

  • 10 mm long,

  • Non- aneurysmal (less than 3.2 cm),

  • Angled less than 60 degrees.

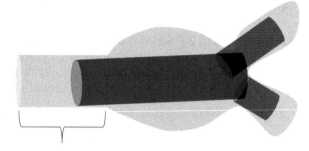

10 mm Long
< 3.2 cm Wide
< 60 Degree of Tortuosity

Device Deployment:

Tortuosity and Vessel Size are issues for device deployment. The general rules are that you have problems if:

• Iliac vessels have an angulation > 90 degrees (especially if heavily calcified)

• Iliac artery diameters < 7 mm (may need a cut down and the placement of a temporary conduit).

Absolute Contraindication to Infrarenal EVAR:

- Landing sites that won't allow for aneurysm exclusion

- Covering a critical artery (IMA in the setting of known SMA and Celiac occlusion, Accessory renals that are feeding a horseshoe kidney, dominant lumbar arteries feeding the cord).

Dealing with the Renals.

There are several anatomy vocab words that are worth knowing for aneurysms near the renals.

- *"Para-Renal"* - which is an umbrella term for aneurysms near the renals

- *"Juxta-Renal"* - Aneurysm that has a "short neck" (proximal landing zone < 1 cm) or one that encroaches on the renals.

- *"Supra-Renal"* - Aneurysm that involves the renals and extends into the mesenterics.

- *"Crawford Type 4 Thoracoabdominal Aortic Aneurysm"* - Aneurysm that extends from the 12th intercostal space to the iliac bifurcation with involvement of the origins of the renal, superior mesenteric, and celiac arteries.

Treating these types of aneurysms requires all kinds of fancy stuff; snorkels, chimney technique, etc… All is beyond the scope of the exam. Just know that it can be done, but it's not easy.

Complications:

The most feared/dreaded (testable) complication of an aortic stent graft is paraplegia secondary to cord ischemia. You see this most commonly when there is extensive coverage of the aorta (specifically T9-T12 Adamkiewicz territory), or a previous AAA repair. "Beware of the hair pinned turn" - famously refers to the morphology of Adamkiewicz on angiogram.

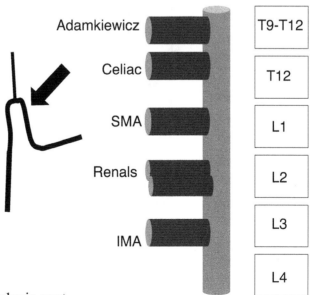

Symptoms of possible / developing paraplegia post procedure. **Next Step = CSF drainage.**

AAA pre/ post Endograft

After an aneurysm has been treated with an endograft, things can still go south. There are 5 described types of endoleaks that lend themselves easily to multiple choice questions.

- **Type 1:** Leak at the top (A) or the bottom (B) of the graft. They are typically high pressure and require intervention (or the sac will keep growing).
- **Type 2:** Filling of the sac via a feeder artery. This is the **MOST COMMON** type, and is usually seen after repair of an abdominal aneurysm. The most likely culprits are the IMA or a Lumbar artery. The majority spontaneously resolve, but some may require treatment. Typically, you follow the sac size and if it grows you treat it.
- **Type 3:** This is a defect/fracture in the graft. It is usually the result of pieces not overlapping.
- **Type 4:** This is from porosity of the graft. (*"4 is from the Pore"*). It's of historic significance, and doesn't happen with modern grafts.
- **Type 5:** This is endotension. It's not a true leak and it may be due to pulsation of the graft wall. Some people don't believe in these, but I've seen them. They are real.

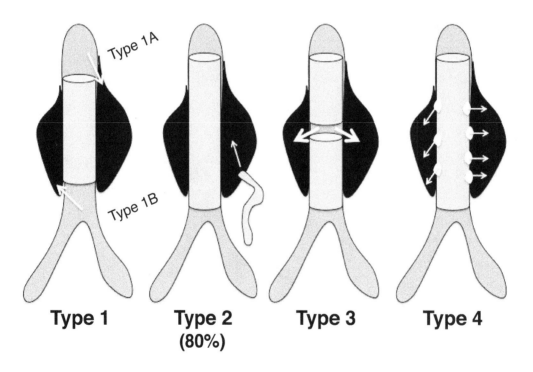

Treatment: *The endoleaks that must be emergently treated are the high flow ones - Type 1 and Type 3.* Most IR guys / vascular surgeons (real doctors) will watch a Type 2 for at least a year (as long as it's not enlarging). Most Type 4s will resolve within 48 hours of device implantation.

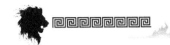 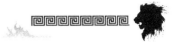

There's a bunch of reasons you might want to do this. The big ones are probably stopping a bleed and killing a tumor.

Which agent do you want? Unfortunately just like picking a catheter these types of questions tend to fall into the mind reading category.

In general you are going to choose the agent based on the desired outcome, and the need to minimize risk. The most classic thinking goes something like this:

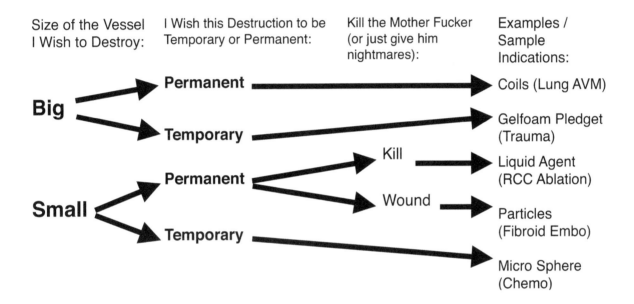

Another way to think / groups the agent is the general class. I think this is the most helpful to talk about them in an introductory sense. After I introduce them, we will revisit what to pick based on a multiple choose vignette.

Mechanical	Particulate	Liquid Agents
Coils	PVA - Particles *(permanent)*	Sclerosants
Vascular Plugs *(Amplatzer)*	Gelfoam *(temporary)*	Non-Sclerosants
	Autologous Blood Clot *(temporary)*	

Mechanical Agents:

Coils:

These are typically used to permanently occlude a large vessel. They come in all kinds of different sizes and shapes. You can deploy them with a "push" via a coaxial system, or if you don't need exact precision you can "chase" them with a saline bolus.

It gets complicated and beyond the scope of the exam (probably), but there are a variety of strategies for keeping these in place. Just know you can pack these things behind an Amplatzer, or you can use scaffolding techniques to hook small coils to a large one

 Buzzword "Accurate Deployment" = Detachable Coil

Trivia: Remember never deploy these with a side-hole + end-hole catheter. You want end-hole only for accurate deployment.

Trivia: Never pack coils directly into an arterial pseudoaneurysm sac - *more on this later in the chapter.*

> **THIS vs THAT:**
> **Coils vs Micro-Coils**
>
> **Coils:** Deployed via standard 4-7F catheter
>
> **Micro:** Deployed via Micro-Catheter. If you try and deploy them through a standard cath they can ball up inside the thing and clog it.

Amplatzer Vascular Plug (AVP)

This is a self expanding wire mesh that is made of Nitinol (thermal memory James Bond shit). You mount this bomb on the end of a delivery device/wire. When deployed it shrinks in length and expands in width.

Best Use = High Flow Situations, when you want to kill a single large vessel. If you are thinking to yourself - I'm gonna need a bunch of coils to take that beast down the answer is probably an amplatzer plug.

Particulate Agents:

These are grouped into:

- *Temporary:* Gelfoam, Autologous Blood Clot

- *Permanent:* PVA Particles

Best Use = Situations where you want to block multiple vessels. Classic examples would be fibroids and malignant tumors.

THIS *vs* THAT:
Gelfoam Powder vs
Gelfoam Pledgets/Sheets

Powder causes occlusion at the capillary level **(tissue necrosis)**

Pledgets/Sheets cause occlusion at the arteriole or larger level (tissue infarct is uncommon)

You are Doing it Wrong / Avoiding Reflux = An easy way to ask this would simply be "When do you stop deploying the agent?"

The classic teaching is to stop embolization when the flow becomes "to and fro." If you continue to pile the particulate agent in until you get total occlusion you risk refluxing the agent into a place you don't want it to go.

THIS vs THAT: Coils vs PVA Particles

In many cases if you can use coils, you can also use appropriately sized particles.

Size is one way to pick. Coils are good for medium to small arteries. PVA is good for multiple small arteries or capillaries.

Smaller particles (less than 300 microns) are going to risk tissue necrosis in many cases - so if you want to preserve the tissue, that's probably the wrong answer.

Another tip for picking between the two is the need for repeat Access. The classic example is the bronchial artery embolization. These things tend to re-bleed. So you should NEVER ever use coils (this will block you from re-accessing).

Bronchial artery embolization = Particles (> 325 micrometers).

Next Step ?

Q: What do you do after placement of an occlusion balloon in the setting of particle embolization ?

A: Test injection to confirm adequate occlusion.

Liquid Agents:

These are grouped into:

- *Sclerosants:* Absolute Alcohol (the one that hurts) and Sodium Dodecyl Sulfate (SDS)

- *Non-Sclerosants:* Onyx (Ethylene–Vinyl Alcohol Copolymer) , Ethiodol

Sclerosants:

As would be expected, the sclerosant agents work by producing near immediate thrombosis / irreversible endothelial destruction. As a result, non-targeted embolization can be fairly devastating. There are three main strategies for not causing a major fuck up (i.e. burning a hole in the dude's stomach, infarcting his bowel, etc…).

(1) Knowing the anatomy really well through careful mapping

(2) Frequent intermittent angiograms during the embolization procedure

(3) Use of Balloon Occlusion to protect non-target sites.

Next Step ?

Q: What do you do prior to deflating the occlusion balloon?

A: Aggressively aspirate (with a 60 cc syringe) to make sure all the poison is out of there.

Non-Sclerosants:

Onyx: Typically used for neuro procedures, hypervascular spine tumors, shit like that. It dries slowly (outside in) and allows for a slower, more controlled delivery.

Ethiodol: This is an oil that blocks vessels at the arteriole level (same as the really small PVA particles). For some reason, hepatomas love this stuff, and it will preferentially flow to the hepatoma. It is also unique in that it is radio-opaque, which helps decrease non-targeted embolization and lets you track tumor size on follow up.

Single Best Answer Classic Scenario

- Autologous Blood Clot = Post-Traumatic High-Flow Priapism (or Priapism induced by the female Brazilian olympic volleyball team)

- Varicocele (Spermatic Vein) = Coils

- Uterine Fibroid embolization (Bilateral Uterine Artery) = PVA or microspheres 500–1000 μm

- Generic Trauma = Gel Foam in many cases.

- Diffuse Splenic Trauma (Proximal embolization) = Amplatzer plug in the splenic artery proximal to the short gastric arteries. **Discussed in detail later in the chapter.

- Pulmonary AVM = Coils

- Hemoptysis (Bronchial artery embolization) = PVA Particles (> 325 μm).

- Hyper-vascular Spinal Tumor = Onyx

- Total Renal Embolization = Absolute ethanol

- Partial or Selective Renal Embolization = Glue (bucrylate–ethiodized oil)

- Segmental Renal Artery Aneurysm = Coils

- Main Renal Artery Aneurysm = Covered Stent (or coils after bare metal stent)

- Peripartum hemorrhage = Gel Foam

- Upper GI Bleed = Endoscopy First (if that fail then in most cases coils)

- Lower GI Bleed = Usually Microcoils

LARGE Vessel - Permanent	small Vessel - Permanent
Coils	Particles
	Liquid Sclerosants
Amplatz Occluder	Thrombin
LARGE Vessel - Temporary	Ethiodol
	small Vessel - Temporary
Gelfoam Pledget / Sheet	
	Microspheres
Autologous Clot	Gelfoam Powder

Post Embolization Syndrome:

Pain, nausea, vomiting, and low grade fever – is basically an expected finding. You don't need to order blood cultures - without other factors to make you consider infection. There is a *rule of 3 days* - it starts within the first 3 days, and goes away within 3 days of starting.

The vignette is most classic for a large fibroid embolization, but it's actually common after a solid organ (e.g. liver) - the tumor just needs to be big. Some texts suggest prophylactic use of anti-pyrexial and antiemetic meds prior to the procedure.

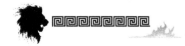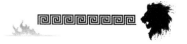
"Threatened Limb" - Acute limb ischemia can be secondary to thrombotic or embolic events. Frequent sites for emboli to lodge are the common femoral bifurcation and the popliteal trifurcation. You can also get more distal emboli resulting in the so called *blue toe syndrome*.

As crazy as this may sound to a Radiologist, physical exam is actually used to separate patients into 3 categories: viable, threatened, or irreversible. This chart (or something similar) is how most people triage.

Category		Capillary Return	Muscle Paralysis	Sensory Loss	Arterial Doppler	Venous Doppler
1 - Viable	Not Threatened	Intact	None	None	+	+
2a -Threatened	Salvageable	Intact/Slow	None	Partial	-	+
2b - Threatened	Salvageable if immediate intervention	Slow/ Absent	Partial	Partial	-	+
3 - Irreversible	NOT Salvageable *Amputation	Absent	Complete	Complete	-	-

Know who you can and can't treat

"Critical Limb Ischemia" – This is described as rest pain for two weeks (or ulceration, or gangrene).

General Idea on Treatment: An important point to realize is that lysis of a clot only re-establishes the baseline (which was likely bad to start with). So after you do lysis, consider additional therapy (angioplasty, surgery, stenting, etc...). If there is combined inflow and outflow disease, you should treat the inflow first (they just do better).

Surgery vs Thrombolysis: If it has been occluded for less than 14 days, thrombolysis is superior, if more than 14 days, (surgery is superior).

ACR Appropriate: Embolism Above / Below the Common Femoral Artery

- Isolated suprainguinal embolism probably should be removed surgically.
- Fragmented distal emboli should have endovascular thrombolytic therapy

---

Ankle – Brachial Index (ABI)

The idea behind the ABI is that you can compare the blood pressure in the upper arm, to that of the ankle and infer a degree of stenosis in the peripheral arteries based on that ratio. In a normal person, ratios are usually slightly greater than 1. In patients with occlusive disease, they will be less than that - with a lower number correlating roughly with the extent of disease.

ABI		
1.0	Normal	No Symptoms
0.75-0.95	Mild	Mild Claudication
0.5-0.75	Moderate	Claudication
0.3-0.5	Moderate - Severe	Severe Claudication
< 0.3	Severe or "Critical"	Rest Pain

How they do it: You take blood pressures in both arms, and both ankles. You only use one of the arm measurements (the higher one). For the actual ratios, opinions vary on this - most people do it by dividing the higher of either the dorsalis pedis or posterior tibial systolic pressure (at the ankle) by the higher of either the right or left arm systolic pressure.

False Numbers? Arterial calcifications (common in diabetics with calcific medial sclerosis) make compression difficult and can lead to a false elevation of the ABI. This is when you will see ratios around 1.3 — those are bullshit, means the exam is non-diagnostic.

Toe Pressures: As above, diabetics will have noncompressible vessels - which makes ABIs worthless. What you can do is look at the toe pressure. The reason this works is because the digital arteries are not as affected by this disease process. A normal systolic toe pressure is greater than 50 mm Hg, and the ratio (toe-brachial index) should be more than 0.6. *The testable trivia is that if the toe pressures are less than 30 mm ulcers are less likely to heal.*

Segmental Limb Pressures: A modification to the standard ABI involves pressures at the thigh, calf, and ankle — if there is a pressure drop of more than 20-30 you can infer that this is the level of disease. This allows you to sorta sorta sorta guess where the level of disease is.

Spectral Waveform Analysis:

The normal pulsatile wave is the result of the pumping action of the left ventricle transmitted to the aortic root and then to the foot. As the LV contracts you have a jet of blood that dynamically expands the aortic root. As the bolus of blood travels towards the feet the vessels will continue to expand along the path — like a cartoon snake that has eaten a mouse (or your neighbors cat). The wave falls as the cardiac cycle enters diastole.

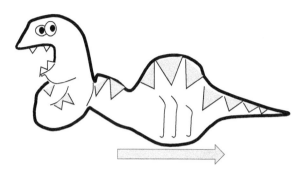

There is a secondary event which is the rebound off the high resistance tibial vascular tree. This is why the normal wave has an up-down-up look to it — "triphasic" they call it. This bounce back or rebound effect demonstrates normal arterial compliance. As the vessel hardens you lose this. With progressive disease there is less and less compliance to the point where the primary wave barely even stretches the vessel.

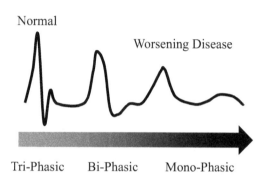

Ulcer Location Trivia *(dinosaur IR guys love this - it really gets their dicks hard):*

- Medial Ankle = Venous Stasis
- Dorsum of Foot = Ischemic or Infected ulcer
- Plantar (Sole) Surface of Foot = Neurotrophic Ulcer

Who are Rutherford and Fontaine? These are "useful" categories and classifications of signs and symptoms of peripheral arterial disease.

False Numbers? Arterial calcifications (common in diabetics) make compression difficult and can lead to a false elevation of the ABI.

Post-Operative Bypass Vocabulary:

- **Primary Patency** – Uninterrupted patency of the graft with no procedure done on the graft itself (repair of distal vessels, or vessels at either anastomosis does not count as loss of primary patency).
- **Assisted Primary Patency** – Patency is never lost, but is maintained by prophylactic interventions (stricture angioplasty etc..).
- **Secondary Patency** – Graft patency is lost, but then restored with intervention (thrombectomy, thrombolysis, etc..).

" Where to Access ? "

One simple way to ask a threatened leg treatment question is to ask for the best route of access per lesion. Again, like many IR questions, this falls into the "depends on who you ask" , and/or "read my mind" category. If forced to choose, this is how I would guess:

Lesion	Access
Iliac	First Choice - Ipsilateral CFA. If that is down also (which it often is), I'd pick the contralateral CFA
CFA	Contralateral CFA
SFA	Ipsilateral CFA
Fem-Pop Graft	Ipsilateral CFA
Fem-Fem Cross-Over	First Choice - Direct Stick. Second choice-inflow CFA

If you are presented with other scenarios, the rule most people use is "shortest, most direct approach."

When would you use the contralateral CFA ? There are two general situations:

1. The Ipsilateral CFA is occluded.

2. The patient is very very fat. Even fatter than your normal acute leg patient. These are the guys/gals who got the milkshake (instead of the diet coke) with the baconator. As a point of gamesmanship, if the question header specifically mentions that the patient is obese they are likely leading you towards contralateral access.

 *Gamesmanship:* Watch out for "retrograde" vs "antegrade" access terminology in the distractors. The nomenclature for a downward (towards the toe) access is "antegrade." The terminology is based on the directions of the arterial flow.

• *Antegrade* access = towards the toes.

• *Retrograde* access = towards the heart.

General Procedural Trivia / Possible "Next Steps"

There are a whole bunch of ways to do this. In the most generic terms, you jam the catheter into the proximal clot and infuse TPA directly into the mother fucker. Every 6-8 hours you check to see if you are making progress. People call that "check angiography."

What if you can't cross the clot with a wire? If they spell that out in the vignette, they are trying to tell you that this clot is organized and probably won't clear with thrombolysis.

What if there is no clearing of the clot during a "check angiogram"? If they specifically state this, they are describing *"lytic stagnation,"* which for most reasonable people is an indication to stop the procedure.

The patient develops "confusion"? Neuro symptoms in a patient getting TPA should make you think head bleed. Next step would be non-con CT head.

The patient develops "tachycardia and hypotension"? This in the setting of TPA means the patient is bleeding out. Next step would be (1) go to the bedside and look at the site. Assuming he/she isn't floating in a lake of their own blood (2) CT abdomen/pelvis and probably stopping the TPA.

End Point? Most people will continue treating till the clot clears. Although continuing past 48 hours is typically bad form.

Venous Treatment

Varicose Vein Treatment: Just know that "tumescent anesthesia" (lots of diluted subcutaneous lidocaine) is provided for ablation of veins. Veins are ablated using an endoluminal heat source. A contraindication to catheter-based vein ablation is DVT (they need those superficial veins).

DVT: The primary complications of DVT are acute PE and chronic post thrombotic syndrome (PTS). There are several clinical predictive models to keep everyone who comes in the ER from getting a CTPA - *"Wells Score"* is probably the most famous. Recently described is this *"Thrombus Density Ratio"* as a superior predictor of PE in patients with known DVT on CTV. The density of thrombus on CTV has been shown to be higher in patients with both DVT and PE relative to just DVT. Thrombus Density Ratio of 46.5 (thrombus HU / normal vein HU) = probable PE.

Phlegmasia alba (painful white leg) and **Phlegmasia cerulea dolens** (painful blue leg) - archaic physical diagnosis terms that are high yield for the exam of the future. Phlegmasia alba = massive DVT, without ischemia and preserved collateral veins. Phlegmasia cerulea dolens = massive DVT, complete thrombosis of the deep venous system, including the collateral circulation. These are described as extreme sequella of May-Thurner - but can occur in any situation where you get a punch of DVT (pregnancy, malignancy, trauma, clogged IVC filter, etc..)

Post Thrombotic Syndrome (PTS): This is basically pain and stuff (venous ulcers) after a DVT. Risk factors include being old (>65), a more proximal DVT, recurrent or persistent DVT, and being fat. PTS is usually diagnosed between 6 months and 2 years after DVT. VEINES-QOL is the scoring system used to diagnose and classify severity of PTS. Catheter-directed intrathrombus lysis of iliofemoral DVT is done to prevent post thrombotic syndrome. This is not needed as much with femoropopliteal DVT as it will recanalize more frequently and have less severe post thrombotic syndrome.

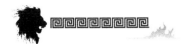
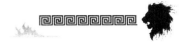
An IVC filter is used in the following situations:

• Proven PE while on adequate anticoagulation

• Contraindication to anticoagulation with clot in the femoral or iliac veins

• Needing to come off anticoagulation – complications. There are a few additional indications that are less firm (basically, we think he/she might get a DVT and we can't anti-coagulate).

Vocab:

• *Permanent Filters:* Do Not Come Out
• *Retrievable Filters:* Can Come Out, But Do Not Have To
• *Temporary Filter:* Come out, and have a component sticking outside the body to aide in retrieval

Position *(before submission)***:**

The device is usually placed infrarenal with a few exceptions (see below chart).

> *Why Not Leave Them In?*
>
> Depending on who bought you lunch (gave you a free pen), thrombosis rates vary.
>
> In general (for the purpose of multiple choice) about ***10% of the permanent filters thrombose within 5 years***.

Why isn't it always just positioned suprarenal? A supra-renal filter has a theoretic increased risk of renal vein thrombosis. There is zero evidence behind this - like most things in medicine.

Indication	Filter Placement	Rationale
Pregnancy	Supra-renal	To avoid compression
Clot in the Renals or Gonadals	Supra-renal	Get above the clot
Duplicated IVCs	Either bilateral iliac, or supra-renal (above the bifurcation)	Gotta block them both
Circumaortic Left Renal	Below the lowest renal	Risk of clot by passing filter via the renals

MEGA-Cava: If the IVC is less than 28 mm, then any filter can be placed. If it's bigger than that, you might need to place a bird's nest type of filter which can be used up to 40 mm. You can also just place bilateral iliac filters.

Random Trivia:

* A "Gunther Tulip" has a superior end hook for retrieval
* A "Simon-Nitinol" has a low profile (7F) and can be placed in smaller veins (like an arm vein).
* All filters are MRI compatible

Prior to placing the Filter:

You need to do an angiographic run. Where I trained, the classic pimping question for residents on service was to "name the 4 reasons you do an angiogram prior to filter placement!" The only answer that would not result in "additional training" (more weekend PICC workups) was:

1. Confirm patency of the IVC

2. Measure the size of the IVC

3. Confirm that you are dealing with 1 IVC

4. Document the position of the renal veins

Complications/Risks:

* *Malposition:* The tip of the filter should be positioned at the level of the renal vein. If it's not, honestly it's not a big deal
* *Migration:* The filter can migrate to another part of the IVC, the heart, or even the pulmonary outflow tract. If it goes to the heart, you need surgery. If it's just superior, you need to snare it out.
* *Thrombosis:* Although the incidence of PE is decreased, the **risk of DVT is increased**. Caval thrombosis is also increased, and you should know that clot in the filter is a contraindication to removal (you need to lyse it, before you remove it).
* *IVC Perforation:* A strut going through the caval wall is common and doesn't mean anything. However, aortic penetration, ureteral perforation, duodenal perforation, or lumbar vessel laceration can occur (rarely) from a strut hanging out of the cava – this is a bigger problem.
* *Device Infection:* A relative contraindication to IVC filter placement is bacteremia.

Positioning the Filter:

Renals on an IVC Gram: There are two ways to show the renals on an IVC Gram. There is the nice way where they opacify normally and it's obvious, and there is the sneaky way where you see the *"steaming effect"* of unopacified blood allowing you to infer the position.

Obviously the sneaky way is more likely to show up on the exam.

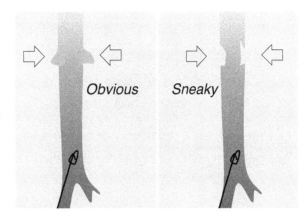

The Tip: For standard anatomy, the standard answer for a cone shaped filter is to put the apex at the level of the renals. Some people think the high flow in this location helps any clot that might get stuck in the filter dissolve.

What if there is clot in the IVC? The filter should be positioned above the most cranial extension of the clot. As mentioned in my glorious IVC Filter position chart, if the clot extends beyond the renals you need a suprarenal filter.

What if you fuck up the deployment (severe tilt, legs won't open, etc...) ? If it's retrievable, you may be able to snare it and restart. If it's permanent you are kind of hosed. Some people will try and stick a second filter above the retarded one.

Filter Removal:

The longer these things stay in, the more likely they will thrombose. Prior to removal you should perform an angiogram of the IVC. The main reason to do this is to evaluate for clot.

- More than 1 cm³ of clot = Filter Stays In

- Less than 1 cm³ of clot = Filter Comes Out

You snare the filter but when you pull on it you meet resistance ? In the real world, people will yank that mother fucker out of there. The IVC is the Rodney Dangerfield of vessels - no respect. For multiple choice? Stop and assume that it can't be retrieved.

Angiogram should also be done after removal of the filter to make sure you didn't rip a hole in the IVC. **If you did rip a hole in it -** *Next Step* - Angioplasty balloon with low pressure insufflation to to create tamponade. If that doesn't work, most people would try a covered stent graft. If you created a **wall injury/dissection ?** Again - answers will vary, but the classic answer is systemic anticoagulation.

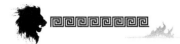 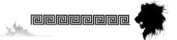

Generally speaking there are two types of "permanent" access options for dialysis; (1) the arterio-venous fistula and (2) the arterio-venous graft.

AV Fistula - This is a subcutaneous anastomosis between an artery and adjacent native vein (for example the radial artery to the cephalic vein). All things equal, the preferred access (over the graft).

AV Graft - This is also a subcutaneous anastomosis between an artery and adjacent native vein. Except this time the distance between the vessels is bridged with a synthetic tube graft.

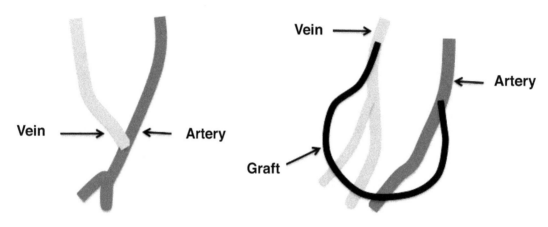

Arteriovenous Fistula   Arteriovenous Graft

What are the pros and cons of each types?

Pros of AV Graft:	Cons of AV Graft:
- Ready for use in 2 weeks - Easier to declot (clot is usually confined to the synthetic graft)	-Less overall longevity -Promotes hyperplasia of the venous intima at or downstream from the graft vein anastomosis, resulting in stenosis and eventual obstruction -More infections (foreign graft material)

Pros of AV Fistula:

- Lasts Longer & More Durable
- Much less prone to development of venous neointimal hyperplasia at or downstream from the artery-vein anastomosis.
- Fewer infections

Cons of AV Fistula:

-Needs 3-4 Months to "Mature" (vein to enlarge enough for dialysis)

Why do grafts/fistulas need treatment (politics and greed) ? The primary reason is "slow flows." It's important to understand that nephrologists get paid per session of dialysis. If they can do a session in 1 hour or 4 hours they make the same amount of money. Therefore they want them running fast. So, really "slow-flow" is referring to slow cash flow in the direction of the nephrologist's pocket.

For the purpose of multiple choice I'd go with:

< 600 cc/min for graft = diagnostic fistulogram

< 500 cc/min for fistula = diagnostic fistulogram

Having said that, you may find different numbers different places - the whole issue is controversial based on the real motivation people have for treating these. Some texts say a fistula can maintain patency with rates as low as 80 cc/min, and grafts can maintain patency with rates as low as 450 cc/min. Also remember medicare won't pay for two treatments within 90 days, so make sure you treat on day 91.

Why do grafts/fistulas need treatment (actual pathophysiology)? Its a violation of nature to have a AF Fistula / Graft pulsating in your arm. Your body won't tolerate it forever. Neointimal hyperpasia develops causing an ever-worsening stenosis. If they don't get treated, they will eventually thrombose. All fistulas/grafts must die.

"Working it Up"

The only thing worse then actually doing a fistulogram is having to talk with and examine the patient prior to the procedure. Nearly all the IR texts and any program worth its snuff will "work them up" starting with physical exam.

Patient arrives in the IR department for "slow flows." *Next Step = Physical Exam*

This is the buzzword orientated algorithm that I would suggest for dealing with physical exam / history related fistula/graft questions:

LOOK	"Arm Swelling" "Chest Wall Collaterals" "Breast Swelling"	Central Venous Stenosis
LOOK	"Discolored Hand" "Pale Colored Hand" "Pallor of the Hand"	Dialysis-Associated **Steal Syndrome** (DASS)
LISTEN	"High-Pitched Bruit" "Bruit in Systole Only" "Discontinuous Bruit"	Localized Stenosis
FEEL	"Water Hammer Pulse" "Diminished Pulse"	Pre Stenosis Post Stenosis

What is normal? A normal graft has an *easily compressible pulse*, a *low-pitched bruit* that is present *in both systole + diastole*, and a *thrill* that is palpable with compression *only at the arterial anastomosis*.

Localizing a Stenosis - *Classic Example - Straight Forearm Graft:*

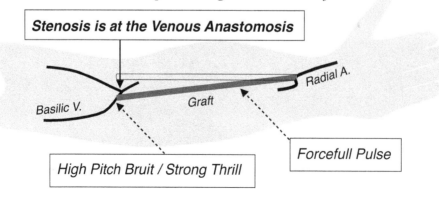

GRAFTS:

Where is the problem (usually) in grafts? The most common site of obstruction is venous outflow (usually at or just distal to the graft-to-vein anastomosis). This is usually secondary to intimal hyperplasia.

What about the normal thrill and bruit in a graft ? There should be a thrill at the arterial anastomosis, and a low pitched bruit should be audible throughout the graft.

What if the bruit is high pitched? High Pitch = Stenosis, Low Pitch = Normal

What are you thinking if I tell you the dude has a swollen arm and chest ? This is classic for central venous stenosis.

FISTULAS:

Where is the problem (usually) in fistulas? It's more variable - you are less likely to be asked this. If you are forced - I'd say venous outflow stenosis - typically junta-anastomotic or runoff vein (AV anastomosis stenosis is uncommon).

If you fix a stenotic area - they are good to go right ? Nope - they reoccur about 75% of the time within 6 months.

What about the "thrill" in the fistula, is this a helpful finding? Yes - there should be a continuous thrill at the anastomosis. If it is present only with systole then you are dealing with a stenosis. Also, if you can localize a thrill somewhere else in the venous outflow - that is probably a stenosis.

What if the fistula is very "pulsatile" ? This indicates a more central stenosis - the fistula should be only slightly pulsatile.

Should there be a bruit ? A low pitched bruit in the outflow vein is an expected finding.

"Steal Syndrome" –The classic story is "**cold painful fingers**" during dialysis, relieved by manual compression of the fistula. Too much blood going to the fistula leaves the hand ischemic. The issue is usually a stenosis in the native artery distal to the fistula. *Fixing this is typically surgical* (DRIL = Distal Revascularization and Interval Ligation of Extremity, or Flow Reduction Banding).

ACCESS and TREATMENT:

Contraindications ? Infection is the only absolute one. If you fuck with an infected fistula or graft the patient could get endocarditis. If you don't fuck with it, the patient will probably still get endocarditis but infectious disease will have to blame it on someone else at the QA meeting.

What if it's "Fresh" ? A "relative contraindication" is a new graft or fistula. "New" to most people means less than 30 days. Significant stenosis prior to 30 days strongly suggests a surgical fuck up ("technical problem" they call it). Not to mention that a new dilating anastomosis is high risk for rupture. Those grafts are doomed to never reach long-term patency.

Access less than 30 days old with stenosis. *Next Step = Send them back to the surgeon.*

What about "long segments" ? You will read some places that stenotic segments **longer than 7 cm** respond poorly to treatment. Some people even consider this a **"relative contraindication."** If the question writer actually spells out the length of the stenosis greater than 7 cm he/she probably wants you to say send them back to surgery. In reality there are plenty of stubborn IR guys that will try and treat multiple long lesions because there is no better way than to prove one's manhood.

What about a contrast allergy? You can use CO_2 for runs.

What direction do you access the graft ? Access is typically directed towards the venous anastomosis - unless you are thinking arterial is the problem (which is much less common). Remember the lingo "antegrade" and "retrograde" refers to the direction of blood flow. *Antegrade is the typical route for venous problems*, and retrograde is the typical route for arterial inflow issues.

How do you typically look at the arterial anastomosis ? The move most places teach is to obstruct the venous outflow (with a clamp, blood pressure cuff, angioplasty balloon, finger - or whatever) which allows the contrast to reflux into the artery.

What are the moves for angioplasty of a narrow spot ? Give them heparin (3000-5000 units). Exchange your catheter for a 5 or 6 F sheath over a standard 0.035-inch guidewire. Dilate the narrow spot with a 6-8 mm balloon with multiple prolonged inflations. Remember to never take that balloon off the wire when you are doing diagnostic runs - as you might need to rapidly put it back if you caused a tear.

When do you place a stent ? There are two main reasons (1) you are getting bad elastic recoil, or (2) you have recurrent stenosis within 3 months of angioplasty.

Does Nitro have a role? You can use a vasodilator (like nitroglycerin) to distinguish between spasm and stenosis. The spasm should improve. The stenosis will be fixed.

What is considered a Successful Treatment? (1) Improved Symptoms (arm swelling better, etc..), or (2) less than 30% residual stenosis.

What about Aneurysms ? Small ones get monitored for size increase, but the classic teaching is that these are *managed surgically.*

General Vascular Access Trivia: Remember that PICC lines should not be put in dialysis (or possible dialysis – CKD 4 or 5) patients because they might need that arm for a fistula.

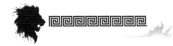
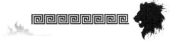
TIPS (Transjugular Intrahepatic Portosystemic Shunt) -

What is this portal hypertension? The portal vein gives you 70-80% of your blood flow to the liver. The pressure difference between the portal vein and IVC ("*PSG*", portosystemic gradient) is normally 3-6 mm Hg. Portal HTN is defined as pressure in the portal vein > 10mm Hg or PSG > 5 mm Hg. The most common cause is EtOH (in North America).

What does portal hypertension look like? On ultrasound we are talking about an enlarged portal vein (>1.3-1.5 cm), and enlarged splenic vein (>1.2 cm), big spleen, ascites, portosystemic collaterals (umbilical vein patency), and reversed flow in the portal vein.

Who gets a TIPS ? Accepted indications include:

- Variceal hemorrhage that is refractory to endoscopic treatment

- Refractory ascites.

- Budd Chiari (thrombosis of the hepatic veins) ** *most authors will include this*

Preprocedural steps for TIPS? You need two things. (1) An ECHO to evaluate for heart failure (right or left). (2) Cross sectional imaging to confirm patency of the portal vein.

How is a TIPS done? The real answer is do an IR fellowship.

First thing you do is measure the right heart pressure. If it is elevated (10-12 mmHg) you stop (absolute contraindication). A normal right heart pressure is around 5 mmHg.

If it is normal, you proceed with the procedure. Access the jugular vein on the right, go down the IVC to the hepatic veins, opacify the veins, do a wedge pressure (don't blow the capsule off), use CO_2 to opacify the portal system. Then stick "Crotch to Crotch" from the hepatic veins to the portal vein (usually right to right). Then put a *covered* stent in and balloon it up.

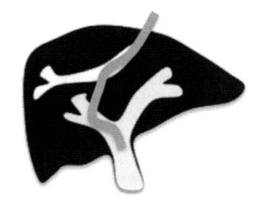

Lastly check pressures and make you sure you didn't over do it (usually want a gradient around 9-12 — **"less than 12"**).

Which direction do you turn the catheter when you are moving from the right hepatic vein, to the right portal vein?

You want to turn <u>anterior.</u>

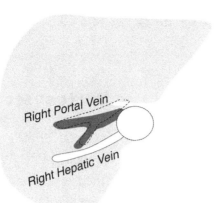

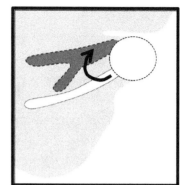

Keeping Score

While you are busy pretending you are a surgeon, why not pretend that you are a medicine doctor also? For the purpose of multiple choice, anything that resembles "Real Doctor" work is always high yield. *"Score Calculation"* is the poster child for the kind of fringe knowledge board examiners have traditionally loved to ask (this was definitely true for the old oral boards). The two highest yield scores are the MELD and the Childs-Pugh.

What is this "MELD" Score ? This was initially developed to predict three month mortality in TIPS patients. Now it's used to help prioritize which drunk driving, Hep C infected, Alcoholic should get a transplant first. MELD is based on liver and renal function - calculated from bilirubin, INR, creatinine. MELD scores greater than 18 are at higher risk of early death after an elective TIPS.

What about this "Childs-Pugh" Score ? This is the "old one," which was previously used to determine transplant urgency prior to the MELD. It works for TIPS outcomes, too, but is *"less accurate" than a MELD.* This score assesses the severity of liver disease by looking at the bilirubin, albumin, PT, ascites, and hepatic encephalopathy. The trivia to know is that *class B & C are risk factors of variceal hemorrhage.*

MELD	Child Pugh
Bilirubin	Bilirubin
INR	PT
creatinine	Albumin
– – –	Ascites, Hepatic Encephalopathy
Greater than 18 = High Risk Death	Class B and C are High Risk

Trivia = "Simplest prognostic measure" = Serum Bilirubin. > 3 mg/dL is associated with an increase in 30-day mortality after TIPS.

What are the contraindications for TIPS? Some sources will say there is no "absolute" contraindication. Others (most) will say <u>severe heart failure</u> (<u>right</u> or left), - but especially right. That the whole reason you check the right heart pressure at the beginning of the procedure. If you are forced to pick a contraindication and right heart failure is not an option, I would choose biliary sepsis, or isolated gastric varices with splenic vein occlusion. Accepted (by most) "relative" contraindications include cavernous transformation of the portal vein, and severe hepatic encephalopathy.

The main acute post procedural complications of TIPS include: Cardiac decompensation (elevated right heart filling pressures), accelerated liver failure, and worsening hepatic encephalopathy.

Evaluation of a "Normal TIPS"

Because the stent decompresses the portal system, you want to see flow directed into the stent. Flow should reverse in the right and left portal vein and flow directly into the stent. Flow in the stent is typically 90-190 cm/s.

Stenosis / Malfunction:

- Elevated maximum velocities (> 200 cm/s) across a narrowed segment.
- Low portal vein velocity (< 30 cm/s is abnormal).
- A temporal increase (or decrease) in shunt velocity by more than 50 cm/s is also considered direct evidence.
- "Flow Conversion" with a change of flow in a portal vein branch from towards the stent to away from the stent.
- An indirect sign of malfunction is new or increased ascites.

TIPS Follow-Up

These things tend to fail (50% primary patent within 1 year for a bare metal stent), so they need tight follow up.

Worsening Ascites, Bleeding, Etc (things that make you think the TIPS isn't working)

Next Step = Venogram with pressures

PSG >12 mmHg. *Next Step = Treat the stenosis (angioplasty + balloon)*

Trivia: The stenosis usually occurs in the hepatic vein, or within the TIPS tract.

Addressing Hepatic Encephalopathy – Dropping the gradient too low increases the risk of HE. If the TIPS is too open you may need to tighten it down with another stent.

What is an alternative to TIPS for treatment of refractory ascites? There is a rarely indicated thing called a "peritoneovenous shunt." This stupid thing has a high rate of infection and thrombosis, and can even lead to DIC. It's designed to allow drainage of the ascites through a tunneled line all the way up to the systemic circulation (jugular).

—

BRTO (Balloon-Occluded Retrograde Transverse Obliteration).

TIPS and BRTO are brother and sister procedures. Where the TIPS takes blood and steers it away from the liver (to try and help the side effects of portal hypertension), the BRTO does the opposite - driving more blood into the liver (to try and help with the side effects of extra hepatic shunting). The inverted indications and consequences are highly testable:

TIPS	BRTO
Treat Esophageal Varices	Treat Gastric Varices
Place a shunt to <u>divert blood around liver</u>	Embolize collaterals to <u>drive blood into liver</u>
Complication is worsening hepatic encephalopathy	Complication is worsening esophageal varices and worsening ascites
Improves esophageal varices and ascites	Improves hepatic encephalopathy

"***The Moves***": The general idea is that you access the portosystemic gastrorenal shunt from the left renal via a transjugular or transfemoral approach. A balloon is used to occlude the outlet of either the gastrorenal or gastro-caval shunt. Following balloon occlusion, a venogram is performed. A sclerosing agent is used to take the vessels out. After 30-50 minutes you aspirate the remaining sclerosing agent and let down the balloons.

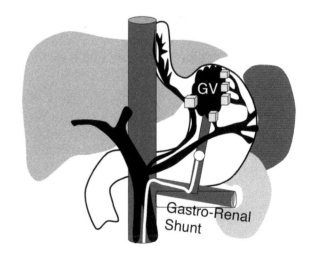

Trivia: The most common side effect of BRTO is gross hematuria.

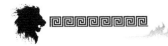 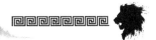
Biliary Duct Anatomy Trivia:

The ductal anatomy mimics the segmental anatomy. The simple version is at the hilum. There are two main hepatic ducts (right and left) which join to make the common hepatic duct. The right hepatic duct is made of the horizontal right posterior (segment 6 & 7) and vertical right anterior (segment 5 & 8). The left duct has a horizontal course and drains segment 2 and 4.

For whatever reason, IR guys love to grill residents about ductal variants (of which there are many). There was a dinosaur GI guy where I trained who also obsessed over this stuff. Apparently, obscure anatomic trivia tickles a psychopathology common to Academic Radiologists. As a result, I would know the 2 most common variants. The right posterior segment branch draining into the left hepatic duct is the most common. The second most common is trifurcation of the intrahepatic radicles.

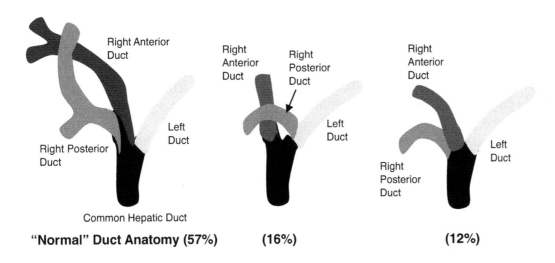

"Normal" Duct Anatomy (57%)   **(16%)**   **(12%)**

Biliary Drainage:

The role of **PTC** (Percutaneous Transhepatic Cholangiogram) and **PTBD** (Percutaneous Transhepatic Biliary Drainage) is centered around situations when ERCP and endoscopy have failed or are not possible (Roux-en-Y).

Things to do before the procedure:

- Check the coags - correct them if necessary (vitamin K, FFP, etc...).

- Most institutions give prophylactic antibiotics (ascending cholangitis is bad).

Approaches:

There are two approaches: right lateral mid axillary for the right system, or subxyphoid for the left system. Realistically, diagnostic cholangiogram and PTBD is usually done from the right. The left is more technically challenging (although better tolerated by the patient because the tube isn't in-between ribs) and usually there is a hilar stricture that won't allow the left and right system to communicate.

"The Moves" - Right-Sided Approach

Line up on the patient's right flank / mid axillary line. Find the 10th rib. Don't go higher than the 10th rib - always below (avoiding the pleura can save you a ton of headaches). Prior to jamming the needle in, most reasonable people put metal forceps (or other metal tool) over the target and fluoro to confirm you are over the liver and below the pleural reflection.

> When I say "Below the 10th Rib," I mean caudal to the 10th rib, not actually under the rib. Always puncture at the TOP EDGE OF A RIB to avoid the intercostal artery (which runs under the rib).

Now the fun begins. The basic idea is to pretend the patient is a voodoo doll of the Attending (or childhood tormentor) that you hate the most. Proceed to blindly and randomly jam a chiba needle in and inject slowly under fluoro as you pull back (but not all the way out). Obviously less sticks is better and it's ideal to do in less than 5 (most places will still consider less than 15 ok). Once you get into a duct the system will opacify. You then can pick your target (posterior is best for best drainage). You stick again, wire in, and place the catheter into the duodenum.

A non-dilated system can be very difficult and there is an old school trick where you stick the gallbladder (on purpose) and retrograde fill the system. The problem with that is you have to keep a drain in the gallbladder as well.

> ### In the Duct?
>
> - *Ducts* = Flow Towards the Hilum
> - *Vein* = Flow Cranially towards the Heart
> - *Artery* = Flow Towards the Periphery

The Moves" - **Left Sided Approach**

This time you use a sub-sternal / subxyphoid approach with ultrasound. Most people aim for the anterior inferior peripheral ducts. Otherwise the moves are pretty much the same.

Catheter / Stent Choice - Bare Bones of Trivia:

Most stent placement is preceded by a period of biliary decompression with an internal-external drain. Plastic stents are cheaper but have a short patency period. Metal stents will stay patent longer but can't be removed. Metal stents are not usually used in benign disease unless the patient has a long life expectancy.

Internal-External drains are the standard for crossing lesions. They have superior stability to a straight drain or pigtail. They offer the advantage of possible conversion to an internal only drain (save those bile-salts).

Some testable trivia is that many centers will manually punch some additional side holes in the proximal portion of the tube to make sure that drainage adequate.

The key is to NOT position any side holes outside the liver (proximal to liver parenchyma).

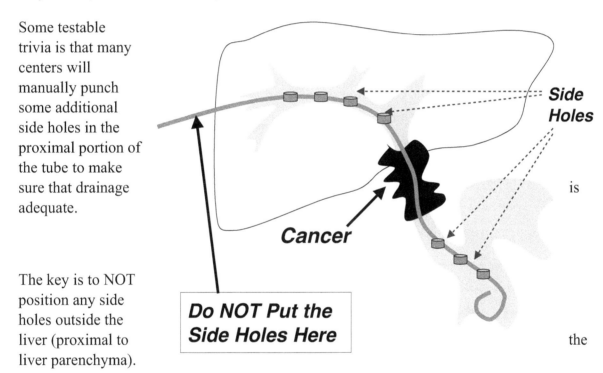

Side Holes

is

Cancer

Do NOT Put the Side Holes Here

the

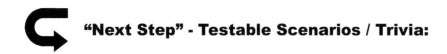 **"Next Step" - Testable Scenarios / Trivia:**

- **There is extensive ascites**. *Next Step* = Drain it prior to doing the PTC.

- **There is a small amount of ascites**. *Next Step* = Opinions are like assholes (everyone has one), so you'll hear different things for this. I think most people would look to make sure the liver still abuts the peritoneum at the puncture site. If it does, then they will do a right sided approach. If it doesn't then they will use ultrasound and go substernal on the left.

- **Right Approach with no filling of the left ducts**. *Next Step* = Slowly and carefully roll the patient on their side (right side up). The right ducts are dependent - so this is actually fairly common. Now obviously if there is a known obstruction you don't need to roll them. The rolling is to prove it's not a real obstruction.

- **You do your contrast run and the patient instantly goes into a full rigor**.
  Next Step = Look around the room for the person you are going to blame for injecting too forcefully. "Rigor" is a multiple choice buzzword for cholangitis. Yes... full on biliary sepsis can happen instantly with a forceful injection. This is actually pretty easy to do if the patient has strictures or an obstructive neoplastic process. In those cases you will want to have your Scapegoat / "Not Me" (tech, med student, resident, fellow, drug rep, non-english-speaking international observer) do the injection. For the purpose of multiple choice some good next step options would be: aggressive resuscitation, place a drain, and inform the primary team / ICU that the Scapegoat gave the patient biliary sepsis.

> **Forceful Injection = ICU Visit for Cholangitis**
> **Buzzword = "Rigors after Injection"**

- **You encounter (or expect stones)**. *Next Step* = Dilute contrast to 200-250 mg/ml to avoid obscuring filling defects.

- **You can't cross the obstruction with a wire**. *Next Step* = Place a pigtail drain and let the system cool down for like 48 hours. Try again when there is less edema.

Cholecystostomy:

This is done when you have a super sick patient you can't take to the OR, but the patient has a toxic gallbladder. In cases of acalculous cholecystitis (with no other source of sepsis), 60% of the time cholecystostomy is very helpful. It's a "temporizing measure." You have to give pre-procedure antibiotics. There are two approaches:

- *Transperitoneal* – This is preferred by many because it's a direct approach, and avoids hitting the liver. The major draw back is the wire / catheter often buckles and you lose access (and spill bile everywhere). This is typically not the first choice. However in patients with liver disease or coagulopathy it may be preferred (depending on who you ask). *If the question writer specifically states (or infers) that the patient has an increased risk of bleeding this is probably the right choice.* Otherwise, if forced to choose, pick the Transhepatic route

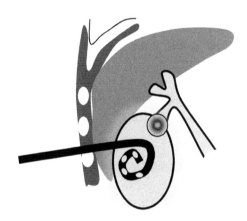

- *Transhepatic* – The major plus here is that when you cross the liver it stabilizes the wire and **minimizes the chance of a bile leak**. This is the route most people choose.

    o *Trivia* = Typically you go through *segments 5 and 6* on your way to the gallbladder

    o *Trivia* = This route transverse the "bare area" / upper one third of the gallbladder (hypothetically).

Important Trivia:

- Prior to the procedure, make sure the bowel isn't interposed in front of the liver/ gallbladder. If a multiple choice writer wanted to be sneaky he/she could tell you the patient has *"Chilaiditi Syndrome"* - which just means that they have bowel in front of their liver. Some sources will list this as a contraindication to PC.

- Even if the procedure instantly resolves all symptoms, you need to leave the tube in for 2-6 weeks (until the tract matures), otherwise you are going to get a bile leak.

- After that *"at least 2 week"* period you should *perform a cholangiogram* to confirm that the cystic duct is patent before you pull the tube.

- Most places will *clamp the tube for 48 hours prior to removal*. This helps confirm satisfactory internal drainage.

Managing Bile Leak – Bile leak is bad as it can lead to massive biliary ascites and chemical peritonitis. Most people will try and place a tube within the bile ducts to divert bile from the location of the leak (this usually works).

General Biopsy Pearls

There are two primary techniques for sampling tissue:

(1) Fine Needle Aspiration — *Cytology*

(2) Cutting Needle ("Core") — *Biopsy*

Fine Needle Aspiration:

This is for situations when you only need a few cells. It is typically performed through a 21 or 22G Chiba needle. Vacuum aspiration with a 20 cc syringe is applied as you pass the needle back and forth through the target.

Trivia: Apply "gentle" suction as you remove the needle. If you suck too hard a tiny sample could get lost in the syringe. If you forget to apply suction the sample will stay in the patient.

The needle is small so the risks are small.

Cutting / Core Needle

This is for situations when you need a larger sample. There are lots of devices but the most basic mechanism involves a needle with two parts; an outer shaft for cutting, and an inner stylet.

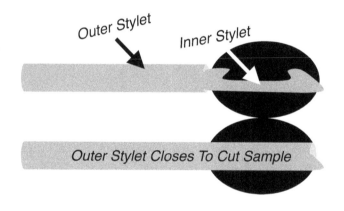

Trivia: For the purpose of multiple choice, the target is "cut" where the outer shaft is advanced.

Trivia: The general rule is pick the shortest length needle that will reach the target.

Trivia: "Automated Systems" fire both the inner and outer components to take the sample. The key point is that with these systems the sample is taken from tissue 10-20 mm in front of the needle.

Conventional Liver Biopsy -

You can do targeted approaches (for a specific lesion) or you can do non-targeted approaches (sampling). General pearls include: trying to cross the capsule only once, <u>biopsy the subcapsular masses through an area of uninvolved liver, and avoid the diaphragm.</u>

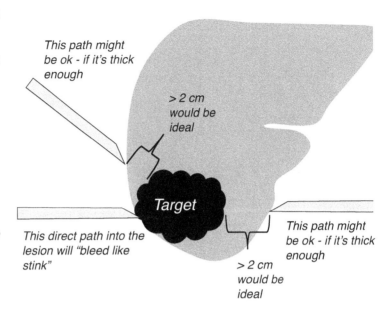

This path might be ok - if it's thick enough

> 2 cm would be ideal

Target

This direct path into the lesion will "bleed like stink"

This path might be ok - if it's thick enough

> 2 cm would be ideal

If given the choice, you want to biopsy peripheral lesions through 2-3 cm of normal liver prior to hitting the target.

This is done to avoid a blood bath.

Next Step: There is ascites = Drain it prior to doing the biopsy

Trivia: Mild shoulder pain (referred pain) is common after liver biopsy.

Trivia: Prolonged Shoulder Pain (> 5 mins) = Possible Bleed *"Kehr Sign"*.

Next Step: Prolonged Shoulder Pain (> 5 mins) = Re-evaluation with ultrasound. Always look behind the liver (Morrison's pouch) to see if blood is accumulating. Bleeding after liver biopsy occurs more from biopsy of malignant lesions (compared to diffuse disease).

Contraindications: Uncorrectable coagulopathy, thrombocytopenia (< 50,000), infections in the right upper quadrant – are contraindications for a conventional biopsy.

Trivia: Biopsy of carcinoid mets is controversial and death by carcinoid crisis has occurred after biopsy.

Next Step: Massive ascites or severe coagulopathy = *Transjugular approach*

Transjugular Liver Biopsy

The rationale is that the liver capsule is never punctured, so bleeding is less of a risk. Obviously this is a non-targeted biopsy for the diagnosis of infectious, metabolic, and sometimes neoplastic processes (classic example = grading chronic hep C).

Specific Indications:

- **Severe Coagulopathy**

- Massive ascites

- Failure of prior percutaneous liver biopsy

- Massive obesity *("Fat Even By West Virginia Standards")*

- Patients on mechanical ventilation

- Need for additive vascular procedures like TIPS

Procedural Trivia:

The general technique is to access the hepatic veins via the IVC (*via the right jugular vein*). Most people will tell you to biopsy through the *right hepatic vein* while angling the sheath anterior.   The reason this is done is to get the biggest bite of tissue, and avoid capsular perforation (which was the entire point of this pain in the ass procedure).

Trivia: Right Sided Jugular Route is the superior route (better than left IJ, or femoral)

Trivia: Biopsy via the Right Hepatic Vein by angling anterior. Never perform an anterior biopsy from the middle hepatic vein.

Trivia: This procedure has the added benefit of allowing you to measure hepatic venous pressures - which can guide therapy or assess varix bleeding risk.

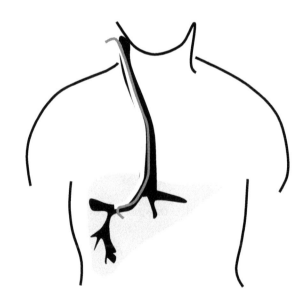

Hepatic / Splenic Trauma –

Embolization is a potential method for dealing with significant trauma to the hepatic or splenic arteries. Opinions on the exact role of angiography vary between institutions, so "read my mind" questions are likely.

I think the most likely type of indication question might actually be *who does NOT go to angio?*

The most accepted contraindication in a bleeding patient is probably a very busted-up unstable dude who needs to go straight to the OR for emergent laparotomy.

> **Indications**
> *agreed upon by most:*
>
> • Continuous hemorrhage (active extrav) in a patient who is borderline stable post resuscitation
>
> • Early ongoing bleeding after a surgical attempt to gain primary hemostasis
>
> • Rebleeding after successful initial embolization
>
> • Post traumatic pseudo-aneurysm and AVFs (even if they aren't currently bleeding).

 Tools and Strategy - Hepatic Considerations:

• Gelfoam, pledgets, particles, and/or microcoils are typically used.

• Massive non-selective hepatic artery embolization is usually avoided to reduce the risk of large volume tissue necrosis.

• *What's the main issue with tissue necrosis?* Hepatic abscess development (which is fairly common in a major liver injury anyway).

• *Trivia:* Coils should NOT be placed in the pseudoaneurysm sac. This can lead to a late rupture. The strategy is to occlude the distal and proximal parent vessels. You'll want to perform "completion angiography" to prove the thing is occluded prior to catheter removal.

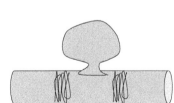
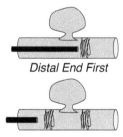

Distal End First

"Sandwich Technique" to exclude arterial pseudo aneurysm

Then Pull Back

• Hepatic surface is bleeding from more than one spot. Next Step = Gelfoam or particles.

• Hepatic Pseudoaneurysms can be treated at the site of injury (with the sandwich technique) because they are not end arteries (no collaterals). Plus the liver has a dual blood supply.

Tools and Strategy Continued - Spleen Considerations:

- Splenic laceration (without active extravasation) is NOT considered an indication to angio (by most people). Remember to use your mind reading powers to confirm the question writer agrees.

- The spleen does not have a dual blood supply, and is considered an "end organ" unlike the liver. So if you go nuts embolizing it you can infarct the whole fucking thing.

- Focal Splenic Abnormality. *Next Step* = Selective Embolization treatment

- Multiple Bleeding Sites. *Next Step* = Use a proximal embolization strategy, and drop an Amplatzer plug into the splenic artery proximal to the short gastric arteries. The idea is to maintain perfusion but reduce the pressure to the spleen (slower blood will clot), with the benefit of preserved collateral supply and less infarction risk.

- *Trivia:* Even with this proximal embolization strategy the patient usually does not require vaccination post embolization, as a lot of functional tissue should remain.

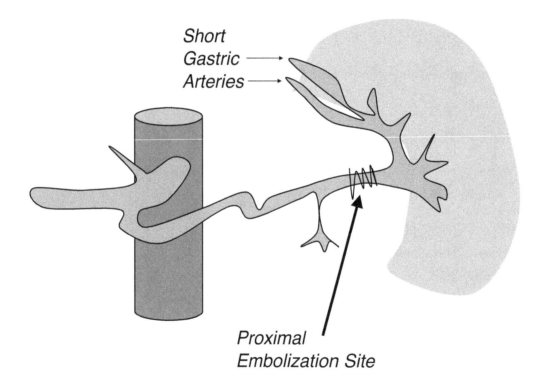

HCC Treatment:

You will read in some sources that transplant is the only way to "cure" an HCC. Others will say transplant, resection, or ablation are "curative" if the tumor is small enough. Arterial embolization (TACE) is typically used in situations where the tumor burden is advanced and the patient cannot undergo surgery.

Transarterial Chemoembolization (TACE) – Most people will consider this first line for palliative therapy in advanced cases. The mechanism relies on HCC's preference for arterial blood. High concentration of chemotherapy within Lipiodol (iodized oil transport agent) is directly delivered into the hepatic arterial system. The tumor will preferentially take up the oil resulting in a prolonged targeted chemotherapy. The Lipiodol is usually followed up with particle embolization, with the goal of slowing down the washout of the agent.

Absolute Contraindication = Decompensated (acute on chronic) Liver failure.

Trivia: Some sources will list portal vein thrombosis as a contraindication (because of the risk of liver infarct). Others say portal vein thrombosis is fine as long as an adjustment is made to limit the degree of embolization and you can document sufficient hepatic collateral flow. Simply read the mind of the question writer to know which camp they are in.

Trivia = TACE in Patients with a biliary stent, prior sphinctertomy, or post Whipple are all high risk for biliary abscess.

Trivia = *"Sterile cholecystitis"* or *"chemical cholecystitis"* are buzzwords that when used in the setting of TACE should lead you to believe that the agent was injected into the *right hepatic artery prior to the takeoff of the cystic artery* (artery to the gallbladder) .

Trivia = TACE will prolong survival better than systemic chemo

Trivia: Unfortunately, repeat TACEs can result in a ton of angio time and therefore a ton of radiation. Patient do sometimes get *skins burns* (usually *on their left back* because of the RAO camera angle).

RFA: Tumor is destroyed by heating the tissue to 60 degrees C (140 F). Any focal or nodular peripheral enhancement in the ablation lesion should be considered residual / recurrent disease. Sometimes, on the immediate post treatment study you can have some reactive peripheral hyperemia – but this should decrease on residual studies. Important trivia is that RF ablation is indicated in patients with HCC and colorectal mets (who can't get surgery).

TACE + RFA: As a point of trivia, it has been shown that TACE + RFA for HCC lesions larger than 3cm, will improve survival (more so than either treatment alone). This is still not curative.

Yttrium-90 Radioembolization - An alternative to TACE is using radioactive embolic materials (Y-90). The primary testable trivia regarding Y-90 therapy is understanding the pre-therapy work up. There are basically two things to know:

(1) *Lung Shunt Fraction* - You give Tc-99 MAA to the hepatic artery to determine how much pulmonary shunting occurs. A shunt fraction that would give 30 Gy in a single treatment is too much (Y-90 is contraindicated).

(2) *The take off of the right gastric.* The fear is that you get non-targeted poisoning of the stomach, leading to a non-healing gastric ulcer. To help prevent reflux of the Y-90 (poison) into places you don't want (basically anywhere that's not liver) prophylactic embolization of the right gastric and the GDA is performed. The right gastric origin is highly variable, and can come off the proper hepatic or the left hepatic.

Trivia Review:

• Shunt Fraction > 30 Gy to the Lungs = No Y-90

• Before you give the poison, embo the right gastric (which has a variable take off) and GDA - so you don't put a hole in the stomach.

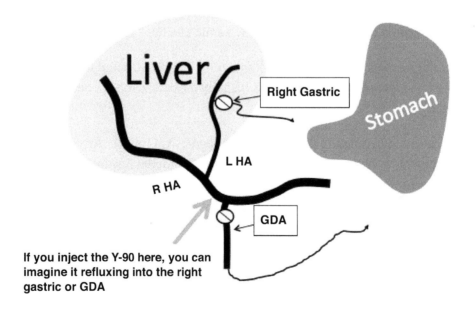

Liver **Right Gastric** **Stomach**

L HA

R HA

GDA

If you inject the Y-90 here, you can imagine it refluxing into the right gastric or GDA

Generalized Tumor Treatment Trivia (Regardless of the Organ)

RFA

- Tumors need to be less than 4 cm or you can't "cure" them. You can still do RFA on tumors bigger than 4 cm but the buzzword you want for this is "debulking".

> - Cure = < 4 cm
> - Debulk = > 4 cm

- You always need a burn margin of 0.5-1.0 cm around the tumor. So your target is the tumor + another 1 cm of healthy organ.

- A key structure (something you don't want to burn up) that is within 1 cm of the lesion is considered by most to be a contraindication to RFA. Some people won't cook lesions near the **vascular hilum**, or near the gallbladder. Be on the look out for **bowel**. It is possible to cook bowel adjacent to a superficial lesion. If they are asking you if a lesion is appropriate for RFA and it's superficial look for adjacent bowel - that is probably the trick.

- RFA requires the application of a "Grounding pad" on the patient's leg. Blankets should be jammed between the arms/body and between legs to prevent closed circuit arcs/burns.

- *"Hot Withdrawal"* supposedly can reduce the risk of tumor seeding. Basically you leave the cooker on as you remove the probe to burn the tract.

- *"Heat Sink"* - this is a phenomenon described exclusively with RFA. Lesions that are near blood vessels 3mm or larger may be difficult to treat (without getting fancy) because the moving blood removes heat away from the lesion.

- You can overcook the turkey. Temperatures at 100 C or greater tend to carbonize the tissue near the probe, reducing electrical conductance (resulting in suboptimal treatment). Around 60 C is the usual target.

- ***"Post Ablation Syndrome"*** - Just like a tumor embolization you can get a low grade fever and body aches. The larger the tumor, the more likely the syndrome (just like embolization).

  - Low Grade Fever and Body Aches Post Ablation. *Next Step* = Supportive Care

  - Persistent Fever x 2-3 weeks post ablation. *Next Step* = Infection workup.

Microwave

Similar to RFA is that it cooks tumors. The testable differences are that it can generate more power, can cook a bigger lesion, requires less ablation time, it's less susceptible to heat sink effect, and it does NOT require a ground pad.

Cryoablation

Instead of burning the tumors, this technique uses extreme cold in cycles with thawing. The freeze-thaw cycles fuck the cells up pretty good. The cold gun is generated by the compressing argon gas. I actually knew a guy who constructed a similar device shortly after an industrial accident left him unable to survive outside of subzero environments.

Trivia = Thawing is what actually kills the cancer cells

Trivia = If you are planning on treating immediately after biopsy, most sources will advise you to place the probes first, then biopsy, then treat. If you try and place the probes you make a bloody mess then you might not get accurate probe placement. Just don't biopsy the probe. Seriously, if you crack the probe and the high pressure gas leaks out - shit is gonna explode (better have your medical student ready as a shield).

Trivia: It hurts less than RFA - so patients need less sedation

Trivia: The risk of bleeding is higher than with RFA - because you aren't ablating the small vessels

Treatment Response

RFA Treatment Response:

Size:

- Week 1-4: It's ok for the lesion to get bigger. This is a reactive change related to edema, tissue evolution, etc...

- Month 3: The lesion should be the same size (or smaller) than the pre-treatment study.

- Month 6: The lesion should be smaller than pre-treatment.

Contrast Enhancement:

- Central or Peripheral Enhancement is NEVER normal in the lesion post treatment.

- You can have "benign peri-ablational enhancement" - around the periphery of the ablation zone. This should be smooth, uniform, and concentric. It should NOT be scattered, nodular, or eccentric (those are all words that mean residual tumor).

Time Interval

- Multiphase CT (or MR) at 1 month. If residual disease is present at this time, *Next Step =* Repeat treatment (assuming no contraindications)

- Additional follow up is typically at 3-6 months intervals.

TACE Treatment Response

On follow up CT, you need to have pre and post contrast imaging including washout. The iodized oil is going to be dense on the pre-contrast. The more dense oil is in the tumor the better outcome is likely to be. The necrotic tissue should not enhance. If there is enhancement and/or washout in or around the tumor, then you have viable tumor that needs additional treatment. Beam hardening from the iodized oil can cause a problem.

"Zone of Ablation" is the preferred nomenclature for the post-ablation region on imaging.

Also, Dude, "Chinaman" is not the preferred nomenclature. Asian-American

Cryoablation Treatment Response

Post therapy study is typically performed at 3 months, with additional follow ups at 6 months and 12 months.

A good result should be lower in density relative to the adjacent kidney. On MR, a good result is typically T2 dark and T1 iso or hyper.

Size: Just like RFA, ablated lesions can initially appear that they grew in size relative to the pre-treatment study. With time they should progressively shrink (usually faster than with RFA). An increase in size (after the baseline post treatment) should be considered recurrent tumor.

Enhancement: Any nodular enhancement (>10HU change from pre-contrast run) after treatment should be considered cancer.

Vocab

"Residual tumor" or *"Incomplete Treatment"* = Vocab words used when you see focal enhancement in the tumor ablation zone of a patient for their first post therapy study.

"Recurrent tumor" = Word used when you see focal enhancement in the tumor ablation zone that is new from the first post therapy study.

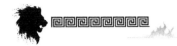 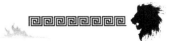
G Tubes:

A "G- Tube" is a gastric tube, placed directly into the stomach. They are primarily used as an attempt to prolong the suffering of stroked out Alzheimer Patients with stage 4 sacral decubitus ulcers.

Traditional method (Radiographically Inserted Gastrostomy - RIG):   The basic idea is that you put an NG tube down and pump air into the stomach until it smushes flat against the anterior abdominal wall. Then you spear it and secure it with 4 "T-Tacks" to tack the stomach to the abdominal wall in the gastric body. Then spear it again, wire in and dilate up to the size you want. Typically, the T-Tacks are removed in 3-6 weeks. Other things that you can do is give a cup of barium the night before to outline the colon.

If the patient has ascites. *Next Step* = Drain that first.

The Ideal Target:

Left of Midline *(lateral to the rectus muscle to avoid inferior epigastric)*

Mid to Distal Body

Equal distance from the greater and less curves - *to avoid arteries*

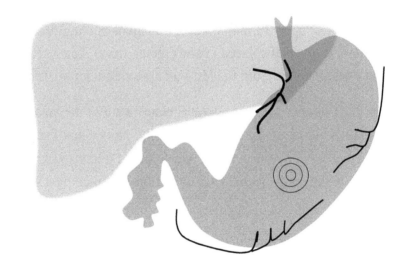

Anatomy Trivia: The cardia of the stomach is actually the most posterior portion.

There is another method often called a *"PIG"* because of the *P*eroral route. In that version you stab the stomach and tread a wire up the esophagus. Then you grab the wire, slip the tube over it, and advance the tube over the wire into the stomach all the way out the stabbed hole.
Then it's back to the nursing home for Grandma.

Honestly, it's probably best to do it with a scope, but since we are Radiologists my official statement is that only a Radiologist can do this procedure well.

How long does Granny need to wait before she can have her ensure via the G-Tube? Depends on who you ask. Some people will say 12-24 hours fasting post placement. Other people will say use it right away. It depends on the brand and practitioners bias. To know the correct answer for the exam - simply read the mind of the person who wrote the question.

Esophageal Stents

Probably the most common indication for one of these is esophageal cancer palliation. These are usually placed by GI, but that doesn't mean you won't get asked about them.

In the real world, most people don't even size these things. The overwhelming majority of lesions can be covered by one stent. Having said that, for the purpose of multiple choice you need a stent with *a length at least 2 cm longer than the lesion on each side*. You do the procedure through the mouth. I imagine it would be great fun to try and place a stent through the nose - if you really hated the person. You give them some oral contrast to outline the lesion. An amplatz wire is dropped down into the stomach. The stent (usually self expanding) is deployed over the wire.

Post Angioplasty? Most people don't angioplasty after deployment of the stent. However, if the tumor is bulky and near the carina, some sources will suggest doing a pre-stent angioplasty test up to 20 mm to see if this invokes coughing / stridor. The concern is that a large tumor may get displaced against the carina and cause a respiratory emergency. If the patient doesn't cough from the test you are safe to deploy the stent (probably).

Upper 1/3 Cancer: Most esophageal cancers are in the lower 1/3. If the question specifically tells you it's higher up (or shows you), they may be leading you towards a *"don't cover the larynx dumbass!"* question. The way to avoid this is to have endoscopy do the case so they can identify the cords. If that isn't an option then placing a smaller device might be an alternative.

Stent Drops into the Stomach: Most people will just leave the motherfucker alone. However, if the patient is symptomatic, endoscopic removal is the textbook answer.

Stent Occludes. *Next Step* = Esophagram. The most common cause is food impaction - which sometimes can be cleared with a soda. If that fails, the next step is endoscopy. If it's not food but instead tumor overgrowth, sometimes you can place a second stent. It depends on a lot of factors and asking that would be horse shit.

Gamesmanship:

• Acute obstruction is likely food

• Worsening symptoms over time is likely tumor.

GI Bleed

You can split GI bleeds into two categories upper (proximal to ligament of Treitz) and lower.

Upper GI:

Some testable trivia is that 85% of upper GI bleeds are from the left gastric, and often *if a source cannot be identified, the left gastric is taken down prophylactically.* If the source of bleeding is from a *duodenal ulcer, embolization of the GDA* is often performed. About 10% of the time, an upper GI bleed can have bright red blood per rectum.

"Pseudo-Vein" Sign – This is a sign of active GI bleeding, with the appearance of a vein created by contrast pooling in a gastric rugae or mucosal intestinal fold. If you aren't sure if it's an actual vein, the "pseudo-vein" will persist beyond the venous phase of injection.

Dieulafoy's Lesion - This is a monster artery in the submucosa of the stomach which pulsates until it causes a teeny tiny tear (not a primary ulcer). These tears can bleed like stink. It's typically found in the lesser curvature. It's not exactly an AVM, more like angiodysplasia. Sometimes you can treat it with clips via endoscopy. Sometimes it needs endovascular embolization.

When I say pancreatic arcade bleeding aneurysm, you say celiac artery stenosis.

There is a known association with celiac artery compression (median arcuate ligament) and the dilation of pancreatic duodenal arcades with pseudoaneurysm formation.

Gamesmanship: It is classically shown with an angiographic run through the SMA, showing a dilated collateral system and retrograde filling of the hepatic artery.

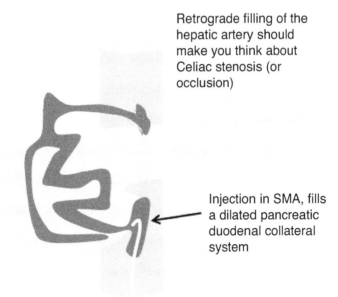

Retrograde filling of the hepatic artery should make you think about Celiac stenosis (or occlusion)

Injection in SMA, fills a dilated pancreatic duodenal collateral system

Upper GI Bleed "Next Step" Algorithm

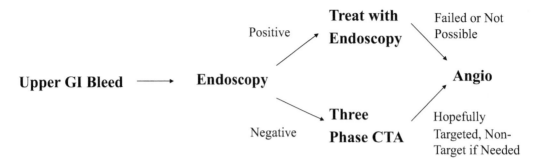

Lower GI:

The work-up for lower GI bleeds is different than upper GI bleeds. With the usual caveat that algorithms vary wildly from center to center, this is a general way to try and answer next step type questions regarding the workup.

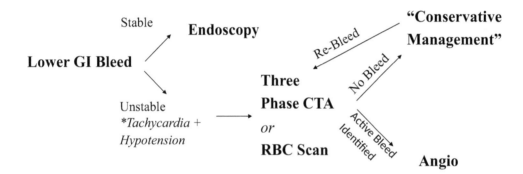

ACR Appropriateness specifically states that in a STABLE patient with lower GI bleeding that endoscopy is first line.

ACR Appropriate:
Intermittent / Obscure GI Bleeding

— GI Bleeding that continues (or recurs) despite negative upper endoscopy and colonoscopy is described as *"obscure GI bleeding."* The actual culprit is often from the small bowel (arteriovenous malformation).

— There is no clear consensus on the optimal study to interrogate the small bowel.

— ACR Appropriateness Criteria rank CT angiography and capsule endoscopy as the most appropriate choices in this situation. Tc-99m RBC scan is considered as a "reasonable alternative" for localization - but only in the setting of active bleeding. Remember GI bleed scan only works if there is active bleeding.

High Yield Trivia is that **nuclear scintigraphy (RBC bleeding scan) is more sensitive than angiography**.

Bleed Scan = 0.1 mL/min
CTA = 0.4 ml/min
Angiography = 1.0 mL/min

Causes with Angiographic Buzzwords:

 •**Angiodysplasia** - Right Sided Finding. *"Early Draining Vein."* Embolization of angiodysplasia rarely stops a re-bleed and these often need surgery.

 •**Diverticulosis** - Left Sided Finding (usually). More commonly venous. If arterial, *"filling the diverticulum first"* is classic.

 •**Meckles** - Usually shown on Meckles scan (^{99m}Tc-Na-pertechnetate). The feeding artery (vitelline) has a classic look with *"extension beyond the mesenteric border,"* *"no side branches"* and *"a corkscrew appearance"* of the terminal portion.

Technical Aspects / Trivia:

You will want runs of all 3 vessels (SMA, Celiac, IMA). Some old school guys will say to start with the IMA because contrast in the bladder will obscure that territory as the procedure continues. That's not really an issue anymore with modern DSA and starting with the SMA will typically be the highest yield. You have to sub select each vessel. Runs in the aorta are not good enough and that would never be the right answer.

What if you don't see bleeding? You can try **"provocative angiography"** - which is not nearly as interesting as it sounds. This basically involves squirting some vasodilator (nitro 100-200 mcg) or thrombolytic drug (tPA 4 mg) into the suspected artery to see if you can make it bleed for you.

What if you do see it bleeding? Administer some street justice. Anyone who trained in the last 30 years is going to prefer microcoils and PVA particles. Old guys might use gel-foam. Alcohol should not be used for lower GI bleeds (causes bowel necrosis).

Microcoils: Good because you can see them. Good because you can place them precisely. Bad because they deploy right where you drop them. So you need to go right up next to that bleed to avoid a large bowel infarct.

Trivia = Inability to advance the micro-catheter peripherally is the most common cause of microcoil embo failure

I say "non-selective embolization of bowel with microcoils," you say "bowel infarct"

PVA: Good because they are "flow directed." So you don't need to be as peripheral compared to the microcoils. Bad because you have less control.

Trivia: Particles must be <u>300-500 microns</u>. Particles that are smaller will/could cause bowel infarct.

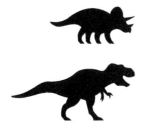

But Prometheus my Geriatric Attending says to use Vasopressin?
Between me and you this argument was settled in 1986 by a lady named Gomes. Her study showed coils stopped GI bleeds 86% of the time, compared to 52% for vasopressin and the shit we have today is way better making the disparity even greater. Having said that, some Dinosaurs still do it.

For the purpose of multiple choice, this is what I would know:

- Vasopressin works as a vasoconstrictor

- Vasopressin does not require superselection. You can squirt it right into the main trunk of the artery.

- Vasopressin sucks because the re-bleed rates are high (once the drug wears off)

- Vasopressin can actually cause non-occlusive mesenteric ischemia (NOMI)

- Vasopressin should NOT be used with large artery bleeding (i.e. splenic pseudoaneurysm), bleeding at sites with dual blood supply (classic example is pyloroduodenal bleed), severe coronary artery disease, severe hypertension, dysrhythmias, and after an embolotherapy treatment (risk of bowel infarct).

Post Embolization: You need to do angiography post embolization to look for collateral flow (if there is a dual supply). The classic example is: after performing an embolization of the GDA (for duodenal ulcer), you need to do a run of the SMA to look at the inferior pancreaticoduodenal (collateral to the GDA). You might have to take that one out too, but obviously that would increase the risk of bowel infarct.

Trivia - Risk of bowel infarct is way lower for upper GI bleeds (because of the extensive collateral supply), relative to bleeds distal to the ligament of Trietz.

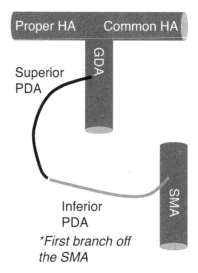

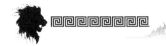 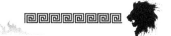
General Tactics:

In general, there are two methods, you can use a trocar or you can use the seldinger technique (wire guided).

- *Trocar:* You nail it with a spinal needle first. Then adjacent to the needle (in tandem) you place a catheter.
- *Seldinger:* One stick with a needle, then wire in, dilate up and place a catheter.

Drain Size: The grosser and thicker stuff will need a bigger tube. If forced I'd go with:

- 6-8 F for clear fluid

- 8-10 F for thin pus

- 10-12 F for thick pus

- 12F+ for collections with debris or in collections that smell like a Zombie farted.

Drain Type: You pretty much always use a pigtail. I wouldn't guess anything else.

 Trivia / Gamesmanship

- Any "next step" question that offers to *turn doppler on prior to sticking it* with a needle is always the right answer. Trying to trick you into core needling a pseudoaneurysm is the oldest trick in the book.

- Decompressing the urinary bladder prior to a pelvic abscess drainage is often a good idea.

- Collection has pus. Next step = aspirate all of it (as much as possible) prior to leaving the drain

- You can't advance into the cavity because it's too fibrous/thick walled. *Next Step ?* I'd try a hydrophilic coated

- Family medicine want you to put a 3 way on that 12 F drain. Next step = don't do that. You are reducing the functional lumen to 6F.

Trivia / Gamesmanship Continued

- Family medicine wants you to hold off on antibiotics till after you drain this unstable septic shock patient's abscess. Next step = don't do that. Antimicrobial therapy should never be withheld because some knuckle head is worried about sterilizing cultures. (1) Cultures almost never change management from the coverage they were on anyway, (2) the trauma of doing the drainage will seed the bloodstream with bacteria and make the sepsis worse.

- Family medicine wants to know how many cc to flush this complex (but small) abscess with? Remember that *"flushing"* and *"irrigation"* are different. Flushing is done to keep the tube from clogging with viscous poop. Irrigation is when you are washing out the cavity (the solution to pollution is dilution) for complete cavity drainage. Going nuts with the irrigation can actually cause a bacteremia. The vignette could say something like "waxing and waning fever corresponding to flush schedule." The next step would be to train the nurses / family medicine to limit the volume to less than the size of the cavity.

- You irrigate the abscess with 20 cc of fluid but when you aspirate back you only get 5ccs. Next Step? Stop irrigating it! You have a big problem. The fluid (which is dirty) is being washed into a location that is not able to be sucked back out by the tube. So you are creating a new pocket of infection that isn't being drained.

- Catheter started out draining but now is stopped. Next Step = (1) confirm that it is in the correct location and not kinked - might need imaging if not obvious at bedside, then (2) try flushing it or clearing an obstruction with a guidewire. If the catheter is clogged for real then you'll need to exchange it - probably for a larger size. If the tract is mature (older than a week) you can probably get a hydrophilic guidewire through the tract into the collection to do an easy exchange.

- Remove the catheter when: (1) drainage is less than 10cc / day, (2) the collection is resolved by imaging (CT, Ultrasound, etc...), and (3) there is no fistula.

- Persistent Fever > 48 Hours post drainage. The patient should get better pretty quickly after you drain the abscess. If they aren't getting better it implies one of two things (1) you did a shitty job draining it, or (2) they have another abscess somewhere else. Either way they need more imaging and probably another drain.

- The drainage amount spikes. This is a bad sign. In a normal situation the drainage should slower taper to nothing and then once you confirm the abscess has resolved you pull the drain. Spikes in volume (especially on multiple choice exams) suggest the formation of a fistula. Next step is going to be more imaging, possibly with fluoro to demonstrate the fistula (urine, bowel, pancreatic duct, bile duct, etc...).

Pelvic Abscess Drainage - *tubo-ovarian abscess, diverticular abscess, or peri-appendiceal*

General Ideas for Choosing the Correct Route:

(1) All things equal, pick the shortest route

(2) Avoid bowel, solid organs, blood vessels *(inferior epigastrics are classic)*, nerves

(3) Try not to contaminate sterile areas

(4) Choose the most dependent position possible *(usually posterior or lateral)* to facilitate drainage

Routes

Most abscesses in the pelvis are layering in a dependent position so anterior routes are typically not easy. In general there are 4 routes; transabdominal, transgluteal, transvaginal, and transrectal. I'm gonna try and cover the pros/cons and testable trivia for each route.

Transabdominal - The pull of gravity tends to cause infection to layer in the more posterior spaces. As a result transabdominal approaches tend to be long, and therefore violate one of the 4 general ideas. If you are shown an abscess where this would be the best, shortest route then remember to watch out for the inferior epigastrics. For sure there will be an option to stick the trocar right through one of them. Make sure you ID them before you choose your answer.

Transgluteal - The transgluteal approach is done for a variety of posterior targets. The patient is positioned prone for targeting.

Avoid the sciatic nerve and gluteal arteries by:

- Access through the sacrospinous ligament

- Medial as possible

- Inferior to the piriformis

Disadvantages: Legit risk of artery/ nerve injury. Prone to catheter kinking. Gotta use CT (radiation).

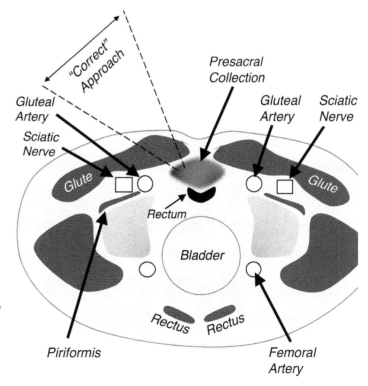

423

Endoluminal Routes: There is a subset of perverts who prefer to biopsy and drain things through the vagina (tuna purse) and/or the rectum.… Not that there's anything wrong with that. Well actually the primary disadvantage of both of these "endoluminal routes" is catheter stability. Many catheters are literally pooped out within 3-4 days. Although advocates for these routes will argue that (a) they are more fun to do, and (b) most collections resolve within 3 days.

Transvaginal: Biopsy and/or drainage through the vagina (pink taco) has the advantage of providing a very short safe route that can be guided by transvaginal ultrasound, allowing for no radiation and very accurate placement. This was the classic in office route for drainage of infected gynecologic fluid collections (PID related). The procedure is done in the lithotomy position. Catheter size is traditionally limited to 12F (or smaller). You should never do this to a patient under the age of 14 - not even Jared from Subway would try that.

Although controversial, it is possible (and well described in the literature) to drain / biopsy adnexa cysts through the vagina (penis fly trap).

Vaginal prep / cleansing prior to the procedure is controversial and unlikely to be tested.

Transrectal: Of the three routes (gluteal, vaginal, rectal) transrectal is supposedly the least painful - although in my literature review the psychological pain was not discussed (this kinda thing would really fuck with my machismo). Essentially this route offers all the advantages of the transvaginal route (ultrasound guidance, very short / safe route) plus the added advantage of pre-sacral access. Depending on what you read, people will argue this is first line (over trans-gluteal) for pre-sacral collection but that is highly variable.

Choosing between transgluteal and trans-rectal for a pre-sacral collection would be the worst "read my mind" question ever. If forced into that scenario I would set aside the psychologic trauma to the alpha male ego and use (1) the size of the collection - *do you think that will drain before he/she poops the catheter out ?*, and (2) is the transgluteal route safe - *are the vessels nerves obviously in the way?*

Prep with a cleansing enema is not controversial and is endorsed pretty much everywhere.

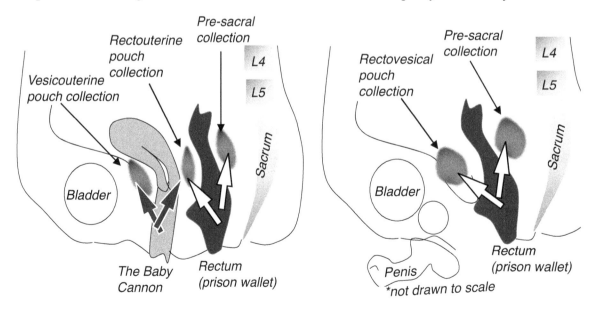

424

Diverticular Abscess

There are a few pearls / special considerations that we should discuss regarding the diverticular abscess.

Size: The typical threshold for a diverticular abscess to be drained is 2 cm. Anything smaller than that will be more trouble than it is worth.

Tube Choice: Remember the grosser and thicker stuff will need a bigger tube. Diverticular abscesses form because of a perforated diverticulum. Thus, you can come to the logical conclusion that you need a tube capable of draining shit. For the purpose of multiple choice, anything smaller than 10F is probable NOT the right answer.

Gas: If the abscess is gas producing (they would have to tell you the bulb suction fills rapidly with gas), the correct ***next step*** is to treat the collection like a pleural drain in a patient with an air leak (i.e. put on water seal).

Liver Abscess

Lots of etiologies for these, but don't forget to think about the appendix or diverticulitis. The draining of these things is somewhat controversial with some authors feeling the risk of peritoneal spread out weighs the benefits and reserving the drainage for patient's with a poor prognosis. Other authors say that everyone and their brother should get one, and consider it first line treatment.

A pearl to draining these things is to not cross the pleura (you'll give the dude an empyema). If there is a biliary fistula, prolonged drainage will usually fix it (biliary drainage or surgery is rarely needed).

Trivia: Biopsy / Aspiration of Echinococcal cysts can cause anaphylaxis. Surgical removal of the presumed echinococcal cysts should be discussed with surgery before attempting the procedure in IR (you want to be able to blame it on them, if shit goes bad).

Renal Abscess

Renal abscess is usually secondary to ascending infection or hematogenous spread. The term *"perinephric abscess"* is used when they perforate into the retroperitoneal space. When they are small (< 3-5 cm) they will resolve on their own with the help of IV antibiotics.

Indications for aspiration or drainage include a large (> 3-5 cm), symptomatic focal fluid collection that does not respond to antibiotic therapy alone.

The strategy is to use ultrasound and stick a pig tail catheter in the thing. After a few days if the thing is not completely drained you can address that by upsizing the tube. If you create or notice a urine leak, you'll need to place a PCN. There are really only relative contraindication – bleeding risk etc…, and the procedure is generally well tolerated with a low complication rate.

Perirenal Lymphocele

This is seen in the setting of a transplant. When they are small you typically just watch them. However, on occasion they get big enough to cause local mass effect on the ureter leading to hydronephrosis. You can totally aspirate them, but they tend to recur and repeated aspiration runs the risk of infecting the collection. For multiple choice I would say do this: Aspirate the fluid and check the creatinine. If it's the same as serum it's probably a lymphocele (*if it's more then it's a urinoma*). Either way you are going to drain them with a catheter. However, if it's a lymphocele you might sclerose the cavity (alcohol, doxy, povidine-iodine).

*Urinomas (that are persistent) of any size are drained.

Pancreas Drainage

Remember that necrotizing pancreatitis is bad, but infected necrotizing pancreatitis is a death sentence. So, be careful draining something that is NOT infected already (otherwise you might make it infected). If you aren't sure if it's infected, consider aspirating some for culture (but not placing a tube).

Indications: General indications include infected collections or collections causing mass effect (bowel or biliary obstruction).

Progression to surgery: If you can get 75% reduction in 10 days, the drain is good enough. If not, the surgeons can use the tract for a video-assisted retroperitoneal debridement (which still avoids open debridement).

Pancreatic Cutaneous Fistula: Other than pancreatic pseudocysts, most pancreatic collections are either brown or grayish. When the fluid is clear, you should think about pancreatic fluid, and send a sample for amylase to confirm. If this lasts more than 30 days then you have yourself a *"persistent pancreatic fistula."* Nice job idiot... you could have just left it alone. That will teach you to let those medicine docs pressure you into doing stuff that's not indicated. It may be possible to treat that with octreotide (synthetic somatostatin) to inhibit pancreatic fluid, although in these cases extended drainage is usually needed.

You've Been Talked into Draining the Pseudocyst — Which Route:

General Rule: If the pseudocyst communicates with the pancreatic duct drainage will be prolonged (6-8 weeks in most cases). You can try and use somatostatin to slow it down.

Most Cases: Transperitoneal with CT guidance — avoid organs, avoid going through the stomach twice.

Can't Avoid the Stomach or Patient has a known Duct Communication (so they gonna have a tube for a long time) - Transgastric Approach — so it drains into the stomach

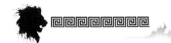 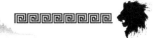

Percutaneous Nephrostomy (PCN) –

There are 3 main reasons you might subject someone to this:

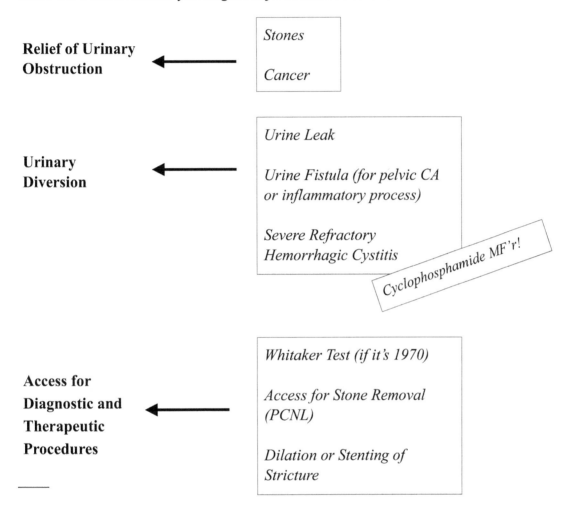

Relief of Urinary Obstruction ← *Stones*

Cancer

Urinary Diversion ← *Urine Leak*

Urine Fistula (for pelvic CA or inflammatory process)

Severe Refractory Hemorrhagic Cystitis

Cyclophosphamide MF'r!

Access for Diagnostic and Therapeutic Procedures ← *Whitaker Test (if it's 1970)*

Access for Stone Removal (PCNL)

Dilation or Stenting of Stricture

____

PCN Contraindications (Absolute):

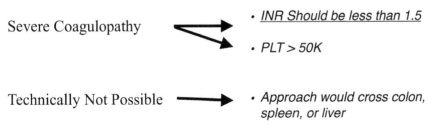

Severe Coagulopathy
- *INR Should be less than 1.5*
- *PLT > 50K*

Technically Not Possible →
- *Approach would cross colon, spleen, or liver*

Technical Stuff:

- Prior to the procedure, it would be ideal if you normalized the potassium (dialysis). Certainly anything about 7 should be corrected prior to the procedure.

- Hold anti-platelet drugs for at least 5 days prior to the procedure.

- The lower pole of a posteriorly oriented calyx is ideal. The reason you use a posterior lateral (30 degrees) approach is to attack along **Brodel's Avascular Zone** (area between the arterial bifurcation).

30 Degrees off sagittal (towards the back)

- Skin entry site should be 10 cm lateral to the midline (not beyond the posterior axillary line). You don't want to go too medial unless you want to try and dilate through the paraspinal muscles. You don't want to go too lateral or you risk nailing the colon.

- Choosing a lower target minimizes the chance of pneumothorax. Additional benefit of the posterior calyces approach is that the guidewire takes a less angled approach (compared to an anterior calyces approach).

- Direct stick into the collecting system without passing through renal parenchyma is NOT a good move (high risk of urine leak).

- Dilated System = Single Stick: Ultrasound and stick your ideal target (low and posterior), then use fluoro to wire in, dilate up, and then place the tube. Alternatively you can do the whole thing under CT.

- Non-Dilated System = Get your partner to do it (these blow). If forced to do = Double Stick. Ultrasound and stick anything you can. Opacify the system. Then stick a second time under fluoro in an ideal position (low and posterior), then wire in, dilate up, and then place the tube. Alternatively you can do the whole thing under CT.

- The posterior calyces (your target) will be seen "end on" if you use contrast. The anterior ones should be more lateral. If you use air, you should just fill the posterior ones (which will be non-dependent with the patient on their belly. Air is useful to confirm.

- You place the drain and get frank pus back. *Next Step* = Aspirate the system

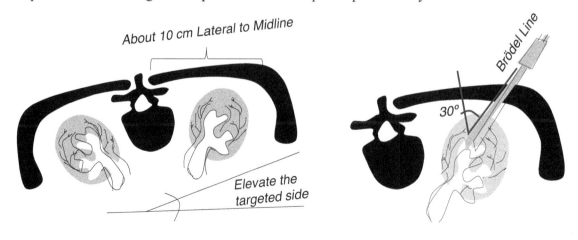

Special Situations:

Nephrostomy on Transplant - The test writer will likely write the question in a way to make you think it's crazy to try one of these. Transplant is NOT a contraindication. In fact it's technically easier than a posterior / native kidney.

Testable Transplant Trivia:

• Anterolateral Calyx Should be Targeted (*instead of posterior*)

• Entry site should be LATERAL to the transplant to avoid entering the peritoneum

• Middle to Upper Pole (*instead of a lower pole*)

Percutaneous Nephrostolithotomy – This is done to remove stones in conjunction with urology. The idea is very similar with a few differences. The most testable difference is that the **site is often the upper pole (instead of lower pole) to make stone access easier.** The tube / hole is bigger and there is more risk of bleeding.

"Tube Fell Out" - The trick to handling these scenarios is the "freshness" of the tube. If the tract is "fresh," which usually means less than 1 week old, then you have to start all over with a fresh stick. If the tract is "mature," which usually means older than 1 week, you can try and re-access it with a non-traumatic wire.

Catheter Maintenance: Exchange is required every 2-3 months because of the crystallization of urine in the tube. Some hospitals / departments will do exchanges more frequently than 2 months and that is because of how well this pays… uh I mean they do it for excellent patient care.

"Encrusted Tube" - If this thing gets totally gross it can be very difficult to exchange in the normal fashion. The most likely "next step" is to use a hydrophilic wire along the side of the tube (same tract) to maintain access.

Ureteral Occlusion - Sometimes urology will request that you just kill the ureters all together. This might be done for fistula, urine leak, or intractable hemorrhagic cystitis. There are a bunch of ways to do it. The most common is probably a sandwich strategy with coils. The sandwich is made by placing large coils in the proximal and distal ends of the "nest", and small coils in the middle. Big Coils = Bread, Small Coils = Bacon.

Nephroureteral Stent (NUS)

This is used when the patient needs long-term drainage. It's way better than having a bag of piss strapped to your back.

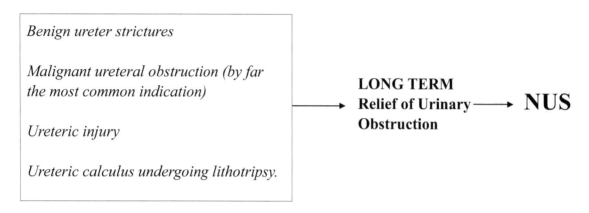

Benign ureter strictures

Malignant ureteral obstruction (by far the most common indication)

Ureteric injury

Ureteric calculus undergoing lithotripsy.

→ **LONG TERM Relief of Urinary** → **NUS**
Obstruction

Technically they can be placed in a retrograde (bladder up) or an antegrade (kidney down) fashion. You are going to use the antegrade strategy if (a) you've got a nephrostomy tube, or (b) retrograde failed.

Can you go straight from Nephrostomy to NUS ? Yes, as long as you didn't fuck them up too bad getting access. If they are bleeding everywhere or they are uroseptic you should wait. Let them cool down, then bring them back to covert to the NUS.

Who should NOT get a NUS ? Anyone who doesn't have a bladder that works (outlet obstruction, neurogenic bladder, bladder tumors, etc..). It makes no sense to divert the urine into a bladder that can't empty.

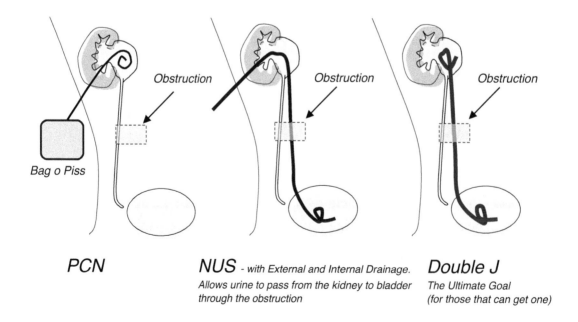

PCN
Bag o Piss

NUS - with External and Internal Drainage.
Allows urine to pass from the kidney to bladder through the obstruction

Double J
The Ultimate Goal (for those that can get one)

Obstruction

430

Internal NUS - Double J:
This is the ultimate goal for the patient. The testable stipulation is that this will require the ability to do retrograde exchanges (via the bladder).

"The Safety" - A safety PCN – is often left in place after the deployment of a double J PCN. The point is to make sure the stent is going to work.

The typical protocol:

1. Place the double J and the safety

2. Cap the safety - so that the internal NUS is draining the patient

3. Bring the patient back in 24-48 hour and "squirt the tube" (antegrade nephrostogram). The system should be non-obstructed.

4. If it's working you pull the safety.

5. If it's NOT working you uncap the safety and just leave it as a PCN.

——-

Suprapubic Cystostomy –

Done to either (a) acutely decompress the bladder or (b) decompress long-term outflow obstruction *(neurogenic bladder, obstructing prostate cancer, urethral destruction, etc..)*

The best way to do it is with ultrasound in the fluoro suite. The target is midline just above the pubic symphysis at the junction of the mid and lower thirds of the anterior bladder wall. You chose this target because:

• The low stick avoids bowel and the peritoneal cavity

• The low 1/3 and mid 1/3 junction avoids the trigone (which will cause spasm).

• The vertical midline is chosen to avoid the inferior epigastric.

Use ultrasound and stick it, confirm position with contrast, wire in and then dilate up. Use a small tube for temporary stuff and a larger tube for more long-term stuff. You can always upsize to a foley once the tract is mature. A 16F foley is ideal for long-term drainage.

Contraindications:

• Buncha Pelvic Surgeries – Extensive scar
• Being a Big Fat Pig/Cow
• Coagulopathy
• Inability to distend bladder
• Inability to displace overlying small bowel

Weapon of Choice

Let's do a rapid review of urinary diversion options.

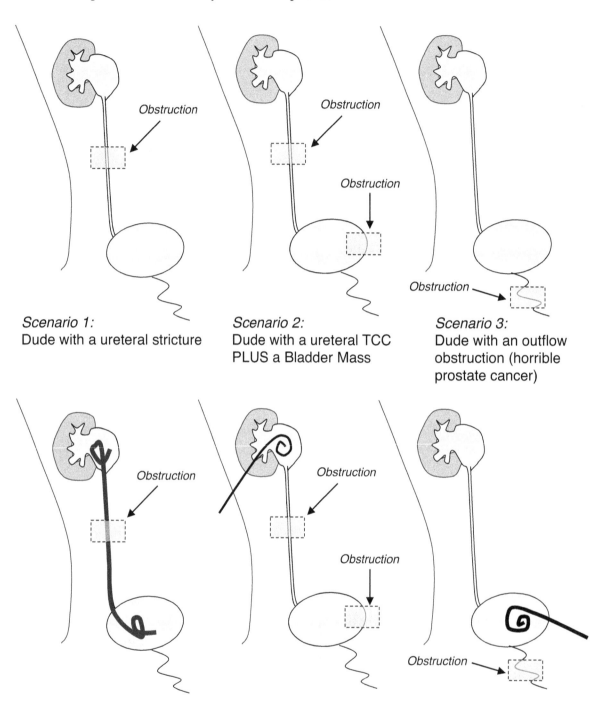

Scenario 1:
Dude with a ureteral stricture

Scenario 2:
Dude with a ureteral TCC PLUS a Bladder Mass

Scenario 3:
Dude with an outflow obstruction (horrible prostate cancer)

*If you can cross the lesion, and the bladder works then internal **Double J** NUS is idea*

*This guy has obstruction at the ureter and the bladder. The only option is to divert at the level of the kidney. He gets a **PCN**.*

*This guy has obstruction at the bladder. He doesn't need to cross the ureter. He gets a **Cystostomy***

Renal Biopsy – This can be done for two primary reasons:

(1) renal failure or (2) cancer biopsy.

Non-Focal: The renal failure workup "non-focal biopsy" is typically done with a 14 - 18 gauge cutting needle , with the patient either prone or on their side (target kidney up). The most obvious testable fact is that **you want tissue from cortex** (lower pole if possible) to maximize the yield of glomeruli on the specimen and minimize complications by avoiding the renal sinus. The complication rate is relatively low, although small AV fistulas and pseudo-aneurysms are relatively common (most spontaneously resolve). Some hematuria is expected. In a high risk for bleeding situation a transjugular approach can be done but that requires knowing what you are doing.

Focal: It used to be thought that focal biopsy should NEVER be done because of the dreaded risk of upstaging the lesion and seeding the track. This has been shown to be very rare (<0.01%). Having said that I think it's still the teaching at least in the setting of pediatric renal masses. This procedure is probably better done with CT. The patient is placed in whatever position is best, but the lateral decubitus with the **lesion side down** is "preferred" , as it stabilizes the kidney from respiratory motion, and bowel interposition. Just like with ultrasound, not crossing the renal sinus is the way to go. Just put the needle in the tumor. If it's cystic and solid make sure you hit the solid part. Some texts recommend both fine needle and core biopsy. The core biopsy is going to give a higher yield. A testable pearl is that if lymphoma is thought likely, a dedicated aspirate should be sent for flow cytometry. As with any renal procedure hematuria is expected (not gross – just a little). Renal colic from blood clots is rare.

ACR Appropriate / SIR Practice Guidelines: Renal Biopsy

— Renal Bx is a procedure with "significant bleeding risk, difficult to detect or control."

— SIR guidelines recommend holding aspirin for 5 days prior to the procedure.

— *Why 5 Days ?* Aspirin irreversibly inhibits platelet function and since platelet lifespan is about 8-10 days, patients with normal marrow will replenish 30-50% of their platelets within 5 days of withholding the willow bark (aspirin).

Renal RFA: Radiofrequency ablation (RFA) is an alternative to partial nephrectomy and laparoscopic nephrectomy. It can be used for benign tumors like AMLs, renal AVMs, and even for RCCs. Angiomyolipomas (AMLs) are treated at 4cm because of the bleeding risk. Sort of a general rule is that things that are superficial you can burn with RFA. Things that are closer to the collecting system it may be better to freeze (cryoablation) to avoid scaring the collecting system and making a stricture. Pyeloperfusion techniques (cold D5W irrigating the ureter) can be done to protect it if you really wanted to RFA. If anyone would ask, RFA has no effect on GFR (it won't lower the GFR).

Things that make you think recurrent/residual disease after therapy:
(1) Any increase in the size beyond the acute initial increase,
(2) Areas of "nodular" or "crescentic" enhancement, or
(3) A new or enlarging bright T2 signal.

There is a paper in AJR (2009) that says that lesions that are < 3cm will appear larger in 1-2 months and lesions >3cm do not grow larger – when successfully treated. So, smaller lesions may initially get bigger but after that – any increase in size should be considered tumor recurrence.

—-

Renal Arteriography: You should always do a non-selective aortogram first to see how many arteries feed the kidney, where they are , etc. Sometimes the aortogram will show you an obvious ostial problem which you can then select down on and address. Otherwise, you need to do selective angiography and look at each vessel. **LAO is the projection of choice for looking at the renals.** Sometimes the stenosis is further out, in fact branch artery stenosis is a cause of hypertension in kids.

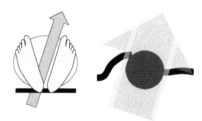

LAO Minimizes Angiographic Overlap from the Aorta

Angioplasty of Renal Arteries: Used to treat hypertension caused by atherosclerosis (usually ostial) or FMD. Risks include thrombosis, and vessel spasm. Calcium channel blockers can be given to decrease the risk of spasm. Heparin should be on board to reduce thrombosis risk. Most people take daily aspirin the day before and every day after for 6 months, to reduce the risk of restenosis.

- *Indications for angioplasty = Renal Vascular HTN or Azotemia*
- *Atherosclerosis at the Ostium = Angioplasty + Stent*
- *FMD - usually mid vessel = Angioplasty Alone*

But Prometheus!?! - I was reading the New England Journal...

Don't read the NEJM. The NEJM is run by a bunch of family medicine doctors who hate all procedures. They published a thing called the **CORAL trial** in 2014, that showed no added benefit from angio + stenting in the setting of renal vascular stenosis compared to high quality medical therapy.

This remains controversial and several prominent IR guys still like to stent, especially if they can measure a pressure gradient in the renal artery. For the purpose of multiple choice, if "high quality medical therapy" is a choice for treated RAS related hypertension, that is probably the right answer — otherwise, pick angio + stent.

Renal Hemorrhage:

Trauma to the kidney (usually iatrogenic from biopsy or diversion procedure) can typically be embolized. The renal arteries are "end arteries," which means that collaterals are not an issue. It also means that infarction is a legit issue so if you want to salvage the kidney you need to try and get super selective. Having said that, don't be an idiot and fuck around trying to get super selective while the patient is bleeding to death. Remember most people have two of these things, plus in a worst case scenario there is always dialysis. Bottom line: if you get into trouble and the patient is crashing, just trash the whole thing.

Next Step: Arterial trauma from the nephrostomy tube placement. Bleeding source is occult on angio. *Next step ?* Remover the nephrostomy tube (over a guidewire), then look again. Often the catheter tamponades the bleed, making it tougher to see.

Gamesmanship: Oral boards guys used to be sticklers for the phrase *"over a wire."* In other words if you just said "I'd remove the PCN" they would ding you. You have to say "I'd remove the PCN *over a wire.*" The only reason I bring this up is the use of possible distractors / fuckery.

Maybe something like this:

Q: The highly skilled Interventionalist grants the Fellow the great privilege of performing a fresh stick nephrostomy. The clumsy, good for nothing Fellow manages to place the tube, but now there is a large volume of bright red blood in the tube and the Patient's blood pressure is dropping rapidly. You start fluids and perform an emergent renal arteriography. The source of bleeding is not seen. *What is the best next step?*

A: Remove the PCN and repeat another angio run
B: Kick the fellow in the shin for using too much fluoro time
C: Call Urology and admit you need help from a "real doctor"
D: Remove the PCN *over a wire* and repeat another angio run. ←

> *Just like a Midget using a urinal... you gotta stay on your toes.*
>
> **Read all the choices!**

Renal Aneurysms

"Look, man. I only need to know one thing: where they are" - Private Vasquez

- *Small Segmental Arteries* = coils

- *Main Renal Artery* = Covered Stent to exclude the aneurysm. Alternatively, you could place a bare metal stent across the aneurysm and then pump detachable coils into the sac.

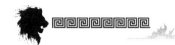 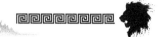
Pleural Drainage – Most everyone has done a few thoracenteses as a resident. I just want to touch on a few testable points.

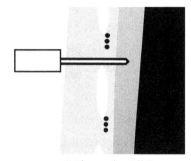

"Above the Rib"
avoid the neurovascular bundle.

• Remember that you go *"above the rib"* to avoid the neurovascular bundle.

• If you pull off too much fluid too fast you can possibly get pulmonary edema from re-expansion (this is uncommon).

• If it's malignant you might end up with a trapped lung (lung won't expand fully)- in other words a thick pleural rind or fibrothorax, can prevent lung reexpansion - makes percutaneous drainage pointless in many cases. A "vacu-thorax" - in the setting of a trapped lung, does not mean anything, and does not need immediate treatment even if it's big. If you really need to fix it, you'll need a surgical pleurectomy / decortication. Pleurodesis (which can be done to patients with recurrent pleural effusions), does NOT help in the setting of trapped lung.

• Pneumothorax is rare but is probably the most common complication (obviously it's more common when done blind).

Additional Trivia related to Chest Tubes:

• Continuous air bubbles in the Pleur-evac chamber represent an air leak, either from the drainage tubing or from the lung itself. In the setting of multiple choice - think about a bronchopleural fistula.

• INR should generally be < 1.5 prior to placement of a chest tube.

• In the paravertebral region, the intercostal vessels tend to course off of the ribs and are therefore more prone to injury if this route is chosen for chest tube placement

Choice of Drainage Catheter			
Parapneumonic Effusion / Empyema		**Malignant Effusion**	
Inpatient	Outpatient	Inpatient	Outpatient
12-14 Fr	10 Fr	14 F	15.5 Indwelling (PleurX etc...)

Lung Abscess: Just remember that you can drain an empyema (pus in the pleural space), but you should NOT drain a lung abscess because you can create a bronchopleural fistula (some people still do it).

Lung RFA – Radiofrequency ablation of lung tumors can be performed on lesions between 1.5cm and 5.2cm in diameter. The most common complication is pneumothorax (more rare things like pneumonia, pseudoaneurysm, bronchopleural fistula, and nerve injury have been reported). The effectiveness of RFA is similar to external beam radiation with regard to primary lung cancer. The major advantage of lung RFA is that it has a limited effect on pulmonary function, and can be performed without concern to prior therapy.

Imaging (CT and PET) should be performed as a follow up of therapy. Things that make you think residual /recurrent disease: nodular peripheral enhancement measuring more than 10 mm, central enhancement (any is bad) , growth of the RFA zone after 3 months (after 6 months is considered definite), increased metabolic activity after 2 months, residual activity centrally (at the burned tumor).

Lung Biopsy – The most common complication is pneumothorax, which occurs about 25% of the time (most either resolve spontaneously or can be aspirated), with about 5% needing a chest tube. The second most common complication (usually self-limiting) is hemoptysis.

The testable pearls include:

• The lower lung zones are more affected by respiratory motion,

• The lingula is the most affected by cardiac motion,

• Avoid vessels greater than 5 mm,

• Try and avoid crossing a fissure (they almost always get a pneumothorax),

• Areas lateral to and just distal to the tip of a biopsy gun will be affected by "shock wave injury", so realize vessels can still bleed from that.

Reducing the Risk of Pneumothorax - Post Biopsy

Enter the lung at 90 degrees to pleural surface

Avoid interlobar fissures

Put the patient puncture side DOWN after the procedure

No talking or deep breathing after the procedure (at least 2 hours)

If the patient is a cougher, consider postponing the procedure - or giving empiric anti-tussive meds

Nonspecific Thoracic Core Biopsy Results - Next Step:

Repeat the biopsy and / or close follow up. Nonspecific biopsy results don't mean shit — especially in the lung.

Biopsy is only helpful when you get an actual result (cancer, hamartoma, etc…). Otherwise - you could have just missed, or targeted the infection behind the cancer.

Chests Tube / Pigtail Placement:

Potential algorithm to deal with pneumothorax post biopsy cases:

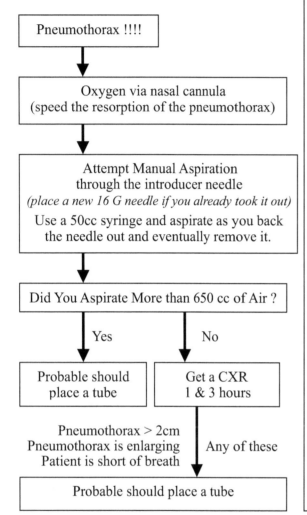

Pneumothorax !!!!

↓

Oxygen via nasal cannula
(speed the resorption of the pneumothorax)

↓

Attempt Manual Aspiration
through the introducer needle
(place a new 16 G needle if you already took it out)
Use a 50cc syringe and aspirate as you back
the needle out and eventually remove it.

↓

Did You Aspirate More than 650 cc of Air ?

Yes → Probable should place a tube

No → Get a CXR 1 & 3 hours

Pneumothorax > 2cm
Pneumothorax is enlarging
Patient is short of breath — Any of these →

Probable should place a tube

Procedural Pearls

You can usually get away with a small-caliber, (6-10 French) catheter. A 10 French Pigtail Catheters would require an 18G needle / 0.035 Amplatz wire. You would need a larger tube if there is fluid (otherwise it will get clogged). You should use CT guidance since you obviously have it available. Most people will tell you to use the so called " *triangle of safety*," located above the 5th intercostal space, mid-axillary line. This has the thinnest muscle, lets you avoid the breast in females (and fat sloppy dudes) - plus keeps you free of the axillary vasculature, diaphragm, liver, and spleen.

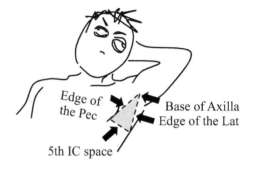

Edge of the Pec

Base of Axilla
Edge of the Lat

5th IC space

Always go along the superior aspect of the rib to avoid the neurovascular bundle along the inferior border of each rib.

Heimlich valves will let the patient remain ambulatory, otherwise you can use a conventional water seal device.

In most cases, the tube can be removed 1–2 days after the procedure.

Obstruction

Detected by noticing (being told) that the water-seal chamber isn't fluctuating with respiration or coughing while the drainage system is set to gravity.

This means either (1) the lung is fully expanded or (2) the tube is clogged — CXR will tell you the difference.

It is controversial to "milk" the tubing - plenty of people still do it. Some people put TPA in the tube - people do lots of crazy shit beyond the scope of the exam…. probably.

Air Leak

Detected by persistent bubbling within the water seal chamber.

Air leak = Air within the pleural space. This is expected after initial insertion of a chest tube, (with an actively resolving pneumothorax). It becomes a problem when it is new or persistent.

Next Step: CXR confirm position of the tube. Inspect the bandage - usually a vaseline bandage covers the insertion site. If everything looks ok - you might be dealing with a bronchopulmonary fistula.

Subcutaneous Emphysema

Typically detected by crepitus on physical exam, or shown on chest x-ray.

Confirm the tube is in the pleural space. Specially, make sure the side holes are ALL within the pleural space. Look for those fucking side holes. Reposition if needed.

If the tube is appropriately positioned, subcutaneous emphysema is self-limited - do nothing.

Thoracic Angio:

This section is going to focus on the two main flavors of pulmonary angio; *pulmonary artery* (done for massive PE and pulmonary AVM treatment) and *bronchial artery* (done for hemoptysis).

Pulmonary Artery

The primary indications for pulmonary arteriography is diagnosis and treatment of massive PE or pulmonary AVM.

Technical Trivia:

The "Grollman" catheter, which is a preshaped 7F, is the classic tool. You get it in the right ventricle (usually from the femoral vein) and then turn it 180 degrees so the pigtail is pointing up, then advance it into the outflow tract. Some people will say that a **known LBBB is high risk**, and these patients should get prophylactic pacing (because the wire can give you a RBBB, and RBBB + LBBB = asystole). An important thing to know is that patients with chronic PE often have pulmonary hypertension. Severe pulmonary hypertension needs to be evaluated before you inject a bunch of contrast. **Pressures should always be measured before injecting contrast** because you may want to reduce your contrast burden. Oh, one last thing about angio... never ever let someone talk you into injecting contrast through a swan-ganz catheter. It's a TERRIBLE idea and the stupid catheter will blow apart at the hub. I would never ever do that....

Next Step: Cardiac dysrhythmias (v-tach) during procedure. *Next Step ?* Re-position the catheter / wire

Pulmonary Embolism – Patients with PE should be treated with medical therapy (anticoagulation with Coumadin, Heparin, or various newer agents), allowing the emboli to spontaneously undergo lysis. In patients who can't get anticoagulation (for whatever reason), an IVC filter should be placed. The use of transcatheter therapy is typically reserved for unstable patients with massive PE.

Massive PE? Just think lotta PE with hypotension.

In those situations, catheter directed thrombolysis, thromboaspiration, mechanical clot fragmentation, and stent placement have all been used to address large clots.

> **Pulmonary Angiography**
> *Relative Contraindications*
>
> **Pulmonary HTN with elevated right heart pressures** (greater than 70 systolic and 20 end diastolic).
>
> *If you need to proceed anyway - they get low osmolar contrast agents injected in the right or left PA (NOT the main PA).*
>
> **Left Bundle Branch Block** - The catheter in the right heart can cause a right block, leading to a total block.
>
> *If you need to proceed anyway - they get prophylactic pacing.*

Pulmonary AVM – They can occur sporadically. For the purpose of multiple choice when you see them think about HHT (Hereditary Hemorrhagic Telangiectasia / Osler Weber Rendu). Pulmonary AVMs are most commonly found in the lower lobes (more blood flow) and can be a source of right to left shunt (**worry about stroke and brain abscess**). The rule of **treating once the afferent (feeding) artery is 3mm** is based on some tiny little abstract and not powered at all. Having said that, it's quoted all the time and a frequent source of trivia that is easily tested. The primary technical goal is to crush the feeding artery (usually with coils) as close to the sac as possible. You don't want that think reperfusing from adjacent branches. Pleurisy (self limited) after treatment seems to pretty much always happen.

Key Trivia:

• HHT Association

• Brain Abscess / Stroke - via paradoxical emboli

• Treat once the afferent (feeding) artery is **3mm**

• Coils in the feeding vessel, as close as possible to the sac

Special Situation - Rasmussen Aneurysm

This is an aneurysm associated with chronic pulmonary infection, classically TB. The trick on this is the history of hemoptysis (which normally makes you think bronchial artery).

"It's a Trap!" - *Admiral Gial Ackbar*

Next Step Strategy to avoid the trap:

Patient blah blah blah hemoptysis….. *Next Step?* Bronchial Artery Angio

• Bronchial Artery Angio is negative, still bleeding. Oh, and his PPD is positive. *Next Step ?* Pulmonary Artery angio to look for Rasmussen Aneurysms

• Rasmussen Aneurysm identified. *Next Step ?* Coil embolization (yes coils for hemoptysis - this is the exception to the rule).

Bronchial Artery

The primary indication for pulmonary arteriography is diagnosis and treatment of massive hemoptysis.

Hemoptysis – Massive hemoptysis (> 300 cc) can equal death. Bronchial artery embolization is first line treatment (bronchial artery is the culprit 90% of the time). Unique to the lung, active extravasation is NOT typically seen with the active bleed. Instead you see tortuous, enlarged bronchial arteries. The main thing to worry about is cord infarct. For multiple choice the most likely bad actor is the *"hairpin-shaped"* anterior medullary artery (Adamkiewicz). Embolizing that thing or anywhere that can reflux into that thing is an obvious contraindication. If present, those bad boys typically arise from the right intercostal bronchial trunk.

Particles (> 325 micrometers) are used (<u>coils should be avoided</u> - because if it re-bleeds you just jailed yourself out).

The vast majority (90%) of bronchial arteries are located within the lucency formed by the left main bronchus. This is right around the T5-T6 Level

There is a ton of vascular variation but the pattern of an intercostobronchial trunk on the right and two bronchial arteries on the left is most common (about 40%)

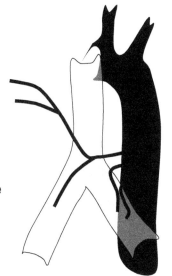
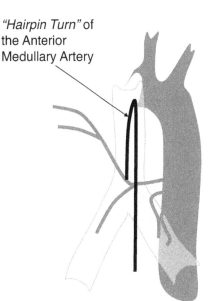

"Hairpin Turn" of the Anterior Medullary Artery

In the lower thoracic / upper lumbar region the primary feeding artery of the anterior spinal cord is the legendary anterior radiculomedullary artery (artery of Adamkiewicz). This vessel most commonly originates from a left sided posterior intercostal artery (typically between T9-T12) , which branches from the aorta. The distal portion of this artery, as it merges with the anterior spinal artery, creates the classic (and testable) "*hairpin*" turn.

It is worth noting that Adamkiewicz can originate from the right bronchus (like 5%).

Occlusion of Central Veins (SVC Syndrome) –

Yes - I know this really isn't a pulmonary thing, but it is in the chest so I'm going to talk about it here.

Acute vs Chronic SVC Occlusion:

- Acute = No Collaterals
- Acute = Emergency

- Chronic = Has Collaterals
- Chronic = Not an Emergency

There are a variety of ways to address occlusion of the SVC. The goal is to return in line flow from at least one jugular vein down through the SVC. Most commonly thrombolysis is the initial step, although this is rarely definitive. The offending agent (often a catheter) should be removed if possible. If the process is non-malignant, often angioplasty alone is enough to get the job done (post lysis).

Technical Trivia:

- Malignant causes: you should do lysis, then angioplasty, then stent.

- Non-malignant causes: may still need a stent if the angioplasty doesn't remove the gradient (if the collateral veins are still present).

- Self-expanding stents should NOT be used, as they tend to migrate.

- The last pearl on this one is not to forget that the pericardium extends to the bottom part of the SVC and that if you tear that you are going to end up with hemopericardium and possible tamponade.

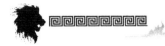 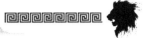
Uterine Artery Embolization (UAE):

Can be used for bleeding or the bulk symptoms of fibroids. Procedure may or may not help with infertility associated with fibroid. If you are paying cash.... it definitely helps.

Patient Selection (not all fibroids were created equal). To do this you need a pre-op MRI/MRA to characterize the fibroids and look at the vasculature.

Subtypes:
* Degenerated leiomyoma are more likely to have a poor response
  (these are the ones that don't enhance).
* "Cellular" Fibroids - the ones with high T2 signal tend to respond well to embolization.
  Most fibroids "Hyaline Subtype" are T2 dark.
* Smaller lesions do better than larger lesions.

Location:
* Submucosal does the best. Intramural does the second best.
* Serosal does the third best (it sucks). It speaks the third most Italian -
* Cervical fibroids do NOT respond well to UAE -- they have a different blood supply.

* Intracavitary Fibroids – Less than 3 cm.
    o Next Step = GYN referral for hysteroscopic resection
* Intracavitary Fibroids – Less than 3 cm , with failed hysteroscopic resection
    o Next Step = IR Embo
* Large Serosal Fibroid, patient wants to be pregnant, no history of prior myomectomy
    o Next Step = GYN referral for myomectomy
* Pedunculated Serosal Fibroid
    o Next Step = GYN referral for resection
* Broad Ligament Fibroid
    o Next Step = Refer to voodoo priest (these don't do well with UAE and are technically challenging to operate on).

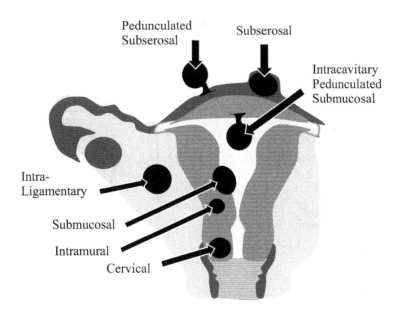

PreTreatment Considerations / Trivia

- Remember fibroids are hormone responsive. They grow with estrogen (and really grow during pregnancy). Gonadotropin-releasing medications are often prescribed to control fibroids by blocking all that fancy hormone axis stuff.
- The testable trivia is to delay embolization for 3 months if someone is on the drugs because they actually shrink the uterine arteries which makes them a pain in the ass to catheterize.
- The EMMY trial showed that hospital stays with UAE are shorter than hysterectomy
- The incidence of premature menopause is around 5%
- **DVT / PE is a known risk of the procedure** (once pelvic vein compression from large fibroid releases – sometimes the big PE flies up). The risk is about 5%.

Contraindications: <u>Pregnancy</u>, Uterine/Cervical <u>Cancer,</u> Active Pelvic Infection, Prior Pelvic Radiation, Connective Tissue Disease, Prior Surgery with Adhesions (relative)

Treatment Trivia
- Occlusion of small feeding arteries cause fibroid infarction (and hopefully shrinkage). Embolic material is typically PVA or embospheres for fibroids (targeting the pre-capillary level). If ask to choose an agent - I'd say **"particles"** - don't pick coils, or glue. For postpartum hemorrhage / vaginal bleeding, gel foam or glue is typically used.
- Most people will say either 500-700 micro or 700-900 micron particle sizes. As a point of trivia smaller particle size does not give you a better result for fibroids -- but can help with Adenomyosis.
- Treatment of adenomyosis with UAE is done exactly the same way, and is an effective treatment for symptomatic relief (although symptoms recur in about 50% of the cases around 2 years post treatment). As above - slightly smaller particles are typically used for this (vs fibroids).
- Fibroids should reduce volume 40-60% after the procedure. If you are treating intracavitary fibroids they should turn to mush and come out like a super gross chunky vegetable soup period mix. You actually want that - if they stay ("retained") inside they can get infected.

Anatomy Trivia:
- Remember the uterine artery is off the anterior division of the internal iliac
- Regardless of the fibroid location, bilateral uterine artery embolization is necessary to prevent recruitment of new vessels
- In most cases, branches of the ovarian artery feed the fibroids via collaterals with the main uterine artery. Uterine artery can be identified by the characteristic **"corkscrew"** appearance of its more disc branches -- named the **Helicine** branches (twisty like a helix)

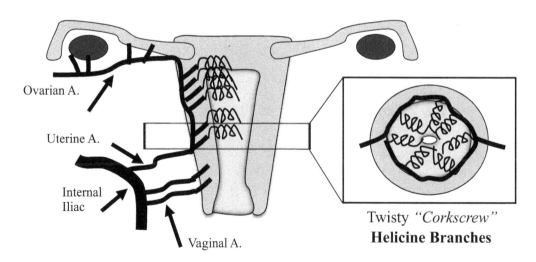

Ovarian A.

Uterine A.

Internal Iliac

Vaginal A.

Twisty *"Corkscrew"*
Helicine Branches

Uterine Artery Embolization Continued:

Post Embolization Syndrome: I mentioned this earlier but just wanted to remind you that it's classically described with fibroid embolization. Remember you don't need to order blood cultures - without other factors to make you consider infection. The low-grade fever should go away after 3 days. Some texts suggest prophylactic use of anti-pyrexial and antiemetic meds prior to the procedure.

- 3 Days or less with low grade fever = Do nothing
- More than 3 Days with fever = "Work it up" , cultures, antibiotics, etc…

Hysterosalpingogram (HSG):

I'm 100% certain no one went into radiology to do these things. You do it like a GYN exam. Prep the personal area with betadine, drape the patient, put the speculum in and find the cervix. There are various methods and tools for cannulating and maintaining cannulation of the cervix (vacuum cups, tenaculums, balloons). Insertion of any of these devices is made easier with a catheter and wire. Once the cervix and endometrial cavity have been accessed, the contrast is inserted and pictures are obtained.

Contraindications: Pregnancy, Active Pelvic Infection, Recent Uterine or Tubal Pregnancy.

Trivia:

- The ideal time for the procedure is the proliferative phase (day 7-14), as this is the time the endometrium is thinnest (improves visualization, minimizes pregnancy risk).
- It's not uncommon for a previously closed tube to be open on repeat exam (sedative, narcotics, tubal spasm – can make a false positive).
- Air bubbles can cause a false positive filling defect.
- **Intravasation** – The backflow of injected contrast into the venous or lymphatic system, used to be an issue during the Jurassic period (when oil based contrast could cause a fat embolus). Now it means nothing other than you may be injecting too hard, or the intrauterine pressure is increased because of obstruction.
- *The reported risk of peritonitis is 1%.*

Fallopian Tube Recanalization (FTR):

Tubal factors (usually PID / Chlamydia) are responsible for about 30% of the cases in female infertility ~ depending on what part of the country you are from sometimes much more (*insert joke about your hometown here*). Tubal obstruction comes in two flavors; proximal / interstitial, or distal. The distal ones get treated with surgery. The proximal ones can be treated with an endoscope or by poking it with a wire under fluoro.

Things to know:
- You should schedule it in the follicular/proliferative phase (just like a HSP) - day 6-12ish.
- You repeat the HSG first to confirm the tube is still clogged. If clogged you try and unclog it with a wire (*"selective salpingography"*).
- Hydrophilic 0.035 or 0.018 guidewire (plus / minus microcatheter) is the typical poking tool
- Repeat the HSG when you are done to prove you did something
- Contraindications are the same as HSG (active infection and pregnancy)

Pelvic Congestion Syndrome

– Women have mystery pelvic pain. This is a real (maybe) cause of it. They blame dilated ovarian and periuterine veins in this case, and give it a name ending in the word "syndrome" to make it sound legit. The symptoms of this "syndrome" include pelvic pain, dyspareunia, menstrual abnormalities, vulvar varices, and lower extremity varicose veins. The symptoms are most severe at the end of the day, and with standing.

Diagnosis ? Clinical symptoms + a gonadal vein diameter of 10 mm (normal is 5 mm).

Treatment ? GnRH agonists sometimes help these patients, since estrogen is a vasodilator. But the best results for treatment of this "syndrome" are sclerosing the parauterine venous plexus, and coils/plugs in the ovarian and internal iliac veins (performed by your local Interventional Radiologist). This is often staged, starting with ovarian veins plugged first, and then (if unsuccessful) iliac veins plugged second.

Trivia: Most optimal results occur when the entire length of both gonadal veins are embolized.

Complications ? Complications are rare but the one you worry about is thrombosis of the parent vein (iliac or renal), and possible thrombus migration (pulmonary embolism).

Will it get better on its own ? The symptoms will classically improve after menopause.

Varicocele

- They are usually left-sided (90%), or bilateral (10%). Isolated right-sided varicoceles should prompt an evaluation for cancer (next step = CT Abd).

When do you treat them? There are three indications: (1) infertility, (2) testicular atrophy in a kid, (3) pain.

Anatomy Trivia (regarding varicoceles): Remember that multiple venous collaterals "pampiniform plexus" or "spermatic venous plexus" drain the testicles. Those things come together around the level of the femoral head, forming the internal spermatic vein. The left internal spermatic vein drains into the left renal vein, and the right internal spermatic vein drains into the IVC. Common variants include: multiple veins on the right terminating into the IVC or renal vein, or one right-sided vein draining into the renal vein (instead of the IVC).

Why Varicoceles Happen: The "primary factor" is right angle entry of the left spermatic vein into the high pressure left renal vein. Nut-cracker syndrome (compression of the left renal vein between the SMA and aorta) on the left is another cause (probably more likely asked).

Basic Idea: You get into the renal vein and look for reflux into the gonadal vein (internal spermatic) which is abnormal but confirms the problem. You then get deep into the gonadal vein, and embolize close to the varicocele (often with foam), then drop coils on the way back, and often an Amplatzer or other occlusion device at the origin.

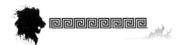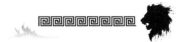
Vertebroplasty

There is a paper in the NEJM that says this doesn't work. Having said that, NEJM doesn't like any procedures. They're run by family medicine doctors. They are equally amoral to the person that will do any non-indicated procedure. Regardless of the actual legitimacy, it's a big cash cow and several prominent Radiologists have made their names on it... so it will be tested on as if it's totally legit and without controversy.

Trivia to Know:

- Indications = Acute to subacute fracture with pain refractory to medical therapy or an unstable fracture with associated risk if further collapse occurs.
- Contraindications = Fractures with associated spinal canal compression or improving pain without augmentation.
- There is a risk of developing a new vertebral fracture in about 25% of cases. The literature says you should *"counsel patients on the need for additional treatments prior to undergoing vertebroplasty.".*
- The cement can embolize to the lungs.
- Risk of local neurologic complications are about 5%.

Lymphangiogram:

1950 called and they want to stage this cancer. Prior to CT, MRI, and US injecting dye into the toes was actually a way to help stage malignancy (mets to lymph nodes, lymphoma, etc..).

Another slightly more modern application is to use this process as the first step in the embolization of the thoracic duct. Why would you take down the thoracic duct? If it's leaking chylous pleural effusions - status post get hacked to pieces by a good for nothing Surgery Resident.

Technical Trivia:

This is done by first injecting about 0.5 cc methylene blue dye in between the toes bilaterally. You then wait half an hour until the blue lymphatic channels are visualized. You then cut down over the lymphatic channels and cannulate with a 27 or 30 gauge lymphangiography needle. An injection with lipiodol is done (maximum 20 ml if no leak). If you inject too much there is a risk of oil pneumonitis. You take spot films in a serial fashion until the cisterna chyli (the sac at the bottom of the thoracic duct) is opacified. At that point you could puncture it directly and superselect the thoracic duct to embolize it, typically with coils.

Standing Waves:

Standing waves are an angiographic phenomenon (usually) that results in a ringed layering of contrast that sorta looks like FMD. A common trick is to try and make you pick between FMD and Standing Waves.

Obviously it's bullshit because in real life standing waves typically resolve prior to a second run through the same vessel, and even if they stayed around they tend to shift position between each run (up or down). FMD on the other hand is an actual physical irregularity of the vessel wall so it's fixed between runs and doesn't go away.

Morphology should be your strategy for multiple choice:

Standing waves are very symmetric and evenly spaced.

FMD is more irregular and asymmetric.

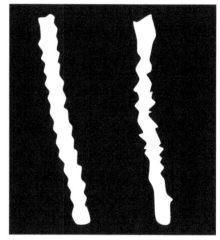

Standing Waves   FMD

"The Lingo"

"Give me a 10 x 6 Balloon" - This means a 10 mm diameter x 6 cm length balloon

"Give me 20 for 30" - This means do an angio run at 20 cc/sec for a total of 30 mL.

"Squirted" - An Angiogram — Oh really? A splenic lac with active extrav? Let's call IR right away and get him squirted.

"Thrash" - A difficult case

"Hot Mess" - I have an admit for you. This lady is a hot mess.

"That poor lady" - A way of feigning sympathy.

"Sick as Stink" - also, "sick AND stinks" be careful not to mess this up.

Artery of Interest	C Arm Angulation	Misc
Aortic Arch	70 Degrees LAO	"Candy Cane"
Innominate (Right Subclavian & Right Common Carotid)	RAO	In the LAO the right subclavian and right common carotid overlap
Left Subclavian	LAO	——
Mesenteric Vessels	Lateral to Steep RAO	——
Left Renal	LAO	Same side as renal
Right Renal	RAO or LAO - depending on who you ask.	This is controversial - a lot of sources will say you can get away with LAO.
Left Iliac Bifurcation	RAO	Opposite side common
Right Iliac Bifurcation	LAO	Opposite side common
Left Common Femoral Bifurcation	LAO	Ipsilateral Oblique
Right Common Femoral Bifurcation	RAO	Ipsilateral Oblique

The Confusing Oblique Views

Normally, views are defined by the direction of the x-ray beam.
However, in Angio it gets a little squirrely. The sidedness refers to the side of the I.I.

RAO: The imaging intensifier is on the right side of the patient.

A reasonable person might call this LPO - but they would be wrong.

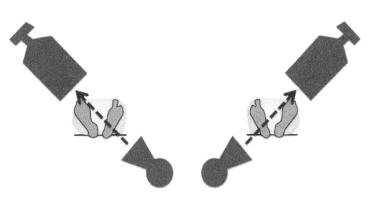

LAO: The imaging intensifier is on the left side of the patient.

A reasonable person might call this RPO - but they would be wrong.

Superficial or Deep? - Understanding Geometry

Sometimes it's difficult to tell if you are superficial or deep to the lesion you are trying to put a needle in under fluoro. You can problem solve by tilting the I.I. towards the patient's head or towards the patient's feet.

If you tilt towards the head, a superficial needle will be shorter but a deep needle will look longer.

If you tilt towards the feet, a superficial needle will be longer but a deep needle will look shorter.

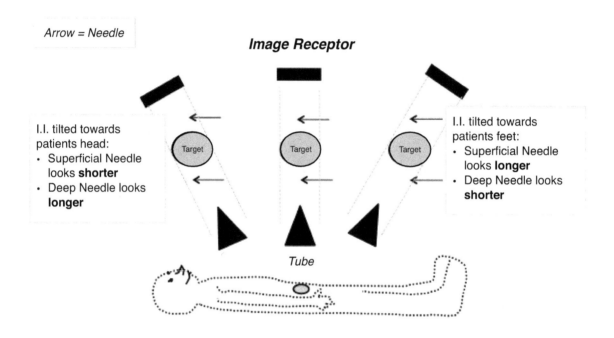

Arrow = Needle

Image Receptor

I.I. tilted towards patients head:
- Superficial Needle looks **shorter**
- Deep Needle looks **longer**

I.I. tilted towards patients feet:
- Superficial Needle looks **longer**
- Deep Needle looks **shorter**

Tube

Air Embolus

Classic Clinical Buzzwords: "Sudden onset shortness of breath" "Whoosh sound" or "Sucking sound" during central catheter insertion.

Next Step: *"Durant's maneuver"* = left-lateral decubitus + head-down positioning. Other verbiage = "right side up" or "left side down", "trendelenburg"

Next Next Step: 100% Oxygen

Medications:

Anti-Coagulation Issues:

- Remember that Platelets Replace Platelets.
- Cryoprecipitate is used to correct deficiencies of fibrinogen.
- Heparin: The half life is around 1.5 hours. Protamine Sulfate can be used as a more rapid Heparin Antidote.
- Protamine can cause a sudden fall in BP, Bradycardia, and flushing
- Coumadin: Vitamin K can be given for Coumadin but that takes a while *(25-50mg IM 4 hours prior to procedure)*, more rapid reversal is done with factors (cryoprecipitate).
- Remember that patients with "HIT" (Heparin Induced Thrombocytopenia) are at increased risk of clotting – not bleeding. If they need to be anti-coagulated then they should get a thrombin inhibitor instead (remember those end in "rudin" and "gatran").
- The Life Span of a Platelet is 8-10 days
- IV Desmopressin can increase factor 8 - may be helpful of hemophilia

Medication	Mechanism	Trivia
Aspirin	Inhibits thromboxane A_2 from arachidonic acid by an irreversible acetylation	Irreversible - works the life of the platelet (8-12 days).
Heparin	Binds antithrombin 3 - and increases its activity.	Monitored by PTT. Can be reversed with protamine sulfate
Plavix (Clopidogrel)	Inhibits the binding of ADP to its receptors - leads to inhibition of GP IIb/IIIa	——
Coumadin	Inhibits vitamin K dependent factors (2,7,9,10)	Monitored by INR. Delay in onset of activity (8-12 hours). Action can be antagonized by vitamin K - but this takes time (4 hours). For immediate reversal give factors (cryopercipitate)
Thrombolytic Agents (TPA)	Act directly or indirectly to convert plasminogen to plasmin (cleaves fibrin)	TPA has a very short biologic half life - between 2-10 mins.

ACR Appropriate: / SIR Practice Guide: Pre-Procedure Hold

— For procedures with a MODERATE risk of bleeding (liver or lung biopsy, abscess drain placement, vertebral augmentation, tunneled central line placement)

— INR should be corrected to < 1.5 prior to the procedure.
— Aspirin need not be held,
— Clopidogrel (plavix) should be held for 5 days.
— Platelet count should be more than 50,000.

Sedation Related:

- "Conscious Sedation" is considered "moderate sedation", and the patient should be able to respond briskly to stimuli (verbal commands, or light touch). No airway intervention should be needed.
- Flumazenil is the antidote for Versed (Midazolam).
- Narcan is the antidote for Opioids (Morphine, Fentanyl).

Local Anesthesia (Lidocaine)

- Maximum Dose is 4-5 mg/kg
- A dirty trick would be to say - "Lido with Epi" - in which case it is 7 mg/kg
- Some basic scrub nurse math:
    - 1% Plain Epi - 10 mg per 1 mL
    - So 1 mg per 0.1 mL
    - And we said Maximum Dose is 5 mg/kg, so it would be equal to 0.5 mL / kg
- Remember that small doses in the right spot can cause a serious reaction.
    - 150 mg in the thecal sac can cause total spine anesthesia and the need for a ventilator.
    - Direct arterial injection can cause immediate seizures.
    - Tinnitus and dizziness are the earliest signs of toxicity.
- Local anesthesia agents have a low potential for allergy - although it can still occur, it's usually a bogus allergy once a real history is taken. Most "allergies" to lidocaine are actually vaso-vagal, or other CV side effects from epinephrine mixed with lidocaine
- There are elaborate mechanisms for testing for a true allergy, or reaction to methylparaben (a preservative).
- So what if the allergy is real? or you can't prove it's false? - Some texts describe using an antihistamine such as diphenhydramine (which can have anesthetic properties).

Green, Steven M., Steven G. Rothrock, and Julie Gorchynski. "Validation of diphenhydramine as a dermal local anesthetic." Annals of emergency medicine 23.6 (1994): 1284-1289.

	Indications	Contraindications
Angiography	Numerous; usually diagnosis of and treatment of vascular disease	Only one absolute which is an unstable patient with multisystem dysfunction (unless angio is life saving). There are numerous relatives including inability to lay flat, uncooperative patient, and connective tissue diseases
Ascending Venography	Diagnosis of DVT, Evaluate Venous malformation or tumor encasement.	Contrast Reaction Pregnancy Severely compromised cardiopulmonary status
Descending Venography	Evaluation of post-thrombotic syndrome; valvular incompetence and damage following DVT	
Venography (Non-inclusive)	Thoracic Outlet Syndrome, Venous Access, Pacer Placement, Eval for fistula	
IVC Filter	Can't get anticoagulation, Failed anticoagulation (clot progression), Massive PE requiring lysis, Chronic PE treated with thromboendarterectomy. Trauma high risk DVT	Total thrombosis of IVC IVC too big or too small *Sepsis is NOT a contraindication, including septic thrombophlebitis*
Fistulography	Making the nephrologist money ("slow flows" they call it).	Absolute: Right to left cardiopulmonary shunt, Uncorrectable coagulopathy, fistula infection. Relative is significant cardiopulmonary disease (a declot invariably causes PE)

	Indications	Contraindications
TIPS	Variceal bleeding refractory to endoscopy. Refractory ascites.	Absolute: Heart Failure (especially right heart failure). Severe encephalopathy. Rapidly progressing liver failure.
Percutaneous Transhepatic Cholangiography (PTC)	Performed prior to percutaneous biliary interventions, Choledochojejunostomy patients (liver transplant) with suspected obstruction	Absolute: Uncorrectable Coagulopathy, Plavix or other anti-platelet agent Relative: Large Volume Ascites (consider para and left sided approach)
Percutaneous Biliary Drainage	Basically CBD obstruction (with failed ERCP), cholangitis, bile duct injury/leak.	No absolute contraindications Relative: Large Volume Ascites (consider para and left sided approach), Coagulopathy
Percutaneous Cholecystosomy	Cholecystitis in patients who are not surgical candidates, Unexplained sepsis when other sources excluded, Access to biliary tree required and other methods failed	No absolute contraindications Relative: Large Volume Ascites (consider para and left sided approach), Coagulopathy
Percutaneous Nephrostomy	Obstructive Uropathy (**Not hydronephrosis**), Urinary diversion (leak, fistula), Access for percutaneous intervention	Uncorrectable coagulopathy, Contrast Reactions

Blank for Scribbles

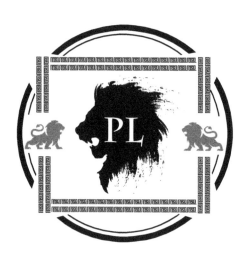

14
MAMMO

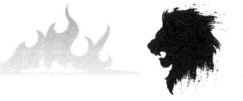

PROMETHEUS LIONHART, M.D.

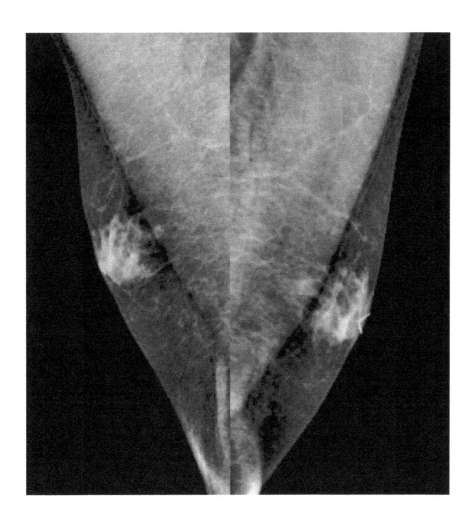

A Brief Overview - For the complete novice:

Many foreign graduates have had little or no experience with mammography. I'll try and give you a very brief overview before I get into the testable trivia.

In America, women are told they need to have screening mammograms done once a year. Because breast cancer is common (and scary), most women will get this done, and will continue to get it done into their 90s. They will literally take people from the ICU who are in cardiogenic shock down to x-ray to keep them up to date on their screening mammograms (usually at the patient's request).

I want you to think about mammograms in two categories: (a) *the screener* - these are the people who are coming in once a year, and have no symptoms other than being female, and (b) *the diagnostic* - these people have a symptom (palpable lump, nipple discharge, breast pain, etc..). These two are handled totally different.

Nomenclature is rigidly controlled with regard to reporting. "BI-RADS" is a book of approved vocabulary words for describing the findings, and a system for reporting results based on a percentage of risk. The basic idea is that you use scary words like "spiculated" to describe things you think are cancer, and benign words like "fat density" to describe things you think are not cancer.

Here are some basic scenarios - I'll explain all the stuff in the chapter and we can revisit some more scenarios at the end of the chapter. This is just for you to get a feel for how this works if you have never been around it before. Don't spaz if you are lost, it will be clear by the end of the chapter and then we will do them again with some quizzing.

(1a) A 50 year old women comes in for a normal annual screening mammogram. She has no symptoms, and is just following the recommendation. She gets two standard views - a cranial caudal view "CC" and a medial lateral oblique view "MLO." The Radiologist is in a hurry because he has 200 of them to read, so he just calls it normal (Bi-Rads 1). The patient returns to the screening pool - and will get imaged again in 1 year. She is relieved to know she doesn't have cancer.

(1b) The same 50 year old returns 1 month later after she feels a lump. This is no longer a screening study but instead a "diagnostic" because she has a symptom. She gets another mammogram - this time with a palpable marker on the image. She also gets compression spot views (smaller paddle) over the palpable area. In the area of the palpable finding, there is a cluster of calcifications. They were present in retrospect on the mammogram performed 1 month prior, but are new from the year before. Because they are calcifications you need magnification views to fully characterize them. On the mag views you describe them as "coarse heterogeneous." Because they are new from the prior year they must be biopsied, but you aren't done yet. Diagnostic mammogram usually includes an ultrasound - not because of the calcifications but because there was a palpable finding. Just remember no FEMALE with a palpable gets out the door without an ultrasound. You ultrasound the area and find no mass. The next step is to biopsy the calcs (which are BR-4, for intermediate suspicion). You recommend stereo to biopsy them (NOT ultrasound) because you couldn't see them with ultrasound. The results yield fibrocystic change, which you agree is a possibility given the BR-4. When you agree that the biopsy results make sense with the imaging / clinical scenario you use the word *"concordant."* "The results were concordant" said the Resident to his Attending. You inform the patient of the results. She is relieved to know she doesn't have cancer.

(2) A 60 year old women comes in for a normal annual screening mammogram. She has no symptoms, and is just following the recommendation. She gets two standard views - a cranial caudal view "CC" and a medial lateral oblique view "MLO." The Radiologist is in a hurry because he has 200 of them to read, but still manages to see a new mass in the medial breast on the CC view. The breasts are pretty dense and it's hard to find it in on the MLO. So the Radiologist calls it an "asymmetry" and BR-0 (BR-0 because more work up is needed). The patient returns in a week for a diagnostic study - she is convinced that she's gonna die of breast cancer. You can hear her crying in the waiting room. She gets a diagnostic study with spot compression over the mass on the CC view, as well as ML and MLO views. You do manage to see the mass on the CC and in the superior breast on the ML view. The mass is well circumscribed, round, and equal density. Because she is getting a diagnostic work up, she gets an ultrasound too. Before you go in the ultrasound room you guess about where the mass is going to be. Since it's medial and superior on the right breast you guess 2 o'clock. You locate it quickly, and find it to be an anechoic cyst - common in women going into menopause. You tell her it's consistent with a benign cyst. She cries with joy and thanks you repeatedly for "saving her life." She sends you cookies and brownies every year at Christmas with very long letters about how you saved her. She uses a lot of religious references that make you uncomfortable. Some years you throw the food away without eating it, other years you give it to the techs. The simple cyst was reported as a BR-2 (essentially 0% chance of cancer).

(3) A 45 year old woman comes in for a normal annual screening mammogram. She has no symptoms and is just following the recommendation. She gets the two standard views - "CC" and "MLO." The Radiologist is in a hurry because he has 200 of them to read, but still manages to see a new mass in both the MLO and CC views. Because this is a screener he still has to give it a BR-0 (you never BR-4 or BR-5 off a screener). She returns for additional imaging as a diagnostic patient with spot compression views. A spiculated, irregular, high density mass is seen. She is placed in an ultrasound room for further characterization. The ultrasound shows an irregular, circumscribed, anti-parallel, hypoechoic mass, with posterior shadowing and an echogenic halo (all the scary bad words). You are certain the mass is a cancer based on these features so you scan the rest of her breast looking for other tumors, and you look in her axilla for abnormal nodes. You find several enlarged lymph nodes in her axilla. You recommend ultrasound guided biopsy of both the mass and the most suspicious lymph node. You give her a BR-5 (>95% chance of cancer). The biopsy results come back as fibrocystic change. This result is not "*concordant*" with the findings you made on mammography and ultrasound so you instead use the word "*discordant*" and recommend surgical excision. "The results were discordant" said the Resident to his Attending. Gross path shows a high grade invasive lesion.

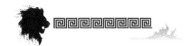
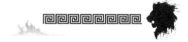

Nipple: The nipple is a circular smooth muscle that overlies the 4th intercostal space. There are typically 5-10 ductal openings. *Inversion* is when the nipple invaginates into the breast. *Retraction* is when the nipple is pulled back slightly. They can both be normal if chronic. If they are new, it should make you think about underlying cancers causing distortion. The nipple is supposed to be in profile so you don't call it a mass. The areola will darken normally with puberty and parity. Nipple enhancement on contrast enhanced breast MRI is normal , *don't call it Pagets!*

Fibroglandular Tissue: The breast mound is fibrous tissue with fat, ducts, and glands laying on top of the anterior chest wall. The axillary extension is called the "*tail of Spence*." The upper outer quadrant is more densely populated with fibroglandular tissue, which is why most breast cancers start there. There is usually no dense tissue in the medial/ inferior breast and retroglandular regions. These are considered "danger zones" and are often where the cancer hides.

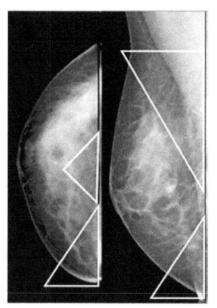

Danger Zones - *where there is usually no dense fibroglandular tissue*

Cooper's Ligaments: These are thin sheets of fascia that hold the breasts up. They are the tiny white lines on mammography and the echogenic lines on US. Straightening and tethering of the ligaments manifests as "architectural distortion" which occurs in the setting of surgical scars, radial scars, and IDC.

Breast Asymmetry: This is common and normal (usually), as long as there are no other findings (lumps, bumps, skin thickening, etc..). *For multiple choice, an asymmetric breast should make you think about the "shrinking breast" of invasive lobular breast cancer.* If the size difference is new or the parenchyma looks asymmetrically dense, think cancer.

Lobules: The lobules are the flower shaped milk makers of the breast. The terminal duct and lobule are referred to as a "terminal duct lobular unit" or TDLU. This is where most breast cancers start.

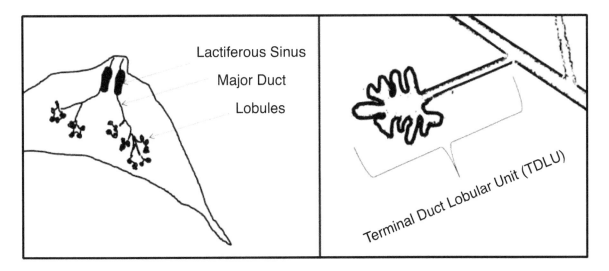

Ducts: The ductal system branches like the roots or branches of a tree. The branches overlap wide areas and are not cleanly segmented like slices of pie. The calcifications that appear to follow ducts ("linear or segmental") are the ones where you should worry about cancer.

Lactiferous Sinus: Milk from the lobules drains into the major duct under the nipple. The dilated portion of the major duct is sometimes called the lactiferous sinus. This thing is normal (not a mass).

Blood Supply / Lymphatic Drainage: The majority (60%) of blood flow to the breast is via the internal mammary. The rest is via the lateral thoracic and intercostal perforators. Nearly all (97%) of lymph drains to the axilla. The remaining 3% goes to the internal mammary nodes.

Axillary Node Levels: The axilla is sub-divided into three separate levels using the pectoralis minor muscle as a landmark. Supposedly drainage progresses in a step wise fashion - from level 1 -> level 2 -> level 3 and finally into the thorax.

Rotter Nodes: These are the nodes between the pec minor and major. They have a fancy name which usually makes them high yield. However, Rotter was German and test writers tend to prefer French sounding trivia. The only exception to this is Nazis. German sounding medical vocab words named after Nazis are fair game. To save you the trouble of looking it up - Rotter died before Hitler took power so he wasn't a Nazi (probably). Since they probably aren't gonna ask the vocab word, the only other conceivable piece of trivia I can imagine being asked would be that these are at the *same level as level 2.*

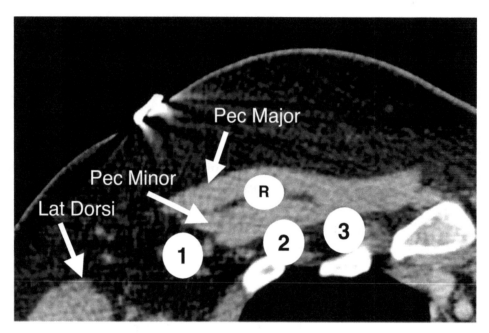

Axillary Lymph Node Levels
Level 1: Lateral to Pec Minor
Level 2: Deep to the Pec Minor
Level 3: Medial and Above Pec Minor
Rotter Node: Between the Pec Minor and Major

Metastasis to the Internal Mammary Nodes: If you can see them on ultrasound they are abnormal. Isolated mets to these nodes is not a common situation (maybe 3%). When you do see it happen, it's from a medial cancer. More commonly, mets in this location occur after disease has already spread into the axilla (in other words - it's spreading everywhere).

Sternalis Muscle: This is an Aunt Minnie. It's a non-functional muscle next to the sternum that can simulate a mass. About 5% of people have one and it's usually unilateral.

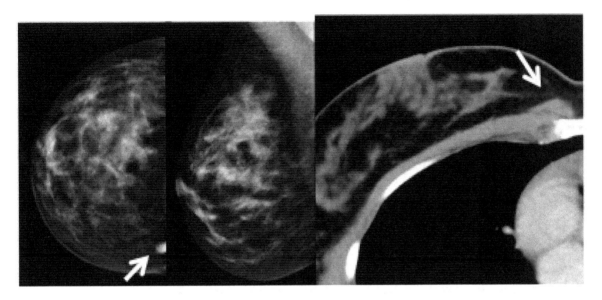

Sternalis - Only on CC, Never on MLO

The main testable trivia is:

1. *WTF is that ?-* Recognize the Aunt Minnie, and don't get tricked into doing a biopsy on it, etc…
2. *How You See It?* It is **ONLY SEEN ON THE CC VIEW**.

Handling this in real life is all about the old gold. Find that thing on the priors (even better is a CT) , CC only, **never on the MLO.**

—-

Breast Development:

The *"milk streak"* is the embryologic buzzword to explain the location of the normal breast and location of ectopic breast tissue. Just know that the **most common location for ectopic breast tissue is in the axilla** (second most common is the inframammary fold). Extra nipples are most commonly in the same locations (but can be anywhere along the "milk streak"). At birth, both males and females can have breast enlargement and produce milk (maternal hormones). As girls enter puberty, their ducts elongate and branch (estrogen effects), then their lobules proliferate (progesterone effects). If you biopsy a breast bud (why would you do that?) you could damage it and potentially fuck up breast development.... and then get sued.

- *Follicular Phase (day 7-14):* Estrogen Dominates. Best time to have both mammogram and MRI.

- *Luteal Phase (day 15-30):* Progesterone Dominates. This is when you get some breast tenderness (max at day 28-30). Breast density increases slightly.

- *Pregnancy:* Tubes and Duct Proliferate. The breast gets a lot denser (more hypoechoic on US), and ultrasound may be your best bet if you have a mass.

- *Perimenopausal:* Shortening of the follicular phase means the breast gets more progesterone exposure. More progesterone exposure means more breast pain, more fibrocystic change, more breast cyst formation.

- *Menopause ("The Floppy Stage"):* Lobules go down. Ducts stay but may become ectatic. Fibroadenomas will degenerate (they like estrogen), and get their "popcorn" calcifications. Secretory calcifications will develop (*but not for 15-20 years post menopause).

- *Hormone Replacement Therapy:* Breasts get more dense (especially estrogen-progesterone combos). Breast pain can occur, typically peaking in the first year. Fibroadenoma (who like to drink estrogen) can grow.

High Yield Trivia Regarding Breast Anatomy / Physiology

- The nipple can enhance with contrast on MRI. This is normal (not Pagets).
- Most cancers occur in the upper outer quadrant.
- Most cancers start in the terminal duct lobular unit (TDLU).
- Majority (60%) of blood flow is via the internal mammary.
- Mets to the Internal Mammary Nodes are uncommon (3%) – seen in medial cancers.
- Axillary Node Levels (1, 2, 3 - lateral to medial)
- Sternalis is usually unilateral, and only on the CC, NEVER on MLO.
- Breast Tenderness is max around day 27-30.
- Mammography and MRI are best performed in the follicular phase (days 7-14).
- Don't Biopsy a prepubescent breast – you can affect breast development
- Perimenopause (50's) is the peak time for breast pain, cyst formation
- Fibroadenomas will degenerate (buzzword popcorn calcification) in menopause
- Secretory Calcifications (buzzword "rod-like) will develop 10-20 years post menopause

Whatcha You Know About Lactation?
Loaded fo-fo on the low where the cheese at?

Density: As mentioned above, the breast gets a lot denser in the 3rd trimester. Mammograms might be worthless, and ultrasound could be your only hope. In other words, ultrasound has greater sensitivity than mammo in lactating patients.

Density Trick: Pituitary Prolactinoma, or meds (classically antipsychotics) can create a similar bilateral increased density.

Biopsy: You can biopsy a breast that is getting ready to lactate / lactating - you just need to know there is **the risk of creating a milk fistula**. If you make one, they will have to stop breast feeding to stop the fistula. The fistula can get infected, but that's not very common.

Galactocele: This is one of those "benign fat containing lesions" that you can BR-2. This is typically seen on cessation of lactation. The location is typically sub-areolar. The appearance is variable, but can have an **Aunt Minnie look with a fat-fluid level**. It's possible to breast abscess these things up.

Lactating Adenoma: These things look like fibroadenomas, and may actually be a charged up fibroadenoma (they like to drink estrogen). Usually these are **multiple.** If you get pressed on follow up recommendation for these I would say 4-6 months postpartum, post delivery or after cessation of lactation -via ultrasound. They usually **rapidly regress after you stop lactation.**

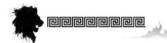 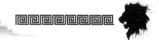
Basics: As I mentioned in the introduction, a screening mammogram starts with two standard views; a cranial caudal view and a medial lateral oblique view.

Technically Adequate?

The first step in reading a mammogram is verifying that the technique is satisfactory. For the purpose of multiple choice there are a few easy ways to test this.

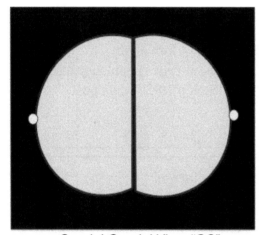

Cranial Caudal View "CC"

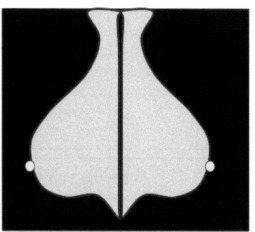

Medial Lateral Oblique View "MLO"

The **Posterior Nipple Line** – this is drawn on the MLO from the nipple to the chest wall. You need to touch pectoralis muscle to be adequate.

Then on CC, you draw a line from the nipple back towards the chest wall. To be adequate **you must be within 1 cm of the length of the posterior nipple line**.

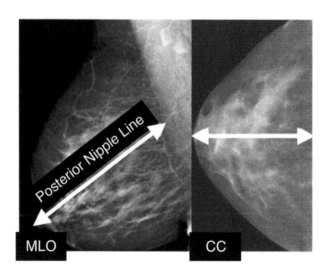

Technically Adequate Cont.

So other points and trivia:

- Ideally, the inframammary fold should be visualized
- *"Camel Nose"* is the buzzword used to describe a breast on MLO that has not be pulled "up and out" by the tech
- The nipple should be in profile in one of two views (to avoid missing the subareolar cancer).
- Relaxed pectoralis muscles are preferred (<u>convex</u>, instead of concave) – showing more breast tissue.

Positioning Trivia:

When do you get a LMO view ? The MLO is the standard, but sometimes you need a LMO. The answer is women with **kyphosis or pectus excavatum**. Or to **avoid a medial pacemaker / central line**.

MLO View Trivia: The MLO view contains the most breast tissue of all the possible views

When using Spot Compression Views: A big point is the recommendation to **leave the collimator open**, giving you a larger field of view, and helping to ensure that you got what you wanted to get. Small paddles give you better focal compression. Large paddles allow for good visualization of land marks.

When using Magnification Views: A CC and ML (true lateral) are obtained. You **get a ML (as opposed to a MLO) to help catch milk of calcium**.

When using a True Lateral View ML vs LM: Using a true lateral is useful for localizing things seen on a single view only (the CC). A trick I use is whatever I said on the screener, is the last letter I'd use on the call backs. In other words, if it's Lateral on the screener you want an ML on the diagnostic. If it's Medial on the screener then you want a LM on the diagnostic. The reason is that you are moving it closer to the receptor. **If you see the area of interest on the MLO only (not the CC), you should pick ML – because most (70%) breast cancers occur laterally**. --- This would make a good multiple choice question.

Mediolateral Oblique View (MLO)	• Primary Image View • Maximized Visualization of the Axillary and Posterior Tissue	• Pectoral Muscle should be seen to the Level of the Nipple • Pectoral Muscle should be Relaxed (convex anterior border)	Motion Artifacts Predominates at the Inferior Part of the Breast (especially in wrinkly floppy stinky saggy ones) secondary to a lack of compression. The "sweep up and out" technique is used by techs to reduce artifact in this location.
Craniocaudal View (CC)	• Primary Image View • Ideally maximizes the posterior medial tissue (the spot that can be missed on the MLO)	• Should have a small amount of skin at the most medial aspect to confirm adequate coverage • Chest wall to nipple should be within 1 cm of the chest wall to pectoral muscle on the MLO.	If you lack adequate coverage at the posterior lateral edge or axillary tail the next appropriate step is an exaggerated lateral CC view (XCCL).

Mediolateral (ML)	90 degree view Can be used to triangulate (medial to the nipple lesions will rise on the true lateral - "muffins rise") Shows the lateral breast (the one closest to the detector) in better detail	**Lateromedial (LM)**	90 degree view Can be used to triangulate (medial to the nipple lesions will rise on the true lateral - "muffins rise") Shows the medial breast in better detail. Remember the posterior medial breast is the toughest is image.

Q: Conan! What is Best in Life ? A: To crush your enemies, and see them driven before you

Q: Conan! What is Best ... View Given the Following Circumstances ?

"Nodule" seen only in CC View	Rolled CC
"Nodule" favored to be in the skin	Tangential (TAN)
"Nodule" favored to be milk of calcium	True Lateral
"Nodule" in the far posterior medial breast	Cleavage View (CV)
Breast Implants	"Eklund Views" or Implant Displaced (MLOID, CCID)
Calcifications	Magnification View

Yes, I'm using the term **"nodule"** deliberately to annoy academic breast imagers who hate that word.
Never pick the word *"nodule"* on the exam !

Basic Artifacts:

Blur: Can be from breathing or inadequate compression (typically along the inferior breast on the MLO). It can be tricky to pick up. The strategy I like to use is to look at Cooper's Ligaments – they should be thin white lines in the fat. If they are thick or fuzzy – it is probably blur (or edema). If there is skin thickening, think edema.

You see blur in 3 scenarios
(1) patient moved,
(2) exposure was too long,
(3) exposure was too short.

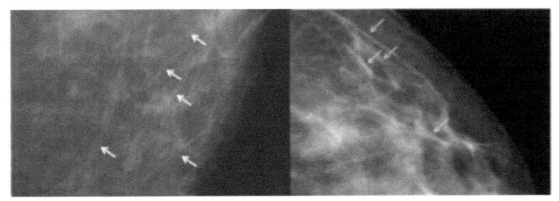

Blur: *"Coopers are too thick"* for normal skin

Grid Lines: Basically mammograms always use a grid (unless it's a mag view). That would make a good multiple choice question actually. No grid on mag views. So, the grid works by moving really fast, and only keeping x-rays that move straight in.

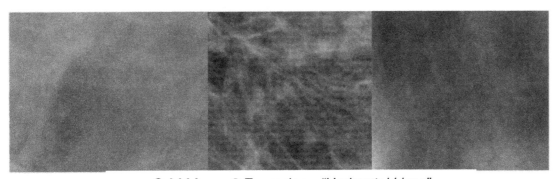

Grid Lines: 3 Examples - *"Horizontal Lines"*

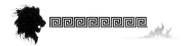
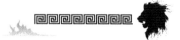
You are trying to find around **3-8 cancers per 1000 mammograms.** Another way to ask this is to say that you are supposed to have a **Positive Predictive Value (PPV$_1$) of around 4%** (in other words anything other than a BR1 or BR2 on a screener). This is demanded by the various regulating bodies.

Be aware that certain areas can sometimes only be seen on a single view. For example, the **medial breast on a CC may not be seen on MLO**, and the **Inferior Posterior Breast on MLO may be excluded from the CC.** That makes these areas "high risk" for missing a cancer.

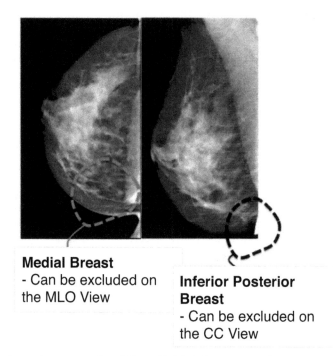

Medial Breast
- Can be excluded on the MLO View

Inferior Posterior Breast
- Can be excluded on the CC View

It's recommended to look at mammograms from 2 years prior (if available) for comparison. Makes it a little easier to see early changes.

Localizing a lesion (only seen in the MLO view): This is a very basic skill, but if you had absolutely no interest in mammography or just terrible training, a refresher might be useful as this is applicable to multiple choice tests. A lesion that is seen in the MLO only will rise on the true lateral (ML) if it is **m**edial on the CC film. A lesion that is seen on the MLO only will fall on the true lateral (ML) if it is **l**ateral on the CC film. The popular mnemonic is *"Lead Sinks, and Muffins Rise"* – L for lateral, and M for medial.

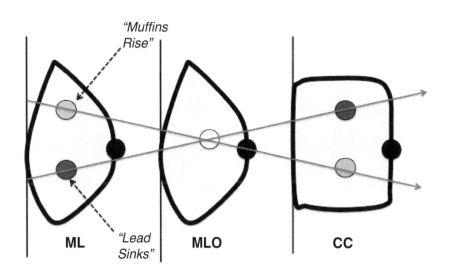

Localizing a lesion (only seen in the CC view): Sometimes you can only see the finding in the CC view. If you want to further characterize it with ultrasound, figuring out if it's in the superior or inferior breast could be very helpful. One method for doing this is a "rolled CC view."

Rolled CC View: This works by positioning the breast for a CC view, but prior to placing the breast in compression you rotate the breast either medial or lateral along the axis of the nipple. Your reference point is the top of the breast.

- If you roll the breast medial; a superior tumor will move medial, an inferior tumor will move lateral.
- If you roll the breast lateral; a superior tumor will move lateral, an inferior tumor will move medial.

In other words, **superior tumors move in the direction you roll** and **inferior tumors move in the opposite direction** you roll. The *"superior"* vs *"inferior"* is inferred based on how it moves when you (the tech) roll the boob.

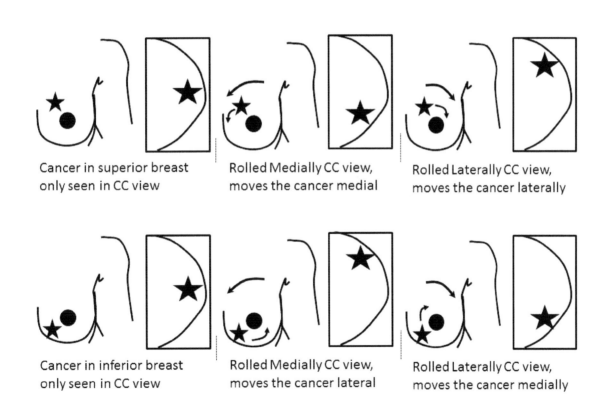

Cancer in superior breast only seen in CC view

Rolled Medially CC view, moves the cancer medial

Rolled Laterally CC view, moves the cancer laterally

Cancer in inferior breast only seen in CC view

Rolled Medially CC view, moves the cancer lateral

Rolled Laterally CC view, moves the cancer medially

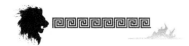 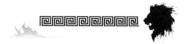

BI-RADS is an acronym for Breast Imaging-Reporting and Data System. It was developed by the ACR to keep everyone on the same page, in a similar way the DSM was developed for psych. You can't have people just calling stuff "breast nodules".

- *BI-RADS Assessment Categories*:
  - 0: Incomplete
  - 1: Negative
  - 2: Benign finding(s)
  - 3: Probably benign — **< 2% Chance of CA**
  - 4: Suspicious abnormality — **2 - 95% Chance of CA**
    - Some people use 4a (low suspicion), 4b (intermediate suspicion), and 4c (moderate suspicion).
  - 5: Highly suggestive of malignancy — **> 95% Chance of CA**
  - 6: Known biopsy – proven malignancy

BI-RADS 0: This is your incomplete workup. They come in for a screener, you find something suspicious. You give it a BI-RADS 0, and bring them back for spots, mags, or ultrasound. You would also BI-RADS 0 anything that required a technical repeat (blur, inadequate posterior nipple line, camel nose, etc.…).

BI-RADS 1: It's normal.

BI-RADS 2: Benign findings. Examples would be cysts, secretory calcifications, fat containing lesions such as oil cysts, lipomas, galactoceles and mixed-density hamartomas.

- *Multiple bilateral well circumscribed, similar appearing masses* - This is BR-2 unless one is growing or different than the rest. The general rule is to not ultrasound these things unless one is palpable.

- *Multiple Foci* – This MRI finding is also a classic BR2.

BI-RADS 3: A key point is that **BR-3 by definition means it has less than 2% chance of being cancer**. This is often a confusing topic. You can only use BR3 on a baseline. You can't call anything BR3 that is new. The typical BR3 scenario: 45 year old comes in for screening and has a focal asymmetry. She gets called back for diagnostic work up with spots and ultrasound. She is found to have mass with imaging features classic for fibroadenoma. This can get a BR-3, and be followed (some places follow for 2 years, in 6 month intervals). Any change over that time ups it to BR-4 and it gets a biopsy.

Things you can BR-3:
• *Finding consistent with fibroadenoma*
• *Focal asymmetry that looks like breast tissue (becomes less dense on compression).*
• *Grouped Round Calcifications*

What if it's palpable? This is a controversial topic. Classic teaching is that palpable lesions can not be BR3. However, recent papers have shown that a palpable lesion consistent with a fibroadenoma has less than 2% chance of cancer. Some people think the new BI-RADS will change this rule. I really doubt they will paint you into a corner on this one - given the controversy.

BI-RADS 4: This is **defined as having a 2-95% chance of malignancy**. Some people will subdivide *this into 4A, 4B, 4C depending on the level of suspicion.* Ultimately you are going to biopsy it, and be prepared to accept a benign result.

BI-RADS 5: This is defined as **> 95% chance of malignancy**. When you give a BR-5, you are saying to the pathologist "if you give me a benign result, I'll have to recommend surgical biopsy." In other words, you **can't accept benign with a BR-5**.

BI-RADS 6: This is path proven cancer.

—

Basic Flow - These are essentially your choices in a work up.

BR 0 - You made a suspicious finding and they need a diagnostic workup

BR 0 - Technical Repeat for Blur, inadequate positioning etc…

BR 1 - Totally Normal

BR 2 - Multiple bilateral, well circumscribed, similar appearing masses

BR 2 - Redemonstration of an unchanged <u>previously worked up</u> thing - a cyst etc…

Screening Mammogram
(no symptoms)

Diagnostic Mammogram
(either a call back,
or someone with
a symptom)

BR 2 - You work it up and it's a benign thing - fat containing lesion, cyst, etc… This returns to screening

BR 3 - Very specific situation where you are dealing with a baseline screener, now called back. Findings meet one of the three things described above; (fibroadenoma, fat with breast tissue, group of round calcs). This gets 2 years of follow up.

BR 4 - Suspicious finding, but you aren't convinced it's cancer. In other words, you would accept a benign result. - This gets a biopsy.

BR 5 - Suspicious finding, that you are convinced is cancer. In other words, you would NOT accept a benign result. - This gets a biopsy.

BI-RADS Terminology

In addition to the "0-6" babysitting, the various regulatory bodies have decided there are only a few words they will trust you with, depending on what modality you are using.

Plain Mammography:

"Mass" – This is a space occupying lesion seen in two different projections

Describing the mass: You need to cover (1) Shape, (2) Margin, (3) Density
   (1) *Shape:* Round, Oval, Irregular - ***"ROI"***
   (2) *Margin:* Circumscribed, Obscured, Microlobulated, Indistinct, Spiculated - ***"COMIS"***
   (3) *Density* (relative to breast parenchyma: Fat Density (radiolucent), Low Density, Equal Density, High Density

Trivia: Of all the possible descriptors - margin is the most reliable feature for determining benign vs malignant.

"Asymmetry" – Unilateral deposition of tissue that doesn't quite look like a mass.
   - *Asymmetry* – This is a density (only seen in one view) that may or may not be a mass, and is often a term used in screeners for BR-0 prior to call back.
   - *Global Asymmetry* – "greater volume of breast tissue than the contralateral side", around one quadrants worth (or more). It's gonna get a call back, and then BR-2'd on a baseline.
   - *Focal Asymmetry* - This is seen in two projections, might be a mass - needs a spot compression.
   - *Developing Asymmetry* – Wasn't there before, now is… or bigger than prior.

Ultrasound:

Describing the mass: You need to cover : (1) Shape, (2) Orientation, (3) Margin, (4) Echo pattern, (5) Posterior acoustic features

   (1) *Shape:* Round, Oval, Irregular (not round or oval)
   (2) *Orientation:* Parallel (wider than tall), Not-Parallel (taller than wide)
   (3) *Margin:* Circumscribed, Indistinct, Angular, Microlobulated, Spiculated
   (4) *Echo Pattern*: Anechoic, Hyperechoic, Hypoechoic, Isoechoic, or Complex *(cystic/ solid)*
   (5) *Posterior Features:* None, Enhancement, Shadowing

MRI:

There has recently been a vocabulary change in the Lexicon, and I'm going to briefly cover the changes.

Background Parenchymal Enhancement:
- This is a newly added BI-RADS "feature." In the literature, they specify that this description is <u>based off the first post contrast sequence</u> (sounds testable to me). The
- Categories are : none, minimal, mild, moderate, and marked.

Lesion Analysis: There are 3 basic categories for this:
- **Foci (< 5 mm):** You don't need to describe shape and margin on these. They are too small.
- **Mass (> 5 mm):** This will have shape, margin, internal enhancement characteristics, & T2.
- **Non-Mass Enhancement:** Distribution, Internal Enhancement, T2

Describing Masses:
- **Shape:** Round, Oval, and Irregular. The word "lobulated" has been removed from the lexicon, so expect that to be a distractor.
- **Margin**: Circumscribed, Irregular, and Spiculated. The word "smooth" has been removed from the lexicon, so expect that to be a distractor.
- **Internal Enhancement Patterns:** Homogenous, Heterogenous, Rim, and Dark Internal Septations. "Enhancing Internal Septations" and "Central Enhancement" are NOT terms in the new vocab - and will likely be distractors.

T2 Signal - This is a new "feature" of the lexicon
- Hyperintense:
    - Greater than parenchyma (on T2)
    - Greater than or equal to fat (on T2)
    - Greater than or equal to water (on T2 Fat Sat)

NME - "Distribution"
- Focal, Linear, Segmental (triangle shaped pointing towards nipple - *suggestive of a duct*), Regional (large area - not a duct), Multiple Regions (two or more regions) and Diffuse.

NME - Internal Enhancement
- Homogenous, Heterogenous, Clumped (looks like cobblestone), Clustered Ring (*this is a buzzword for DCIS or IDC*). "Reticular" and "Dendritic" have been removed and will likely be distractors.

MRI BIRADS Cont..

Kinetic Curves are also described. I'll talk about this more in the Breast MRI Section.

Associated Findings: You are allowed to talk about nipple retraction, skin thickening, edema, invasion of the pec muscles, pre contrast signal, and artifacts.

Implants: When you talk about implants you have to describe the type (silicone vs saline), location (retroglandular vs retropectoral), and luminal features like radial folds, keyhole, linguine, etc... I'll cover this more in the Breast MRI section.

____

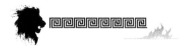 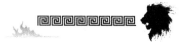

SECTION 5:
CALCIFICATIONS

Calcifications can be an early sign of breast cancer. "The earliest sign," actually, according to some. Calcifications basically come in three flavors: (1) artifact, (2) benign, and (3) suspicious.

Artifacts Simulating Calcifications:

Deodorant: High density material seen in the axilla is the typical appearance. Another trick is to show a speck of high density material that doesn't change position on different views (inferring that it's on the image receptor).

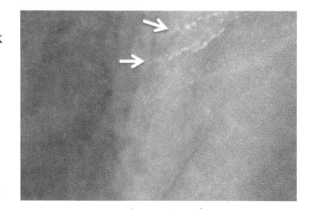

Deodorant Artifact

Zinc Oxide: This is in an ointment old ladies like to put on their floppy sweaty breasts. It can collect on moles and mimic calcifications. If it disappears on the follow up it was probably this (or another dermal artifact).

Metallic Artifact: It's possible for the electrocautery device to leave small metallic fragments in the breast. These will be very dense (metal is denser than calcium). It will also be adjacent to a scar.

Benign vs Suspicious:

The distinction between benign and suspicious is made based on morphology and distribution (those BI-RADS descriptors). Since most breast cancers start in the ducts (a single duct in most cases), a linear or segmental distribution is the most concerning. The opposite of this would be bilateral scattered calcifications.

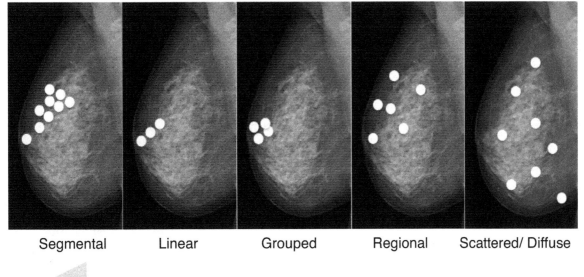

| Segmental | Linear | Grouped | Regional | Scattered/ Diffuse |

More Evil than Ursula (villainous sea witch) from the Little Mermaid →   **Benign**

Benign:

Dermal Calcifications: These are found anywhere women sweat (folds, cleavage, axilla). Just think folds. They are often grouped like the paw of a bear, or the foot of a baby. The trick here is that these **stay in the same place on CC, and MLO views**. This is the so called "**tattoo sign.**" If you are asked to confirm these are dermal calcs, I'd ask for a "tangential view."

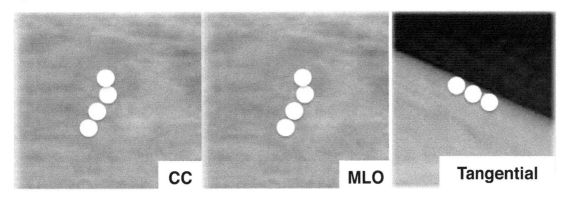

CC   MLO   Tangential

Benign - Continued

Vascular Calcifications: These are parallel linear calcifications. It's usually obvious, but not always.

Popcorn Calcifications: This is an immediate buzzword for degenerating fibroadenoma. The typical look is they begin around the periphery and slowly coalesce over subsequent images.

Secretory (Rod-Like) Calcifications: These are big, easily seen, and point toward the nipple. They are typically bilateral. The buzzword is *"cigar shaped with a lucent center."* Another buzzword is *"dashes but no dots."* The buzz age is *"10-20 years after menopause."* **Don't be an idiot and call these in a premenopausal patient,** they happen because the duct has involuted.

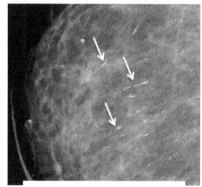

Secretory Calcifications

Eggshell Calcifications: "Fat necrosis" I call them. It can be from any kind of trauma (surgical, or accidental - play ground related). If they are really massive you may see the word **"liponecrosis macrocystica."** As I've mentioned many times in this book, anything that sound Latin or French is high yield for multiple choice. *"Lucent Centered" is a buzzword.*

Dystrophic Calcifications: These are also seen after radiation, trauma, or surgery. These are usually big. *The buzzword is "irregular in shape."* They can also have a lucent center.

Round: The idea is that these things develop in lobules, are usually scattered, bilateral, and benign. When benign (which is most of the time) they *are going to be due to fibrocystic change* (most of the time). The best way I've heard to think about these is the same as a mass.

When masses are bilateral, multiple, and similar they are considered benign (BR-2). When a mass is by itself or different it's considered suspicious. Round calcifications are the same way. They are usually bilateral and symmetric (and benign). If they are clustered together, by themselves, or new, they may need worked up (just like a mass). Remember that if grouped round calcs are on the first mammogram you can BR-3 them.

Benign - Continued

Milk of Calcium:

This has a very characteristic look, and because of that, questions can only be asked in one of two ways: (1) what is it? - shown as CC then ML, (2) what is it due to ?

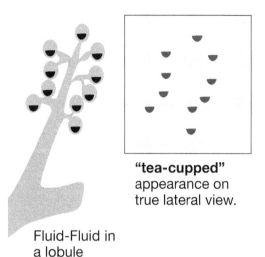

Fluid-Fluid in a lobule

"tea-cupped" appearance on true lateral view.

(1) On the CC view the calcifications look powdery and spread out, on the MLO view they may layer. I suspect they will show you a **ML** view because they should layer into a more linear appearance, with a curved bottom "**tea-cupped**." *For the purpose of gamesmanship if they show you a ML view on a calcs question - look hard for anything that resembles tea-cupping.*

(2) It's fluid-fluid in a lobule - **due to fibrocystic change.**

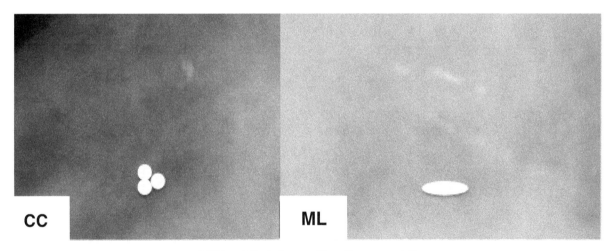

CC   **ML**

Milk of Calcium - Tea Cups on ML

No Calcifications on the Biopsy?

This is a common trick. Apparently **Milk of Calcium needs to be viewed with polarized light to assess birefringence**. Otherwise, you can't see it. I imagine there are several ways to get at that via multiple choice.

Suspicious

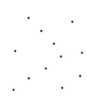 **Amorphous** - These things look like powdered sugar, and you should not be able to count each individual calcification.

Distribution is key with amorphous calcs (like many other types before). If the calcs are scattered and bilateral they are probably benign, if they are segmental they are probably concerning.

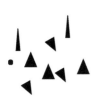 **Coarse Heterogeneous** - These calcifications are countable, but their tips are dull. If you picked one up it would not be poke you.

They are usually **bigger than 0.5 mm.** Distribution and comparison to priors is always important. They can be associated with a mass (fibroadenoma, or papilloma).

 Fine Pleomorphic - These calcifications are countable, and their tips appear sharp. If you picked one up it would poke you. They are usually **smaller than 0.5 mm.** This pattern has the second highest likelihood of malignancy… *probably — see discussion on the following page.*

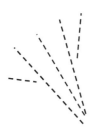 **Fine Linear / Fine Linear Branching** - This is a distribution that makes fine pleomorphic calcifications even more suspicious. The **DDx narrows to basically DCIS** or an atypical look for secretory calcs or vascular calcs. This pattern has the highest likelihood of malignancy.

DDx Amorphous Ca^{+2}	DDx Coarse Heterogeneous Ca^{+2}	DDx Fine Pleomorphic Ca^{+2}
Fibrocystic Change *(most likely)* Sclerosing Adenosis Columnar Cell Change DCIS (low grade)	Fibroadenoma Papilloma Fibrocystic Change DCIS *(low - intermediate grade)*	Fibroadenoma *(less likely)* Papilloma *(less likely)* Fibrocystic Change DCIS *(high grade)*

Suspicious - Continued

Calcifications Associated with Focal Asymmetry/Mass:

When you see increased tissue density around suspicious calcifications, the chance of an actual cancer goes up. This is sometimes called a **"puff of smoke" sign** , or a "warning shot." This is a situation where ultrasound is useful, for extent of disease.

Gamesmanship - Next Step:

Ultrasound is NOT typically used to evaluated pure calcification findings. Exceptions would be (a) if the patient had a mass associated with the calcifications, or (b) if the patient had a palpable finding - then they would get additional evaluation with ultrasound.

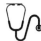 ## Gamesmanship "Highest Suspicion for Malignancy"

Depending on what you read and who you ask, Fine Linear Branching and Fine Pleomorphic Calcifications have the Highest Suspicion for Malignancy. So which one is it?

For sure fine linear branching is the worst. Morphologically it mimics the ductal proliferation of suspicious calcifications (DCIS). The confusion is that some people use fine pleomorphic as an umbrella term under which linear and branching forms exist.

So how to handle this on multiple choice?

• If the answer choices include fine linear branching then that is the correct answer.

• If the answer choices do NOT include fine linear branching but instead have you pick fine pleomorphic vs coarse heterogenous or some other obviously benign calcs (egg shell, etc…) then for sure pick fine pleomorphic.

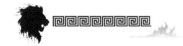
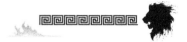

Mondor Disease: This is a thrombosed vein that presents as a tender palpable cord. It looks exactly like you'd expect it to with ultrasound. You don't anticoagulate for it (it's not a DVT). Treatment is just NSAIDS and warm compresses.

Fat Containing Lesions: There are five classic fat containing lesions, all of which are benign: oil cyst / fat necrosis, hamartoma, galactocele, lymph nodes, and lipoma. Of these 5, only oil cyst/fat necrosis and lipoma are considered "pure fat containing" masses.

- **Hamartoma** – The buzzword is "breast within a breast." They have an Aunt Minnie appearance on mammography, although they are difficult to see on ultrasound (they blend into the background).

- **Galactocele** – Seen in young lactating women. This is typically seen on cessation of lactation. The location is typically sub-areolar. The appearance is variable, but can have an Aunt Minnie look with a fat-fluid level. It's possible to breast abscess these things up.

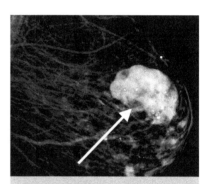

Hamartoma
- "Breast within a Breast"

- **Oil Cyst / Fat Necrosis** – These are areas of fat necrosis walled off by fibrous tissue. You see this (1) randomly, (2) post trauma, (3) post surgery. The peripheral calcification pattern is typically "egg shell." *If you see a ton of them you might think about steatocystoma multiplex* (some zebra with hamartomas).

- **Lipoma** – These are typically radiolucent with no calcifications. Enlargement of a lipoma is criteria for a biopsy.

- **Intramammary Lymph node:** These are normal and typically located in the tissue along the pectoral muscle, often close to blood vessels. They are NOT seen in the fibroglandular tissue.

Practice Point: *Does she need an ultrasound if it's palpable?* Usually a palpable finding is going to get an ultrasound. If you are under 30, most people will skip the mammo and go straight to ultrasound. One of the exceptions is a fat containing lesion definite benign BR-2er on diagnostic mammography.

Pseudoangiomatous Stromal Hyperplasia (PASH): This is a benign myofibroblastic hyperplastic process (hopefully that clears things up). It's usually big (4-6 cm), solid, oval shaped, with well defined borders. Age range is wide they can be seen between 18-50 years old. Follow up in 12 months (annual) is the typical recommendation.

 Pseudoangiomatous Stromal Hyperplasia = Benign thing with a scary sounding name

Fibroadenoma – This is the most common palpable mass in young women. The typical appearance is an oval, circumscribed mass with homogeneous hypoechoic echotexture, and a central hyperechoic band. If it's shown in an older patient, it's more likely to have coarse "popcorn" calcifications – which is a buzzword. On MRI, it's T2 bright with a type 1 enhancement (progressive enhancement).

Phyllodes: Although I clumped this in benign disease, this thing has a malignant degeneration risk of about 10%. They can metastasize - usually hematogenous to the lungs and bone. This is a fast growing breast mass. They need wide margins on resection, as they are associated with a higher recurrence rate if the margin is < 2 cm. It occurs in an older age group than the fibroadenoma (40s-50s). Biopsy of the sentinel node is not needed, because mets via the lymphatics are so incredibly rare (if it does met - it's hematogenous).

Distinguishing Features of Phyllodes Tumor
- *Rapid Growth*
- *Hematogenous Mets*
- *Middle-Age to Older Women*
- *Mimics a Fibroadenoma*

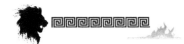 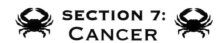 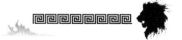
IDC - Invasive Ductal Carcinoma

IDC - Invasive Ductal Carcinoma is by far the most common invasive breast cancer, making up about 80-85% of the cases. This cancer is ductal in origin (duh), but unlike DCIS is not confined to the duct. Instead it "invades" through the duct and if not found by the heroic actions of Mammographers it will progress to distal mets and certain death. Clinically, the most common story is a hard, non-mobile, painless mass. On imaging, the most common look is an irregular, high density mass, with indistinct or spiculated margins, associated pleomorphic calcifications, and an anti-parallel shadowing mass with an echogenic halo on ultrasound.

Invasive Ductal NOS - By far the most common type of breast cancer is the one that is undifferentiated and has no distinguishing histological features. "Not Otherwise Specified" or NOS they call it. These guys make up about 65% of invasive breast cancer.

Less Common (but still testable) IDC Subtypes

IDC Types – (Other than NOS)		
Tubular	Small **spiculated** slow growing mass with a **favorable prognosis.**	Often conspicuous on ultrasound. **Associated with a Radial Scar.** Contralateral breast will have cancer 10-15% of the time.
Mucinous	**Round** (or lobulated) and circumscribed mass	**Uncommon.** Better outcomes than IDC-NOS
Medullary	**Round** or Oval circumscribed mass, without calcifications.	**Axillary nodes can be large even in the absence of mets.** Typically younger patient (40s-50s). Better outcome than IDC-NOS -25% have BRCA 1 mutation
Papillary	**Complex cystic and solid.**	**Axillary nodes are NOT common.** Typically seen in elderly people, favors people who are not white, and is the 2nd most common (behind IDC-NOS).

Multifocal Breast Cancer	Multicentric Breast Cancer
Multiple primaries in the same quadrant (classically same duct system) *Less than 4-5 cm apart from one another*	Multiple primaries in different quadrants *Think of this like "multi-center" clinical trial; multiple discrete un-related sites.*

Synchronous Bilateral Breast Cancer – This is seen in 2-3% of women on mammography, with another 3-6% found with MRI. The risk of bilateral disease is increased in infiltrating lobular types, and multi-centric disease.

DCIS - This is the "earliest form of breast cancer." In this situation the "cancer" is confined to the duct. Histologists grade it as low, intermediate, or high. Histologists also use the terms "comedo", and "non-comedo" to subdivide the disease. If anyone would ask, the **comedo type is more aggressive** than than the non-comedo types.

Testable Trivia:
- 10% of DCIS on imaging may have an invasive component at the time biopsy is done
- 25% of DCIS on core biopsy may have an invasive component on surgical excision.
- 8% of DCIS will present as a mass without calcifications
- Most common ultrasound appearance = microlobulated mildly hypoechoic mass with ductal extension, and normal acoustic transmission

If a test writer wants you to come down on this they will show it in 1 of 3 classic ways:
(1) suspicious calcifications (fine linear branching or fine pleomorphic - as discussed above), (2) non mass enhancement on MRI, or (3) multiple intraductal masses on galactography.

Pagets - Paget's disease of the breast is a high yield topic. It is basically a carcinoma in situ of the nipple epidermis. About 50% of the time the patient will have a palpable finding associated with the skin changes.

Things to know about Breast Pagets:
- Associated with **high grade DCIS (96 %)**
- Wedge biopsy should be done on any skin lesion that affect the nipple-areolar complex that doesn't resolve with topical therapy.
- Pagets is NOT considered T4. The skin involvement does not up the stage in this setting.

Lobular - ILC

Lobular (ILC) : This is the second most common type of breast cancer (IDC-NOS being the most common). It makes up about 5-10% of the breast CA cases.

This pathophysiology lends itself well to multiple choice questions:

Cell decides to be cancer -> Cells lose "e-cadherin" -> Cells no longer stick to one another and begin to infiltrate the breast "like the web of a spider" -> This infiltrative pattern does not cause a desmoplastic reaction so it gets missed on multiple mammograms -> Finally someone (you) notices some architectural distortion without a central mass, on the CC view only. You get fancy and call it a "*dark star.*"

On Ultrasound: The typical look is an ill-defined area of shadowing without a mass.

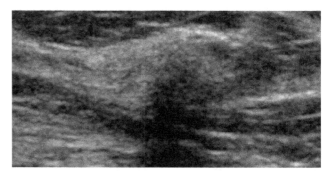

ILC - *Shadowing without discrete mass*

"Shrinking Breast" – This is a buzzword for ILC. The breast isn't actually smaller, it just doesn't compress as much. So when you compare it to a normal breast, it appears to be getting smaller. On physical exam, this breast may actually look the same size as the other one.

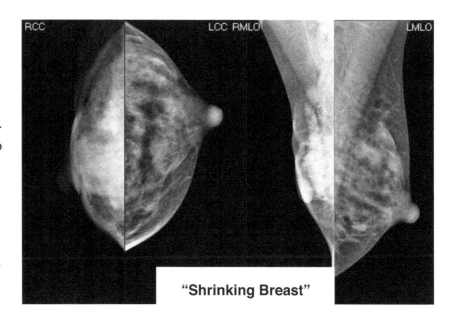

"Shrinking Breast"

Lobular - ILC - Continued

⚖️ **THIS vs THAT: ILC vs IDC:** ILC is more often multifocal. ILC less often mets to the axilla. Instead, it likes to go to strange places like peritoneal surfaces. ILC more often has positive margins, and is more often treated with mastectomy although the prognosis is similar to IDC.

Things to know about ILC:

- It presents later than IDC
- Tends to occur in an older population
- It often is only seen on one view (the CC – as it compresses better)
- Calcifications are less common than with ductal cancers
- Mammo Buzzword = Dark Star
- Mammo Buzzword = Shrinking Breast
- Ultrasound Buzzword = Shadowing without mass
- On MRI – washout is less common than with IDC
- Axillary mets are less common
- Prognosis of IDC and ILC is similar *(unless it's a pleomorphic ILC - which is bad)*
- More often multifocal and bilateral (compared to IDC) - up to 1/3 are bilateral

Dark Star

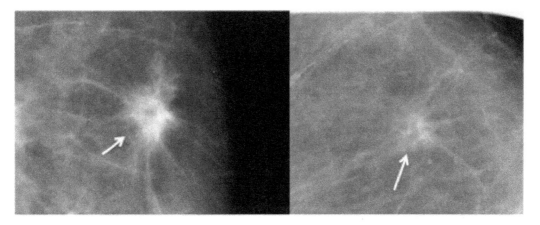

"Dark Star" - Distortion without a central mass

Architectural distortion without a central mass.
The DDx includes: lobular carcinoma, radial scar, surgical scar, and IDC-NOS.

Inflammatory Breast Cancer (IBC) :

IBC an asshole with a notoriously terrible prognosis (at presentation ~30% will have metastases).

Clinical Scenario: The classic clinical scenario is a hot swollen red breast that developed rapidly over 1-3 months. They may even deploy the French sounding word "peau d'orange," - which basically means skin that looks like a delicious ripe grapefruit. Although there may be a mass on the mammogram, in the most classic scenario there isn't a focal palpable mass.

"Skin Thickening" is a mammography buzzword (non-specific). Skin thickening is not (by itself) specific and lots of stuff including CHF can also cause skin thickening. In the case of inflammatory breast cancer the skin thickening is the result of tumor emboli obstructing the lymphatics.

Probably Fuckery: It is likely the question writer will try to make you think mastitis - even though the scenario isn't really classic for that. Remember - mastitis is seen in breast feeding women — that is the most common scenario. If it is just "random woman with a hot swollen breast" - you 100% should think cancer first.   Even if they put them on antibiotics, and she has a history of recurrent infections or whatever — that is all probably bullshit.

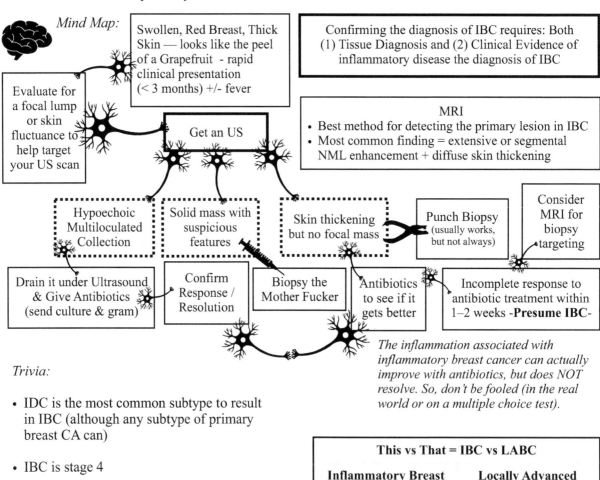

Mind Map:

Swollen, Red Breast, Thick Skin — looks like the peel of a Grapefruit - rapid clinical presentation (< 3 months) +/- fever

Confirming the diagnosis of IBC requires: Both (1) Tissue Diagnosis and (2) Clinical Evidence of inflammatory disease the diagnosis of IBC

Evaluate for a focal lump or skin fluctuance to help target your US scan

Get an US

MRI
• Best method for detecting the primary lesion in IBC
• Most common finding = extensive or segmental NML enhancement + diffuse skin thickening

Hypoechoic Multiloculated Collection

Solid mass with suspicious features

Skin thickening but no focal mass

Punch Biopsy (usually works, but not always)

Consider MRI for biopsy targeting

Drain it under Ultrasound & Give Antibiotics (send culture & gram)

Confirm Response / Resolution

Biopsy the Mother Fucker

Antibiotics to see if it gets better

Incomplete response to antibiotic treatment within 1–2 weeks -**Presume IBC**-

The inflammation associated with inflammatory breast cancer can actually improve with antibiotics, but does NOT resolve. So, don't be fooled (in the real world or on a multiple choice test).

Trivia:

• IDC is the most common subtype to result in IBC (although any subtype of primary breast CA can)

• IBC is stage 4

Treatment: They will try and do chemotherapy prior to surgery because the chance of a positive margin is so high. The standard mastectomy is done for "local control" , which just sounds awful.

This vs That = IBC vs LABC	
Inflammatory Breast Cancer (IBC)	**Locally Advanced Breast Cancer (LABC)**
Rapid onset	Prolonged onset
Younger (mid 50s)	Older (mid 60s)
30% mets at presentation	10% mets at presentation

High Risk Lesions:

There are 5 classic high risk lesions that must come out after a biopsy; Radial Scar, Atypical Ductal Hyperplasia, Atypical Lobular Hyperplasia, LCIS, and Papilloma.

Radial Scar: This is not actually a scar, but does look like one on histology. Instead you have a bunch of dense fibrosis around the ducts giving the appearance of architectural distortion (dark scar).

Things to know:
- *This is high risk and has to come out*
- *It's associated with DCIS and/or IDC 10%-30%*
- *It's associated with Tubular Carcinoma**

Atypical Ductal Hyperplasia (ADH): This is basically DCIS but lacks the quantitative definition by histology (< 2 ducts involved). It comes out (a) because it's high risk and (b) because DCIS burden is often underestimated when this is present. In other words, about 30% of the time the surgical path will get upgraded to DCIS.

Lobular Carcinoma in Situ (LCIS): This is classically occult on mammogram. "An incidental finding" is sometimes a buzzword. The best way to think about LCIS is that it can be a precursor to ILC, but isn't obligated to be. The risk of conversion to an invasive cancer is less when comparing DCIS to IDC. Just like pleomorphic ILC is worse than regular ILC, a pleomorphic LCIS is mo' badder than regular LCIS.

Atypical Lobular Hyperplasia (ALH): This is very similar to LCIS, but histologists separate the two based on if the lobule is distended or not (no with ALH, yes with LCIS). It's considered milder than LCIS (risk of subsequent breast CA is 4-6x higher with ALH, and 11x higher with LCIS). For the CORE, the answer is excision. In the real world, some people do not cut these out, and it's controversial.

Papilloma: A few most commons come to mind with this one. Most common intraductal mass lesion. Most common cause of blood discharge. You typically see these in women in their late reproductive years / early menopausal years (average around 50). The classic location is the subareolar region (1cm from the nipple in 90% of cases).

—*Mammogram:* Often normal - occasionally just showing calcifications.
—*US:* Well-defined smooth walled hypo-echoic mass. Maybe cystic with solid components. Also, tends to have associated duct dilation.
—*Galactography:* Solitary filling defect, with dilated duct.

Multiple Papillomas: These tend to be more peripheral. On mammography it's gonna be a mass(es) or a cluster of calcifications without a mass.

Phyllodes: Yes… I mentioned this already under benign disease. I just wanted to bring it up again to make sure you remember that this thing has a malignant degeneration risk of about 10% (some texts say up to 25%). This is a fast growing breast mass. It occurs in an older age group than the fibroadenoma (40s-50s).

Multiple Masses: Sounds Bad But Actually BR-2

To call multiple masses you need to have multiple (at least 3) bilateral well circumscribed masses without suspicious features. **This gives you a BR-2.**

One common trick is to show multiple unilateral masses, that doesn't fly – they have to be bilateral.

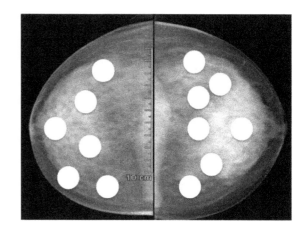

Lymphoma:

Breast Lymphoma		
Primary Breast Lymphoma	**Primary Lymphoma**	**Secondary Lymphoma**
Always , for the purpose of multiple choice, Non Hodgkin (Diffuse Large B-Cell)	Less Common	More Common *most common secondary malignancy or mets to involve the breast*
Usually a hyperdense mass (*Architectural distortion is rare*)	Typical Look: • Usually Solitary • Usually Larger *(compared to secondary)* and most often palpable • Cystic on US	Typical Look: • Inflammatory thickening without a mass (but can look like anything)
"IHC" staining is need to confirm lymphoma		

Do axillary nodes = lymphoma? Bro…. anything can give you axillary nodes

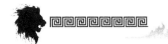 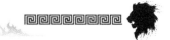
Breast Pain: This is super common and typically cyclic (worse during the luteal phase of the menstrual cycle). Pain in both breasts that is cyclical does not need evaluation. Instead it needs a family medicine referral for some "therapeutic communication." Focal non-cyclic breast pain may warrant an evaluation.

Trivia: The negative predictive value of combined mammogram and US for "focal pain" is right around 100%. When breast cancer is found it's usually elsewhere in the breast (asymptomatic).

Symptoms that are actually worrisome for cancer include: skin dimpling, focal skin thickening, and nipple retraction.

Non-Focal Skin Thickening / Breast Edema: This is usually the result of benign conditions (congestive heart failure, renal failure). For multiple choice tests it will always be bilateral (in the real world you can sleep on one side and have asymmetric edema). As long as the breast isn't red, you can feel confident that it will be benign. On mammography you will see trabecular thickening (diffuse, and favoring the dependent portions of the breast).

Breast Inflammation: The swollen red breast. This finding has a differential of two things: (1) mastitis / abscess, (2) inflammatory breast cancer.

- **Mastitis / Abscess:** This is a swollen red breast which is painful (Inflammatory breast CA is often painless). Patients are usually sick as a dog. Obviously it's associated with breast feeding, and is more common in smokers and diabetics. Abscess can develop (usually Staph A.).

- **Inflammatory Breast Cancer:** As previously discussed, this has a terrible prognosis. The general rule is that a breast that doesn't respond to antibiotics gets a skin biopsy to exclude this. The typical age is 40s-50s. You are going to have an enlarged, red breast with a "peau d'orange" appearance. The breast is often NOT painful, despite its appearance. Mammogram might show a mass (or masses), but the big finding is diffuse skin and trabecular thickening. The treatment is fair game for multiple choice because it is different than normal breast cancer. Instead of going to surgery first, inflammatory breast cancer gets "cooled down" with chemo and/or radiation – then surgery.

The Leaky Tit

Women present with nipple discharge all the time, it's usually benign (90%). **The highest yield information on the subject is that: spontaneous, bloody, discharge from a single duct is your most suspicious feature combo. Serous discharge is also suspicious.** The risk of discharge being cancer is directly related to age (very uncommon under 40, and more common over 60).

Multiple Ducts (Benign)

Single Ducts (Maybe Malignant)
- Papilloma
- DCIS

*Discharge is Bad when it's - Spontaneous, Bloody, and from a Single Duct

Milky Discharge: Milky discharge is NOT suspicious for breast cancer but can be secondary to thyroid issues or a pituitary adenoma (prolactinoma). Any medication that messes with dopamine can stimulate prolactin production - (antidepressants, neuroleptics, reglan).

Causes of Discharge (Not Milky)	
Benign Causes	**Worrisome Causes**
Pre-Menopausal Woman = Fibrocystic Change	Intraductal Papilloma (90%) – single intraductal mass near nipple
Post Menopausal Women = Ductal Ectasia	DCIS (10%) – multiple intraductal masses

Ductal Ectasia – The most common benign cause of nipple discharge in a post menopausal woman. On galactography you will see dilated ducts near the subareolar region, with progressive attenuation more posteriorly.

Papilloma - Discussed previously- this is the most common cause of bloody discharge. As before they can be single or multiple, and carry a small malignant risk (5%).

Galactography

- Ugh… you take a 27 or 30 gauge blunt tipped needle and attempt to cannulate the duct which is leaking. To determine which duct you want - you'll need to have the patient squeeze the breast to demonstrate where it's coming from.

- If you manage to cannulate the duct - gently inject 0.2 - 0.3 cc contrast (rare to need more than 1 cc). You then do mammograms (magnification CC and ML). Filling defect(s) get wire localization.

- *Contraindications:* Active infection (mastitis), inability to express discharge at the time of galactogram, contrast allergy, or prior surgery to the nipple areola complex.

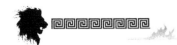 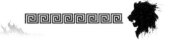

AD: We're talking about unchecked aggression here, Dude. We are talking about distortion of the normal architecture without a visible mass. This manifests in a few ways, including focal retraction, distortion of the edge of the parenchyma, or *radiation of the normal thin lines into a focal point.*

Architectural Distortion vs Summation Artifact: This is the primary differential consideration, with summation of normal vessels, ducts, and ligaments being much more common. The difference is summation should NOT radiate to a central point (AD will).

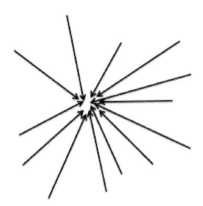 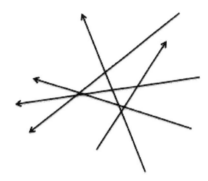

AD - *All lines radiate to a point*   **Summation** - *Lines continue past each other*

Surgical Scar vs Something Bad: Scars should progressively get lighter and harder to see. Some people say that in 5-10 years a benign surgical scar is often difficult to see. Lumpectomy scars tend to stick around longer than a benign biopsy. Basically, look at the priors; if it is a surgical scar, it better be getting less dense. If it's increasing, you gotta stick a needle in it.

Work Up of AD: If you see it on a screener you will want to BR-0 it, and bring it back for spot compression views. If it persists just know you are either going to BR-4 or BR-5 it (unless you know it's a surgical scar). You should still ultrasound it for further characterization (may help you decide between a 4 and a 5).

Ultrasound Trivia: The use of harmonic tissue imaging can make it easier to see some lesions. Be aware that compound imaging can make you lose your posterior features, especially when they are soft to start with – like the shadowing of an ILC. Remember, even if you see nothing, this gets a biopsy. Harmonics can also make not so simple cysts look simple by reducing superficial reverberation.

Things to Know for AD:

- Radiating lines to a single point = AD
- AD + Calcifications = IDC + DCIS
- AD without Calcifications = ILC
- Even with no ultrasound or MRI correlate, AD gets a biopsy.
- Never ever ever ever BR-3 an area of AD.
- Even if it has been there a while, it still needs to be worked up.
- Remember ILC can grow slowly.
- Surgical scars should get less dense with time… not more dense.

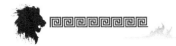 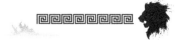

You found a breast cancer – now what? Before you make the patient cry, it's time to stage the disease. Ultrasound her arm pit. About 1 in 3 times you are going to find abnormal nodes.

Unilateral vs Bilateral: This can help you if you are thinking this could be systemic. Unilateral adenopathy should make you worry about a cancer (especially if they have a cancer on that side).

Biopsy It? Some people will recommend biopsy if you have the following abnormal features.

- Cortical Thickness greater than 2.3 mm (some people say 3 mm)
- Loss of Central Fatty Hilum – "most specific sign"
- Irregular Outer Margins.

Staging Trivia: Level 1 and Level 2 nodes are treated the same. Rotter nodes are treated as Level 2. Level 3 and supraclavicular nodes are treated the same.

Special "Sneaky" Situations:

Gold Therapy: Long ago, when the pyramids were still young, rheumatoid arthritis was treated with "chrysotherapy." What they can do is show you an "Aunt Minnie" type picture with very dense calcifications within the node.

Snow Storm Nodes: Another Aunt Minnie look is the silicone infiltration of a node from either silicone leaking or rupture.

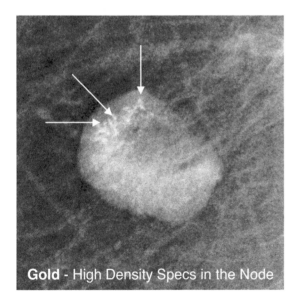

Gold - High Density Specs in the Node

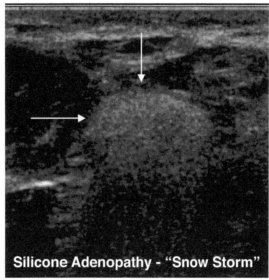

Silicone Adenopathy - "Snow Storm"

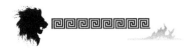 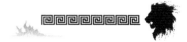
There is no more humiliating way to die for a man than breast cancer. The good news is male breast cancer is uncommon. The bad news is that when it occurs it is often advanced and invasive at the time of diagnosis - Valar Morghulis.

The male breast does NOT have the elongated and branching ducts, or the proliferated lobules that women have. This is key because **men do NOT get lobule associated pathology (lobular carcinoma, fibroadenoma, or cysts).**

Gynecomastia: This is a non-neoplastic enlargement of the epithelial and stromal elements in a man's breast. It occurs "physiologically" in adolescents, affecting about 50% of adolescent boys, and men over 65. If you aren't 13 or 65 it's considered embarrassing and you should hit the gym. If you are between 13-65 it's considered pathology and associated with a variety of conditions (spironolactone, psych meds, marijuana, alcoholic cirrhosis, testicular cancer). There are three patterns (nodular is the most common). Just think **flame shaped, behind nipple, bilateral but asymmetric, and can be painful**. Things that make you worry that it's not gynecomastia include not being behind the nipple, eccentric location, and calcification.

Patterns of Gynecomastia	
Nodular (most common)	"**Flame Shaped**" centered behind the nipple, radiating posterior as it blends into the fat. Breast is often tender. Usually lasts less than 1 year.
Dendritic	Resembles a branching tree. This is a chronic fibrotic pattern. Usually not tender.
Diffuse Glandular	Mammographic pattern looks like a woman's breast (diffuse increase in density). You see this in men receiving estrogen treatment.

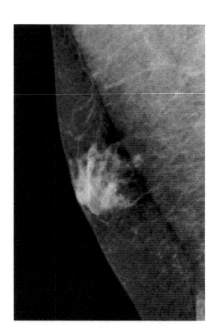
Gynecomastia

Pseudogynecomastia *"Bitch Tits"* – This is an increase in the fat tissue of the breast (not glandular tissue). There will NOT be a discrete palpable finding, and the mound of tissue will not be concentric to the nipple.

Lipoma – After gynecomastia, lipoma is the second most common palpable mass in a man.

Male Breast Cancer: It's uncommon in men, and very uncommon in younger men (average age is around 70). About 1 in 4 males with breast cancer have a BRCA mutation (BRCA 2 is the more common). Other risk factors include Klinefelter Syndrome, Cirrhosis, and chronic alcoholism. The classic description is eccentric but near the nipple. It's almost always an IDC-NOS type. DCIS can occur but is very rare in isolation. On mammography it looks like a breast cancer, if it was a woman's mammogram you'd BR-5 it. On ultrasound it's the same thing, it looks like a BR-5. Having said that, nodular gynecomastia can look suspicious on ultrasound.

Things that make you think it's breast cancer:
- *Eccentric to Nipple*
- *Unilateral*
- *Abnormal Lymph nodes*
- *Calcifications*
- *Looks like breast cancer*

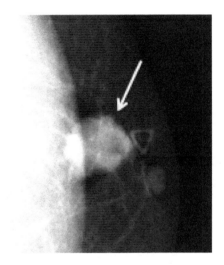

Male Breast CA

Some trivia on calcifications: Micro-calcifications alone are uncommon in men. When you see them they are less numerous, coarser, and associated with a mass (25% of male breast cancers have calcifications).

Should men get screening mammograms? Honestly, women shouldn't even get them (according to the New England Journal of Medicine). This remains controversial, with the bottom line being this: only Klinefelter patients approach the screening range with regards to risk.

As a point of trivia: **males with gynecomastia from gender reassignment on hormone therapy are not high enough risk for screening mammograms**. Obviously, if they have a palpable finding, they can get a diagnostic work up.

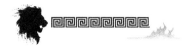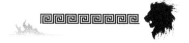
Basic Overview: There are two types , saline and silicone. They both can rupture, but no one really gives a shit if saline ruptures. Saline does not form a capsule, so you can't have intracapsular rupture with saline. There is no additional imaging past mammo for saline rupture, and you just follow up with primary care / plastic surgeon. You can tell it's saline because you can see through it. For silicone you can have both intra and extra capsular rupture. You can only see extra on a mammogram (can't see intra). Extra creates a dense *"snow storm"* appearance on US. Intra creates a *"step ladder"* appearance on US and a *"linguine sign"* on MRI. MRI is done with FS T2 to look at implants.

Big Points:
* You **CAN** have isolated intracapsular rupture.
* You **CAN NOT** have isolated extra (it's always with intra).
* If you see silicone in a lymph node you need to recommend MRI to evaluate for intracapsular rupture

Implant Location: There are two subtypes:
* *Subglandular (retromammary):* Implant behind breast tissue, anterior to pectoral muscle
* *Subpectoral (retropectoral):* Implant between pectoralis major and minor muscles

Silicone Implants

The body will form a shell around the foreign body (implant), which allows for both intracapsular and extracapsular rupture (an important distinction from saline). About 25% of the time you will see calcifications around the fibrous capsule.

Things to know:
* Implants are NOT a contraindication for a core needle biopsy
* Implants do NOT increase the risk for cancer.

Saline Implants

There are also subglandular and subpectoral subtypes. You can tell the implant is saline because you can see through it. Implant folds and valves can also be seen. If it ruptures no one really cares (other than the cosmetic look). The saline is absorbed by the body, and you have a collapsed implant. A practical point of caution, be careful when performing a biopsy in these patients – even a 25g FNA needle can burst a saline implant.

Trivia: Some sources say that "physical exam" is the test of choice for diagnosing saline implant rupture - this is variable depending on what you read / who you ask.

Implant Complications:

Generally speaking, MRI is the most accurate modality for evaluating an implant.

Capsular Contracture: This is the **most common complication of implants**. It occurs secondary to contraction of the fibrous capsule, and can result in a terrible cosmetic deformity. You see it in both silicone and saline implants, but is **most common in subglandular silicone implants**. On mammo it looks like rounding or distortion of the implant (comparisons will show progression).

Gel Bleed: Silicone molecules can (and do) pass through the semi-permeable implant shell coating the exterior of the surface. This does NOT mean the implant is ruptured. The classic look is to show you silicone in the axillary lymph nodes *(remember I showed a case of this under the lymph node section).* Even with axillary lymph nodes, this does NOT mean it has ruptured.

Rupture: As a point of testable trivia, the number one risk factor for rupture is age of the implant. Rupture does not have to be post traumatic, it can occur spontaneously. Rupture with compression mammography is actually rare.

- **Saline:** Saline rupture is usually very obvious (deflated boob). It doesn't matter all that much (except cosmetically), as the saline is just absorbed. On mammo, you will see the "wadded up" plastic wrapper. *They could easily write a question asking you what modality you need to see a saline rupture. The answer would be plain mammo (you don't need ultrasound or MRI).*

- **Silicone:** This is a more complicated matter. You have two subtypes; isolated intracapsular and intracapsular with extracapsular.

    - *Isolated Intracapsular:* This will be occult on physical exam, mammography and possibly ultrasound. You might see a stepladder on Ultrasound. MRI is way more sensitive.

    - *Intracapsular with Extracapsular Rupture:* This is usually obvious on mammogram with dense silicone seen outside the capsule. The contour of a normal intact implant is smooth. Silicone outside the implant can go to lymph nodes. On ultrasound you want to know the buzzword **"snow storm" pattern – which is really echogenic with no posterior shadowing.** A sneaky trick is to show a lymph node with a snow storm appearance on ultrasound. On MRI extracapsular silicon is T1 dark, and T2 bright. Lastly, a very important concept is that *you cannot have isolated extracapsular rupture. If it's extracapsular, then it's also intracapsular.*

Radial Folds - The Mimic of Rupture:

Radial folds are the normal in-foldings of the elastomer shell. They are the primary mimic for the linguine sign of intracapsular rupture. To tell them apart ask yourself *"do the folds connect with the periphery of the implant?"* Radial folds should always do this (linguine does not).

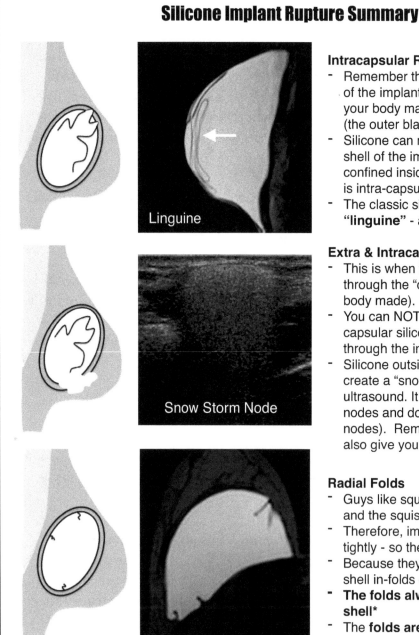

Silicone Implant Rupture Summary

Intracapsular Rupture:
- Remember the "capsule" is not part of the implant. It's the fibrous coat your body makes around the implant (the outer black line in my diagram).
- Silicone can rupture through the shell of the implant, but stays confined inside the fibrous coat - this is intra-capsular rupture.
- The classic sign is the floating **"linguine"** - as in this case.

(image label: Linguine)

Extra & Intracapsular:
- This is when the rupture goes through the "capsule" (the thing your body made).
- You can NOT have isolated extra capsular silicone. It has to make it through the implant shell first.
- Silicone outside the capsule can create a "snow storm" look on ultrasound. It can also infiltrate lymph nodes and do the same (snow storm nodes). Remember *gel bleed* can also give you a node like this.

(image label: Snow Storm Node)

Radial Folds
- Guys like squishy boobs. The bigger and the squishier the better.
- Therefore, implants are not bound tightly - so they can be squishy.
- Because they are loosely bound the shell in-folds creates radial folds
- **The folds always attach to the shell***
- The **folds are thicker** than a rupture, because they represent both layers.

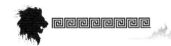
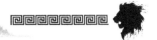
Reduction Mammoplasty and Mastopexy

Reduction Mammoplasty – Yes, there is actually a subpopulation of women who want SMALLER breasts. I know, it sounds impossible to believe , but Mammoplasty is actually done to reduce breast size. I can only pray that the sadistic bastard who developed this procedure has received appropriate punishment (in this life or the next).

Mastopexy – This is a "breast lift," Essentially, **just a removal of skin**. Women get this done to address floppy, saggy, pancake, or "ptotic" boobs.

Normal Findings Post Mastopexy:
  *   *Swirled Appearance Affecting Inferior Breast*
  *   *Fat Necrosis / Oil Cysts*
  *   *Isolated Islands of Breast Tissue*

Keyhole Incision – This is done for both mammoplasty and mastopexy, creating a "swirled" appearance in the inferior aspect of the MLO.

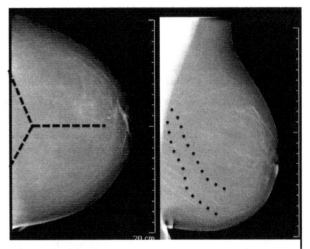

Typical Changes from Mammoplasty

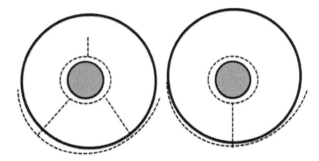

Mammoplasty Keyhole Incision   Mastopexy Keyhole Incision

Surgical Biopsy / Radiation

Terminology:
- **Lumpectomy** – Surgical Removal of Cancer (palpable or not)
- **Excisional Biopsy** – Surgical Removal of **Entire** Lesion
- **Incisional Biopsy** – Surgical Biopsy of a **Portion** of the Lesion

Post Biopsy Changes:

The first post operative mammogram is usually obtained around 6-12 months after biopsy. The key is that **distortion and scarring are worst on this film, and should progressively improve.** On ultrasound, scars are supposed to be thin and linear. If they show you a focal mass like thickening in the scar - you've gotta call that suspicious for local recurrence.

Fat necrosis and benign dystrophic calcifications may evolve over the first year or two, and are the major mimics of recurrence. Fat necrosis can be shown on MR (T1 / T2 bright, and then fat sat drops it out).

Recurrence / Residual Disease:

Numerical Trivia: **Local recurrence occurs 6-8%** of the time when women have breast conserving therapy. The **peak time for recurrence is 4 years** (most occur between 1-7). **Without radiation local recurrence is closer to 35%.** Tumors that recur early (< 3 years) typically occur in the original tumor bed. Those that occur later are more likely to be in a different location than the original primary.

What gets recurrent disease ? Risk of recurrence is highest in the premenopausal woman (think about them having an underlying genetic issue). Other risks include: having an extensive inarticulate component, a tumor with vascular invasion, multi centric tumors, positive surgical margins, or a tumor that was not adequately treated the first go around.

Residual Calcs: Residual calcifications are not good. Supposedly, residual calcifications near or in the lumpectomy bed correlates with a local recurrence rate of 60%.

New Calcs: When it does reoccur, something like 75% of DCIS will come back as calcifications (no surprise). The testable pearl is the **benign calcifications tend to occur early (around 2 years), vs the cancer ones which come back around 4 years.**

Sentinel Node Failure: Sentinel node biopsy works about 95% of the time (doesn't work 5% of the time). So about 5 times in 100 you are going to have a negative node biopsy that presents later with an abnormal armpit node.

Tissue Flap: The cancer is not going to start in the belly fat / muscle. The cancer is going to come from either the residual breast tissue or along the skin scar line. Screening of the flaps is controversial - with some saying it's not necessary. The need for screening of tissue flaps is not going to be asked. If you get asked anything it's "where the recurrence is coming from / going to be?"

Specimen Radiography

If the path report says "close margins" or "positive margins," there is a very high chance you are going to have cancer still in the breast. If you are shown a specimen radiograph, there are two things you need to look at in real life and on multiple choice: (1) is the mass / calcifications on the sample, and (2) is the mass / calcifications near the edge or touching the edge. *If the mass is at the edge, the chance of incomplete excision is going to be near 80%. The "next step" would be to call the surgeon in the OR and tell him/her that.*

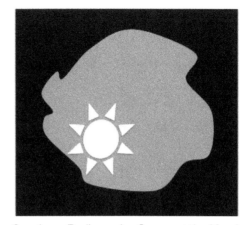

Specimen Radiograph - Cancer at the Margin -High chance of positive margin

Post Radiation Changes:

Practical Point (*the before picture*): The pre-radiation mammogram is very important. If you can identify residual disease on it, the patient has many more treatment options. If you discover the residual disease after the radiation therapy has been given, you've forced the patient to undergo mastectomy.

Radiation Changes: You are going to see skin thickening and trabecular thickening. This is normal post radiation, and should peak on the first post-RT mammogram.

This would be a classic testable scenario:
- Film 1 Post RT: You see skin thickening / trabecular thickening
- Film 2: Skin thickening / trabecular thickening is better
- Film 3: Skin thickening / trabecular thickening is worse * - this is recurrent disease (maybe inflammatory breast CA).

Secondary Angiosarcoma

The primary type is so rare I won't even mention it. The secondary type is seen after breast conservation therapy / <u>radiation therapy</u>. It takes around 6 years post radiation therapy to develop one of these things. Clinically the classic presentation is "red plaques or skin nodules." The challenge with these is that the skin thickening due to the cancer is often confused with post therapy skin thickening.

Staging/ Surgical Planning

Breast Cancer Staging: The staging is based on size from T1-T3, then invasion for T4.
- T1 = < 2 cm.
- T2 = 2-5 cm
- T3 = > 5 cm
- T4 = "Any size" with chest wall fixation, skin involvement, or inflammatory breast CA. *Remember that Pagets is NOT T4.*

Trivia: Axillary Status is the most important predictor of overall survival in breast cancer

Trivia: Melanoma is the most common tumor to met to the breast.

The contraindications for breast conservation are high yield.

Contraindications for Breast Conservation
Inflammatory Cancer,   Large Cancer Size Relative to Breast   Multi-centric (multiple quadrants)   Prior Radiation Therapy, to the same breast   Contraindication to Radiation Therapy (collagen-vascular disease).

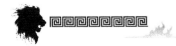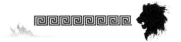
Breast MRI can be used for several reasons: High risk screening, extent of disease (known cancer), axillary mets with unknown primary, diagnostic dilemmas, and possible silicone implant rupture. **The big reason is for high risk screening.**

I'll just briefly go over how it's done, and how it's read.

You need a special breast coil and table set up to make it work. The patient lies belly down with her breasts hanging through holes in the table. You have to position them correctly otherwise they get artifact from their breasts rubbing on the coil. Basic sequences are going to include a T2, and pre and post dynamic (post contrast) fat saturated T1. Remember the breast is a bag of fat - so fat sat is very important. Dynamic imaging is done to generate wash out curves (similar to prostate MRI).

My basic algorithm for reading them is to:

(1) Look at the background uptake. I use this to set my sensitivity when I compare it to prior studies. Ideally you used the same kind of contrast, and imaged at the same time of the month. As I'll mention below, hormone changes with female cycles cause changes in how much contrast gets taken up (less early, and more later).

(2) I look for masses or little dots (foci). MIPS (maximum intensity projections) are helpful just like looking for a lung nodule. If I see a mass or dot I try and characterize it - first by seeing if I can make it T2 bright. Most T2 bright things are benign (lymph nodes, cysts, fibroadenoma). If it's not T2 bright, I look at the features - is it a mass? is it spiculated, etc? These features are more important than anything else. Is it new? Nipple enhancement is ok - don't be a dumb ass and call it Pagets.

(3) Finally I'll look at the wash out curve, but honestly I've made up my mind before I even look at that. I will never let a benign curve back me off suspicious morphology.

(4) I deal with the findings similar to mammo. New masses get BR-4 or BR-5. NMLE (non-mass enhancement) gets BR-4'd if new. T2 bright stuff for the most part (there is one exception of mucinous cancer) gets BR-2'd. Anything with a 4 or a 5 gets biopsy - via MR guided stereo. I never pussy foot out and BR-0 something on MRI - unless it's a technical problem (example inadequate fat sat).

Who gets a screening MRI ?

- *People with a lifetime risk greater than 20-25%*
- *Includes people who got 20 Gy of radiation to the chest as a child*

How do you estimate this risk, to decide who is 20-25%?

- *You use one of the risk models that includes family history (NOT the Gail model). If the question is which of the following is Not one to use ? The answer is Gail. If the question is which of the following do you pick? I'd chose Tyrer-Cuzick, it's probably the best one out now.*

Parenchyma Enhancement:

- *Is it normal ?* – Yes
- *Where is it most common ?* – Posterior Breast in the upper outer quadrant, during the later part of the menstrual cycle (luteal phase - day 14-28)
- *How do you reduce it?* – Do the MRI during the first part of the menstrual cycle (day 7-14).
- *What does Tamoxifen do?* – Tamoxifen will decrease background parenchyma uptake. **Then it causes a rebound.**

Foci:

- *How is it defined?* Round or oval, circumscribed, and **less than 5mm,**

- *Are they high risk?* Usually not. Usually they are benign (2-3% have a chance of being a bad boy).

- *What would make you biopsy one?* Seemed different than the rest, ill-defined borders, or **suspicious enhancement**.

- *Can you BI-RADs 3 one?* If you have a solitary focus (< 5mm) with persistent kinetics on a baseline exam - you can BI-RADS 3 it.

NME (Non-Mass Enhancement):

- *What is NME ?* It's not a mass - but more like a cloud or clump of tissue enhancement.

- *What are the distributions ?* Segmental (triangular blob pointing at the nipple, indicates a single branch), Regional (a bigger triangle), and Diffuse (sorta all over the place).

- *Which one is more suspicious* - homogenous or heterogeneous enhancement of NME ? Heterogeneous is much more suspicious.

Masses:

- These are defined as being 5 mm or larger. They have definable vocabulary for their features (round, oval, indistinct, etc...)

- *When are these bad?* They are bad when you call them bad words. Irregular shape, speculated margins, heterogeneous enhancement, or rim enhancement. Once you say those words you are going to have to biopsy them, because **morphology trumps kinetics**. It doesn't matter what the kinetics shows, you must biopsy suspicious morphology.

- *When is kinetics helpful?* When you are on the fence. If you have benign morphology and you have suspicious kinetics – you probably are going to need to biopsy that also.

Kinetics:

- Breast kinetics are performed in two portions:

    - (1) Initial upslope phase that occurs over the first 2 minutes. This is graded as slow, medium, or rapid (fast).

    - (2) The washout portion which is recorded sometime between 2 minutes and 6 minutes (around about). These are graded as either continued rise "type 1", plateau "type 2", or rapid washout "type 3".

- Risk of Cancer:

    o **Type 1:** Curve: 6%
    o **Type 2:** Curve: 7%-28%
    o **Type 3:** 29% or more.

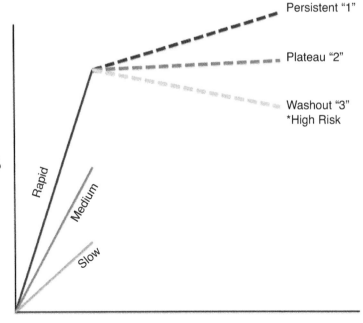

Classic Looks:

- **Fibroadenoma:** These things are classically T2 bright, round, with "non-enhancing septa", and a type 1 curve.

- **DCIS:** Clumped, ductal, linear, or segmental **non-mass enhancement**. Kinetics are typically not helpful for DCIS.

- **IDC:** Spiculated, irregular shaped masses, with heterogeneous enhancement and a type 3 curve.

- **ILC:** Doesn't always show enhancement.

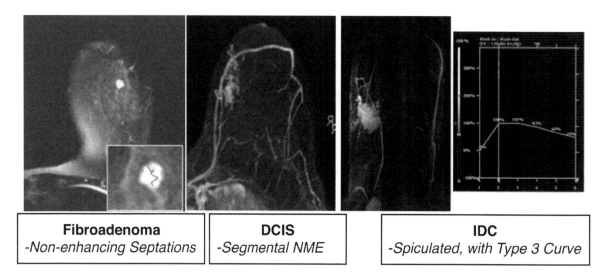

Fibroadenoma	**DCIS**	**IDC**
-Non-enhancing Septations	*-Segmental NME*	*-Spiculated, with Type 3 Curve*

T2 Bright Things:

- Usually T2 Bright = Benign.
- Things that are T2 Bright include: Cysts, Lymph nodes, fat necrosis, Fibroadenoma.
- The exceptions *(anytime I say the word "except" you need to think high yield!)*: **Colloid Cancer**, and Mucinous Cancer can be T2 bright.

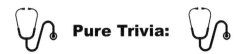 **Pure Trivia:**

- *If you have a patient with known breast CA, how often do you find a contralateral breast CA?* - Answer is 0.1-2% by mammogram, and 3-5% by MRI.

- *Never BR-0 an MRI case.* This is as much workup as you are going to get, so just call it benign or biopsy it. You can actually BR-0 something if you really want to prevent a biopsy – possible lymph node – US and mammo to confirm benign sorta situation. This is still kinda weak. For the purpose of multiple choice, think twice before you BR-0 a MRI case.

- *Spiculated margins* = 80% malignancy. This is the **single most predictive feature of malignancy.**

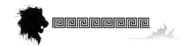 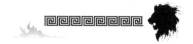
Estrogen: The more exposure to estrogen, the higher your risk of breast cancer. Anything that prolongs this exposure is said to increase risk. For example, an early age to begin menstruating or a late age to have menopause. Hormone replacement therapy with estrogen alone obviously increases exposure. Early maturation of lobules, which can be achieved by getting pregnant young, reduces your risk. Being fat increases estrogen exposure (more aromatase = more estrogen). Being a drunk increases estrogen exposure – via messing with its normal breakdown in the liver.

Estrogen Related Risks
Early Menstruation Late Menopause Late age of first pregnancy / or no kids. Being Fat Being a Drunk Hormone Replacement (with estrogen)

High Risk Lesions: Any of the high risk lesions (ADH, ALH, LCIS, Radial Scar, Papilloma) are associated with an increased risk. These are discussed more in detail later in the chapter.

Density: Density is considered a "medium risk," and is "dose dependent" with the denser you are the more risk you have.

Chest Wall Radiation: Chest wall radiation (usually seen in lymphoma patients) is a big risk factor, especially at a young age. The risk is supposed to peak around 15 years post treatment. **If the child had more than 20 Gy to the chest she is going to qualify for an annual screening MRI – at age 25 or 8 years post exposure** *(whichever is later).*

Relatives with Cancer: A first degree relative with breast cancer increases your lifetime risk from 8% to 13%. Two first degree relatives increases your risk to 21%.

Actual Mutations:

BRCA 1	Chromosome 17. More common than type 2. Increased risk for breast, ovary, and various GI cancers.
BRCA 2	Chromosome 13. Male carriers have a higher risk with 2. Increased risk for breast, ovary, and various GI cancers.
Li Fraumeni	Their p53 does NOT work, and they are high risk for all kinds of rare cancers.
Cowden Syndrome	Risk for breast cancer, follicular thyroid cancer, endometrial cancer, and **Lhermitte-Duclos** (a brain hamartoma).
Bannayan-Riley Ruvalcaba	Associated with developmental disorders at a young age.
NF-1	"Moderate Risk" of breast cancer

Female Cancer Risk Syndromes:

Hereditary Syndromes			
Hereditary Breast and Ovarian Cancer Syndrome -BRCA 1	Breast Cancer (risk 72%) Ovarian Cancer (risk 44%)	Triple Negative (estrogen, progesterone, HER2 negative) - IDC Medullary Subtype is the most common breast CA	Fallopian Tube, Pancreas, Colon Cancers Also at increased risk
Hereditary Breast and Ovarian Cancer Syndrome -BRCA 2	Breast Cancer (risk 69%) Ovarian Cancer (risk 17%)		
Cowden Syndrome	Hamartomas in multiple organs and gross facial and mouth bumps plague these unfortunate souls	Breast CA is the most common malignancy (risk 77%). Increased risk of other breast conditions (fibroadenomas, ADH, fibrocystic changes)	Thyroid Cancer (usually papillary). Also increased risk of various benign thyroid disease. Annual thyroid screening is typically advised. Lhermitte-Duclos (dysplastic gangliocytoma of the cerebellum)
Hereditary Diffuse Gastric Cancer Syndrome	Diffuse Gastric Cancer Risk ~ 70%	Lobular Breast Cancer Risk ~40%	Prophylactic Gastrectomy is recommended.
Li-Fraumeni Syndrome (bad p53)	Cancers literally everywhere.	Breast Cancers are usually seen in 30s-40s with high grade.	

Breast Cancer Risk Models:

There are several risk models, which have pros/cons and differences. I apologize in advance for even suggesting you learn about these…. but it just seems testable to me. I'm sorry…

Gail Model	Oldest and most validated breast cancer risk model	Focuses on personal risk factors, biopsy of ADH, and family history	Doesn't use genetics (it's too old school). Only validated in African Americans.
Claus, BODICEA, and BRCApro		Focus on genetics	Do NOT include personal risk or breast related risk factors.
Tyrer-Cuzick	*"Most Comprehensive"*	Focus on personal risk, biopsy with ADH or LCIS, family history	Does NOT include breast density.

High Yield Take Home Points Regarding Risk:

- Anything that gets you more estrogen increases your risk

- BRCA 1 is more common than BRCA 2 (in women).

- Men with BRCA 2 get more cancer than men with BRCA 1.

- Breast Density is an independent risk factor (denser the breast, the more the risk)

- 20 Gy of Radiation to your chest as a kid buys you a screening MRI – at 25 or 8 years after exposure *(*whichever is later)*

- Cowden Syndrome – Bowel Hamartoma, Follicular Thyroid Cancer, Lhermitte-Duclos, and Breast Cancer

- All current risk models underestimate life time risk.

- Tyrer Cuzick is the most comprehensive risk model, but does not include breast density.

- Exercise *(probably more like not being fat)* reduces the risk of breast cancer

- Tamoxifen and Raloxifene (SERMs) reduce incidence of ER/PR positive cancers. Mortality may not actual be reduced *(sound familiar?)*.

Screening Controversy

A red glow burst suddenly across the enchanted sky as the dark lord of statistics Gilbert Welch published his now infamous and devious work - *"Effect of three decades of screening mammography on breast-cancer incidence,"* in the unscrupulous New England Journal of Medicine.

"I can make things move without touching them. I can make animals do what I want without training them. I can make bad things happen to people who are mean to me. I can make them hurt, if I want..." - Gilbert Welch when asked about his thoughts on screening mammography.

This loathsome, maleficent, and repugnant study (along with several other large heavily powered studies) have brought into question the practice of screening mammograms. I highly recommend you read these *"despicable"* papers, but please wait till after the exam, because the people who write multiple choice questions about mammography are definitely not the same people who wrote these papers.

For the purpose of multiple choice tests, screening mammography saves lots of lives, you should buy pink ribbons, and low grade DCIS in a 95 year old needs a surgical consult.

Bleyer, Archie, and H. Gilbert Welch. "Effect of three decades of screening mammography on breast-cancer incidence." New England Journal of Medicine 367.21 (2012): 1998-2005.

Miller, Anthony B., et al. "Twenty five year follow-up for breast cancer incidence and mortality of the Canadian National Breast Screening Study: randomised screening trial." BMJ: British Medical Journal 348 (2014).

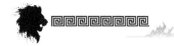 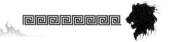

These all make great "next step questions."

Remember scoring is 1-9, with 9 being the most appropriate and 1 being the least.

Breast Cancer Screening:

Variant 1: **High Risk Women.** BRCA (plus untested first degree relatives), History of Chest Radiation, <u>Risk Model Showing 20% or greater lifetime risk</u>

- **Mammo (Highly Appropriate "9"):**

  - Beginning at age 25–30 or 10 years before age of first-degree relative with breast cancer

  - 8 years after radiation therapy, but not before age of 25.

  - Mammography + MRI ? They are complementary examinations, both should be performed.

- **Tomosynthesis (Highly Appropriate "9"):**

  - Beginning at age 25–30 or 10 years before age of first-degree relative with breast cancer

  - 8 years after radiation therapy, but not before age of 25.

  - Mammography + MRI ? They are complementary examinations, both should be performed.

- **MRI (Highly Appropriate "9"):**

  - Mammography + MRI ? They are complementary examinations, both should be performed.

Variant 2: **Medium Risk Women.** Women with person history of Breast CA, lobular hyperplasia, Atypical Ductal Hyperplasia, or <u>Risk Model Showing 15-20% life time risk</u>

- Mammo and Tomo are "9s"

- <u>MRI is a 7</u>. Mammography + MRI ? They are complementary examinations, MRI should NOT replace mammography.

Variant 3: **Average Risk Women.** Women with < 15 % Lifetime Risk

- Mammo and Tomo are "9s"

- MRI is a "3" which means it is NOT appropriate.

Screening for Transgender Women

Screening Annual Mammogram IF:
• Past or Current Hormones (Estrogen & Progestin for > 5 years)
• > 50 years old

Trivia: BMI > 35 = increases Risk

Screening for Transgender Men

Screening Annual Mammogram IF:
• They still have breast tissue (even if they had a reduction mammoplasty)

Breast Pain:

Variant 1: Cyclical, Unilateral or Bilateral. Age < 40.

• No imaging is appropriate.

• Ultrasound is the least inappropriate and it's rated at a "2"

Variant 2: Cyclical, Unilateral or Bilateral. Age > 40.

• No imaging is appropriate.

• Ultrasound, Mammo, and Tomo are the least inappropriate and all rated at a "2"

Variant 3: NON-Cyclical, Unilateral or Bilateral. Age < 40.

• Ultrasound Might Be Appropriate and is rated as a "5."

———-

Stage 1 Breast CA - Initial Workup and Surveillance (No Symptoms)

Newly Diagnosed - rule out mets to the bones, chest, liver, and/or brain

• No imaging is appropriate. (CT, MRI, PET etc… not indicated with initial stage 1)

Surveillance / Rule Out Local Recurrence

• Diagnostic Mammo or Tomo is Appropriate and is rated as a "9."

• Ultrasound might be appropriate and is rated as a "5."

• MRI might be appropriate and is rated as a "5."

Symptomatic Male Breast:

Variant 1: **Any Age with Physical Exam and History Consistent with Gynecomastia or Pseudogynecomastia (bitch tits).**

- No imaging is appropriate.

Variant 2: **Younger than 25 years old with indeterminate palpable.**

- Ultrasound is Appropriate and is rated as an "8."

- Mammo is in the "May Be Appropriate" category as a "5." I would only do this if the ultrasound doesn't answer your question. ** *Page 441, Scenario 4A - has suggested multiple choice strategy.*

Variant 3: **Older than 25 years old with indeterminate palpable.**

- Mammo is Appropriate and is rated as an "8"

- Ultrasound is in the "May Be Appropriate" category as a "5."

Variant 4: **Older than 25 years old with indeterminate palpable. The mammogram was indeterminate or suspicious.**

- Ultrasound is Appropriate and is rated as a "9."

Variant 5: **Physical exam is highly concerning for cancer. Dude has an ulcerative mass, axillary nodes, nipple retraction, etc...**

- Mammo is Appropriate and is rated as an "9"

- Ultrasound is Appropriate and is rated as an "8" - to stage the breast and axilla just like a female breast CA workup.

Random Situations - First/Next Step:

Women > 40 with Palpable

- <u>Mammo is Appropriate</u> and is rated as a "9."

Women > 40 with Mammo Suspicious for CA

- <u>Ultrasound is Appropriate</u> and is rated as a "9."

Women > 40 with Mammo findings of a Lipoma at the Site of a Palpable.

- <u>No additional imaging is appropriate.</u>

Women > 40 with Palpable Findings and a Negative Mammo

- <u>Ultrasound is Appropriate</u> and is rated as a "9."

Women < 30 Initial Evaluation

- <u>Ultrasound is Appropriate</u> and is rated as a "9."

Women 30-39 Initial Evaluation

- <u>Ultrasound is Appropriate</u> and is rated as a "8."
- <u>Mammo is Appropriate</u> and is rated as a "8."

Women < 30 Ultrasound is Suspicious for CA

- Core Biopsy <u>is Appropriate</u> and is rated as a "9."
- <u>Mammo is Appropriate</u> and is rated as a "8."

Women < 30 Ultrasound is Negative

- <u>No imaging is appropriate.</u>

Women < 30 Ultrasound has a B9 finding (like a cyst)

- <u>No imaging is appropriate.</u>

Women < 30 Ultrasound is BR3 able - example fibroadenoma

- <u>Short interval followup</u> - usually Q6 months x 2 years.

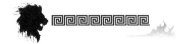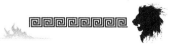
The most common procedures are going to be ultrasound guided and stereotactic biopsy of masses and calcification. I'll try and touch on the testable points.

Ultrasound:

- Overall ultrasound is faster and easier than stereo. If you can see the mass under US - you should do the biopsy under US.

- Usually a 14 gauge automatic spring loaded device is used for masses

- You should put the mass on the far side of the US screen - lets you see the length of the needle better

- Ideally 4 things should line up during the biopsy: the lesion, the transducer, the skin nick, and the biopsy needle

- The needle angle should be parallel to the chest wall (pneumothorax is an embarrassing complication of a breast biopsy)

- Anesthetic should be placed right up to but not into the lesion (especially when the lesions is small).

- You should try and biopsy the deeper part of a lesion first. If you obscure it from bleeding at least you can still get the superficial part.

- If you have two lesions to biopsy, try and hit the smaller one first. If the bigger one bleeds it may obscure the smaller one — it's less likely the other way around.

- If you have a solid and cystic lesion - you should biopsy the solid part.

- About 90% of the time you can make a diagnosis off 1 or 2 passes (though most texts still recommend doing 5).

Next Step Scenario - Like an idiot you injected a bunch of air around the mass, while you were trying to give lidocaine. Now you can't see the mass. What do you do? You have to reschedule. Don't try to biopsy it blind.

Axilla:

- When you biopsy an axillary lymph node you should target the node's cortex.

- Core biopsy is preferred over FNA if you have no clue what it is. If you have known breast cancer and you are nearly certain you are dealing with a met - FNA works fine.

Special Scenario - The Cyst Aspiration

- Indications - Anxiety, pain, uncertain diagnosis.

- Size is NOT an indication for aspiration

- Cysts recur about 70% of the time (this drops to around 15% if you inject air after you aspirate).

The Hypoechoic Mass vs Dirty Cyst Scenario
-Classic "Next Steps" -

Next Step Scenario #1 - You suspect a hypoechoic mass is a debris filled cyst rather than a solid mass... but you aren't totally sure. *What should you do first ?* Aspirate it.

Next Step Scenario #2 - Same hypoechoic mass vs cyst - you aspirate it and you get non-bloody fluid. You also notice the lesion disappeared. *What do you do ?* You should pitch it, no need for cytology. You are done.

Next Step Scenario #3 - Same hypoechoic mass vs cyst - you aspirate it and you get bloody fluid. You also notice the lesion disappeared. *What do you do ?* Send it to cytology and then place a clip.

Next Step Scenario #4 - Same hypoechoic mass vs cyst - you aspirate it and you get purulent "poop like" fluid. The fluid smells like a zombie farted. You also notice the lesion disappeared. *What do you do ?* Send it to the microbiology lab for culture and sensitivity.

Next Step Scenario #5 - Same hypoechoic mass vs cyst - you aspirate it and you get fluid. You also notice the lesion does NOT disappear. *What do you do ?* Proceed to core biopsy of the residual solid mass.

Stereotactic Biopsy *(using a mammogram to localize and target the lesion).*

- This is the preferred move for calcifications. Typically the specimen is x-rayed after the sample to confirm there are calcifications within the biopsied tissue.

- Vacuum assisted devices are typically used for calcifications.

- The biopsy is performed in compression - with slightly less pressure than a normal mammogram. Compressibility of the breast tissue can NOT be less than 2-3cm (some texts say 28 mm). Otherwise you risk throwing the needle through the other side of the breast into the digital receptor. This is called a "negative stroke margin."

> **Gauge Size vs Samples:**
>
> - 10-11 Gauge Needle = 12 Samples
>
> - 7-9 Gauge Needle = 4 Samples

- *Next Step Scenario: What if the breast compresses too small (< 20 mm) ?* You should do a wire localization for excisional biopsy.

- A marker (tiny piece of metal) should be placed after each biopsy. Clip migration can occur (accordion effect). You will need a mammogram in the orthogonal view to evaluate for this post placement.

- QC "Localization and Accuracy Test" to verify system alignment and performance is *performed Daily before patient exams.*

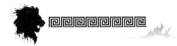 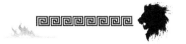

SECTION 18:
MQSA

The U.S. Food and Drug Administration Mammography Quality Standards Act (MQSA) – yes that is a real thing – demands a medical audit and outcome analysis be performed once a year. You are forced to follow up patients with positive mammos, and correlate with biopsy pathology results (so you can see how much benign disease you biopsy and how much fear / anxiety you generate). You have to grade the biopsy with the risk category (you can't accept benign results with a BR-5).

MQSA and Other Crap they could ask:

- 3 months of mammography is required during residency training
- The recall rate should be less than 10%
- Mammography facilities are required to provide patients with written results of their mammograms in language that is easy to understand. Also known as a "lay report," and must be given within 30 days of the study.
- A consumer complaint mechanism is required to be established in mammography facilities to provide patients with a process for addressing their concerns.
- Patients can obtain their original mammograms, not copies, when they are needed.
- For cases in which a facility's mammograms are determined to be substandard and a risk to public health, facilities will notify the patients and their doctors and suggest an appropriate plan of action.
- The "Interpreting Physician" is ultimately responsible for the Quality Control program.
- The required resolution of line pairs is 13 lp/mm in the anode to cathode direction and 11 line pair / mm in the left right direction
- To make it pass image quality; must show 4 fibers, 3 microcalcification clusters, and 3 masses, plus "acceptable artifacts".
- The dose phantom is 50% glandularity, 4.2 cm thick, and is supposed to have a dose less than 3 mGy per image (+ grid).
- Don't get it twisted; there are no patient dose limits in mammography, only a phantom dose. A dense breast can result in a higher patient dose, which could easily exceed 3 mGy/view.
- Typical patient and phantom doses are about 2 mGy per view, or 8 mGy for a bilateral two view (Left CC + MLO, Right CC + MLO) screening examination.
- The typical (average) compressed breast is 6 cm, glandularity of 15 to 20%.
- Digital systems generally uses higher beam qualities which results in lower doses;
- Digital mammography does not use fixed dose (screen-film); can use as much (or little) radiation as deemed appropriate.
- Male Residents must urinate in the sitting position while on the mammography service (standing urination is not allowed per MQSA).

Specific QA Tasks

Processor QC	Daily
Darkroom Cleanliness	Daily
Viewbox Conditions	Weekly
Phantom Evaluation	Weekly
Repeat Analysis	Quarterly
Compression Test	Semi-Annually
Darkroom Fog	Semi-Annually
Screen-Film Contrast	Semi-Annually
Evil Overlord behind MQSA ?	FDA

Appropriate Target Range for Medical Audit

Recall Rate	5-7%
Cancers/ 1000 Screened	3-8

The Privilege to Read a Mammogram

During the last two years of training you have to read	240
Formal Training Requirement	3 months
Documented Hours of Education	60

Male Resident Mammography Specific Trivia
*enforcement may vary per institution

Male residents may urinate in the following position(s) while on the mammo service ?	Seated only. Standing urination is prohibited.
The penis of the male resident should be in what orientation while on the mammo service ?	Tucked posterior and secured with tape* *(Glue - if performing a 3 month focus time)*

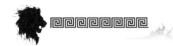 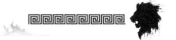
As I promised in the first pages of the chapter, I want to finish by rolling through some scenarios. This is mainly to demonstrate the work flow process and how you handle "next step" type questions.

—

Scenario 1: A 40 year old woman presents for her baseline screening mammogram. You have the great pleasure of reading it. While conducting your normal reading pattern you notice the posterior nipple line is 9cm on the MLO, but only 6 cm on the CC.

What do you do ? - The would be a technical call back

What BR ? - This is a BR-0

—

Scenario 2a: A 50 year old woman presents for her annual screening mammogram. You have the great pleasure of reading it. You notice a mass on two views in the lateral left breast.

What BR ? - This is also BR-0.

Next Step ? Return for diagnostic mammogram, including spot compression views and likely an ultrasound.

Scenario 2b: Same patient returns for the diagnostic mammogram. You can clearly see the mass in two views.

Next Step ? Ultrasound to further characterize

Scenario 2c: You put her in ultrasound and see an obvious shadowing angry, pissed off, mass that is ulcerating through the skin etc…. It 100% for sure cancer.

Next Step? You need to stage. Scan the rest of the breast for multi-focal masses, AND scan the axilla for pathologic nodes.

—

Scenario 3a: A 50 year old woman presents for her annual screening mammogram. You have the great pleasure of reading it. You notice what looks like a mass in the CC view only (can't find it in the MLO). You call it an "asymmetry" because you can only see it in one view.

Next Step ? BR-0, and bring it back with spot compression views

Scenario 3b: Same patient returns for the diagnostic mammogram. After the paddle is applied there does not appear to be any mass. It just looks like normal breast tissue. You look at prior imaging and it looks pretty similar to the priors now.

Next Step? BR-1, and return to screening. This is the classic scenario of a "does not persist" callback.

But Prometheus!? ACR Criteria says....

A common source of confusion is the distinction is between variant 1 and variant 2 ACR criteria for male breasts. The overwhelming majority of male breast path is gynecomastia which will look like a BR-5 mass on ultrasound. The ACR actually says you need no imaging to work it up.

This is how I would handle multiple choice on this:

(Scenario A) If the question specifically says "ACR criteria" and describes a palpable lesion in a male, less than 25, with no other information in the question header to make you believe its gyno:

You need to pick Ultrasound.

(Scenario B) if the question does NOT say "ACR criteria" and describes a palpable lesion in someone with risk factors for gyno (anabolic steroid use, pot smoking, etc....)

Then you should either do no imaging, (if physical exam is a choice pick that), or start with a plain film (mammogram).

(Scenario C) The third possible scenario, which would be the sneakiest way to do this, would be to show you a study obtained at another hospital of a breast ultrasound showing a suspicious lesion in a male around this age and ask you what to do next.

The answer here is always going to be x-ray (mammogram). A work up for cancer on a male breast is NEVER EVER EVER complete without a mammogram ("man" o gram) – with the teaching point being that gynecomastia looks like cancer on ultrasound, but is easily identified as benign on a mammogram

---

Scenario 4a: A 24 year old MALE presents as with a palpable mass in his left breast.

Next Step ? Mammogram (never ultrasound a male breast before you get a mammogram).

Scenario 4b: A mammogram is obtained, and shows a flame shaped density under the nipple, correlating with the palpable marker.

Next Step ? Interview the patient to see if you can come up for a reason for his gynecomastia (psych meds, marijuana use, etc...). You don't want to miss a pituitary tumor. He tells you he smokes pot every day. You tell him that he is a very bad boy - even though there is no evidence that marijuana causes real harm and it's criminalization was based on false propaganda from the hemp industry.

Scenario 4c: After you tell him he is a bad boy for smoking the sticky icky, he still seems worried. He tells you that he got an ultrasound at the outside hospital and they told him he had breast cancer. He pulls a CD out of his pocket and asks you to look at it. You look at the outside images and sure enough there is a shadowing mass in the area of the palpable finding.

Next Step ? BR-2 Gynecomastia. This is the oldest trick in the book - gynecomastia looks like a scary mass on US - that's why you always start with the mammogram.

——

Scenario 5a: Screening mammogram is performed on a 70 year old woman, who has a history of prior lumpectomy 4 years ago. You read in her chart that she refused radiation therapy. She heard on the news that radiation was bad, so she decided on a more holistic approach (bananas) — she also gets yearly thermograms. The area of scarring in the resection bed looks more dense.

Next Step ? BR-0, and recall for spot compressions.

Scenario 5b: The spot compressions show small calcifications in the area of the lumpectomy bed, and the scar is definitely more dense.

Next Step ? Mag views to further characterize the calcifications. You decide they look pointy so you call them fine pleomorphic.

Scenario 5c: You stick her in ultrasound to be complete - it looks like a small mass. You stage the remainder of the breast and axilla - and it looks pretty clean.

Diagnosis ? BR-5 - local recurrence.

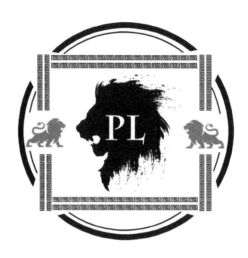

15

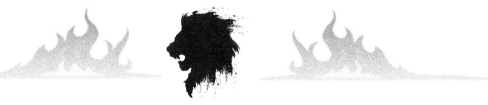

STRATEGY

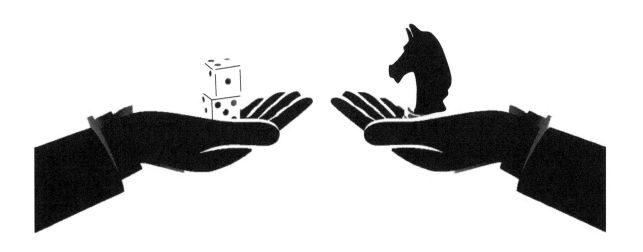

PROMETHEUS LIONHART, M.D.

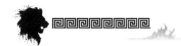 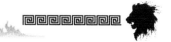
The 3 Kinds of Questions

1. **The ones you know** – you want to get 100% of these right
2. **The ones you don't know** – you want to get 25% of these right (same as a monkey guessing)
3. **The ones you can figure out with some deep thought** – you want to get 60-70% of these right.

If you can do that you will pass the test, especially if you've read my books.

My recommendations:
- For the ones you know, just get them right.
- For the ones you don't know – just say to yourself *"this is one I don't know, Prometheus says just try and narrow it down and guess."*
- For the ones you think you can figure out, mark them, and go through the entire exam. If you follow my suggestion on the first two types of questions you will have ample time left over for head scratching. Other reasons to go ahead and do the whole exam before trying to figure them out is (a) you don't want to rush on the questions you can get right, and (b) sometimes you will see a case that reminds you of what the answer is. In fact it's not impossible that the stem of another question flat out tells you the answer to a previous question.

Let your plans be dark, and impenetrable as night, and when you move, fall like a thunderbolt.
-Sun Tzu

Studying for a C-

For many of you this is the first time you truly do not need an A on the exam. I can remember in undergrad and medical school feeling like I needed to get every question right on the exam to maintain my total and complete dominance.

I felt like if I missed a single question that I wouldn't honor the class, I wouldn't match radiology, and I'd end up in rural West Virginia checking diabetic feet for ulcers in my family medicine clinic. The very thought of a career in family medicine was so horrible that I'd begin to panic.

Panic doesn't help!

Truly this exam is not like that. You can miss questions. You will miss questions. You can miss a lot of questions. You just need to miss less than about 10% of the room. No matter what they tell you, no matter what you read <u>all standardized exams are curved</u>. If they passed 100% - the exam would be called a joke. If they failed 50% the program directors would riot (after first punishing the residents with extra call). The exam will maintain a failure rate around 10-15%. What that means is that you only need to beat 10-15% of the room. You don't need 99th percentile. There is no reward for that. You need 16th percentile. 16th percentile is a C-, that is the goal.

The reason I'm perseverating on this is that you need to avoid panic. If you mark 20-30% of the questions as "not sure" - or Promethean category 2 or 3 - you might begin to freak out. Especially if the inner gunner medical student in you thinks you won't get honors. Chill Out! It's ok to miss questions. Look around the room and know that you studied harder and are smarter than 15% of the room.

Do not flee the exam in tears !

Fate rarely calls upon us at a moment of our choosing.

-Optimus Prime

Exploiting the "Genius Neuron"

Have you ever heard someone in case conference take a case and lead with "It's NOT this," when clearly "this" is what the case was? It happens all the time. Often the first thing out of people's mouths is actually the right answer, but many times you hear people say "it's not" first. Ever wondered why?

I have this idea of a "Genius Neuron." You have one neuron that is superior to the rest. This guy fires faster and is more reliable than his peers and because of this he is hated by them. He is the guy in the front row waving his hand shouting "I know the answer!" You know that guy, that guy is a notorious asshole. So, in your mind he shouts out the answer first, and then the rest of the neurons gang up on him and try and talk him out of it. So the end product is "It's NOT this."

For the purpose of taking cases in conference, this is why you should always lead with "this comes to mind," instead of "it's not." Now, the practical piece of advice I want to give you is to **trust your genius neuron**. Seriously, there is a lot of material on this test. But if you read this book, there will be enough knowledge to pass the test existing somewhere between your ears. You just have to trust that genius neuron.

How?? - Do it like this:

(1) Read the entire question. Look at all the pictures.

(2) Read ALL the answer choices. Never stop at A thinking that is the answer.

(3) Look again at ALL the pictures – now that you see the choices.

(4) Choose the first answer your mind tells you is correct – the one your genius neuron thinks it correct.

(5) After you have finished the test, and you are re-reviewing your answers, NEVER change the genius neuron's answer except for two criteria. (A) You read the question wrong. (B) You are 100% sure that it is another choice, and you can give a reason why. Never change based on your gut feelings. Those secondary gut feelings are the stupid neurons trying to gang up on the smart one. Just like in the real world, the stupid people significantly outnumber the smart ones.

I know this sounds silly, but I really believe in this. This is a real thing. I encourage you to try it with some practice questions.

You either believe in yourself or you don't

       -Captain James T. Kirk.

Dealing with the Linked Question

It is a modern trend for multiple choice tests to have "linked" questions. You may remember that USMLE Step 3 had them, and it is rumored that the CORE Exam has them as well.

These are the questions that prompt you with "this is your final answer, you can't change your answer." When you see this STOP!

If you are 100% sure you are right, then go on. If you had it narrowed down to two choices, think about which one would be easier to write a follow up question about. This might seem obvious, but in the heat of the battle you might get too aggressive. Slow down and think twice on these.

The second point I want to make about these questions is finding some Zen if you miss it. There are a lot of questions on this test, it's ok to miss some. You will still pass (probably). People like you have always studied for the A+, not the C-. So when you miss a question it makes you freak out because you think you blew it. Calm the fuck down. You don't need an A+ this time. You don't need a B. You just need to pass so they don't get any more money from you. Believe me they have taken enough from you already. I just want you to understand that you will miss questions and it's ok. If the second part reveals that you dropped one, don't let it phase you. Just do your best. The most important fight is always your next one.

It isn't the mountains ahead to climb that wears you out; it's the pebble in your shoe

-Muhammad Ali

It's Possible to Know Too Much

If you were to begin studying and begin taking multiple choice practice questions and you plotted your progress as you gained more knowledge you would notice something funny. At first you would begin to get more and more questions right… and then you would start to miss them.

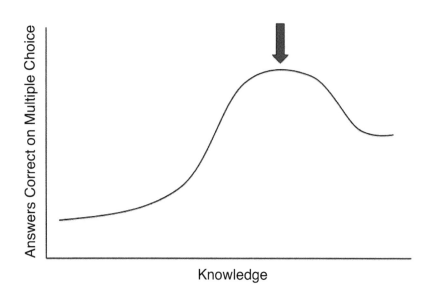

Well how can that be? I will tell you that once you know enough all choices on the exam become correct. Which of the following can occur?… well actually they can all occur - I've read case reports of blah blah blah. That is what happens.

The trick is to not over think things. Once you've achieved a certain level of knowledge, if they give you a gift — take it. It's usually not a trick (usually). Don't look for obscure situations when things are true. Yes… it's possible for you to know more than the person writing the questions. Yes… I said it and it's fucking true. These people don't know everything. You can out knowledge them if you study enough - and that is when you get yourself into trouble.

Take home point - once you've reached the peak (arrow on chart) - be careful over thinking questions past that point.

"Always remember: Your focus determines your reality"

-Jedi Master Qui-Gon Jinn

🏛 8 Promethean Laws For Multiple Choice 🏛

#1 - If you have a gut feeling - go for it ! (trust the genius neuron)

#2 - Don't over think to the extent that you veer from a reflexive answer - especially if choices seem equally plausible (you can know too much).

#3 - Read ALL the choices carefully

#4 - If it seems too obvious to be true (trickery), re-read it and then go with it (even if it seems too easy). Let it happen - it's usually not a trick... usually.

#5 - Add up what you know you know, and compare with what you think you know. Weight your answers by what you KNOW you KNOW.

#6 - If you are torn between two choices, ask yourself "which of these is NOT correct ?" - Sometimes making your brain work backwards will elucidate the solution.

#7 - Do NOT change your answers ! (trust the genius neuron)

#8 - Most Importantly - <u>Don't Panic</u>

Maybe I can't win, maybe the only thing I can do is just take everything he's got. But to beat me, he's gonna have to kill me, and to kill me, he's gonna have to have the heart to stand in front of me, and to do that, he has to be willing to die himself

- Rocky Balboa

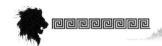 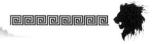
Problem Solving Through MRI

Different programs have variable volume with MRI. Some of you will be excellent at it. Some of you will suck at it. An important skill to have is to understand how to problem solve with different sequences. The best way to do this is to have a list of T1 bright things, T2 bright things, dark things, and things that restrict diffusion.

T1 Bright	T2 Bright	T1 and T2 DARK	Restricts Diffusion
Fat	Fat	Flow Void	Stroke
Melanin (Melanoma)	Water	Fibrosis / Scar	Hypercellular Tumor
Blood (Subacute)	Blood (Extracellular Methemoglobin)	Metal	Epidermoid
Protein Rich Fluid	Most Tumors	Air	Abscess (Bacterial)
Calcification (Hyalinized)			Acute Demyelination
Slow Moving Blood			CJD
Laminar Necrosis			T2 Shine Through

Be able to move through sequences and problem solve.

Think about a Lipoma for example. This will be T1 bright, T2 bright, and fat sat out. Another example might be something with layers in it. What can layer? Fat could layer, water could layer, blood could layer, pus could layer. Fat would be bright/ bright. Water would be dark on T1. Pus would be dark on T2. Blood could do different things depending on it's age. Fat would sat out. Pus may restrict diffusion (like a subdural empyema). You get the idea. Run through some scenarios in your mind. The key point is to know your differentials for this.

Battle Tactics: Peds Neck

This is my suggested strategy. I typically start with cyst vs solid. Then I consider location, morphology, and choice of modality (attempted mind reading of the question writer).

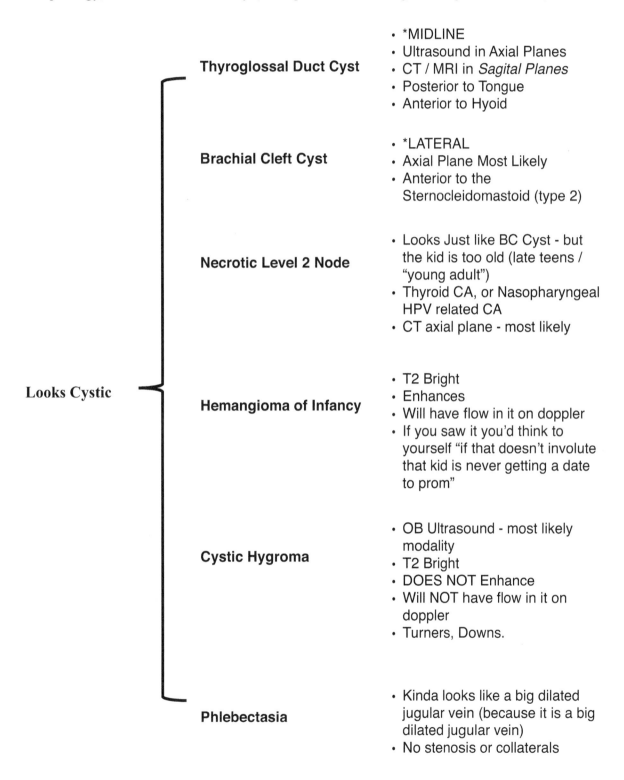

Looks Cystic

Thyroglossal Duct Cyst
- *MIDLINE
- Ultrasound in Axial Planes
- CT / MRI in *Sagital Planes*
- Posterior to Tongue
- Anterior to Hyoid

Brachial Cleft Cyst
- *LATERAL
- Axial Plane Most Likely
- Anterior to the Sternocleidomastoid (type 2)

Necrotic Level 2 Node
- Looks Just like BC Cyst - but the kid is too old (late teens / "young adult")
- Thyroid CA, or Nasopharyngeal HPV related CA
- CT axial plane - most likely

Hemangioma of Infancy
- T2 Bright
- Enhances
- Will have flow in it on doppler
- If you saw it you'd think to yourself "if that doesn't involute that kid is never getting a date to prom"

Cystic Hygroma
- OB Ultrasound - most likely modality
- T2 Bright
- DOES NOT Enhance
- Will NOT have flow in it on doppler
- Turners, Downs.

Phlebectasia
- Kinda looks like a big dilated jugular vein (because it is a big dilated jugular vein)
- No stenosis or collaterals

Looks Solid

Septic Thrombophlebitis

- Jugular Vein with a clot - they will have to prove that has a clot in it - probably with Doppler US
- Lemierre's Syndrome
- Septic Emboli to the lungs
- Recent ENT procedure, or Infection
- Fusobacterium Necrophorum

Ectopic Thyroid

- Back of the tongue or in front of the hyoid
- Tc-MIBI, or I-123

Fibromatosis Coli

- Ultrasound
- "Two Heads" of the Sternocleidomastoid

Rhabdomyosarcoma

- MRI or CT
- Seriously pissed off looking mass (probably in the orbit - maybe in the masticator mass)
- Enhances heterogenous,

Metastatic Neuroblastoma

- MRI or CT
- Soft Tissue Mass,
- Calcifications,
- Restricted Diffusion
- Classic is the orbit

Battle Tactics: Congenital Heart on CXR

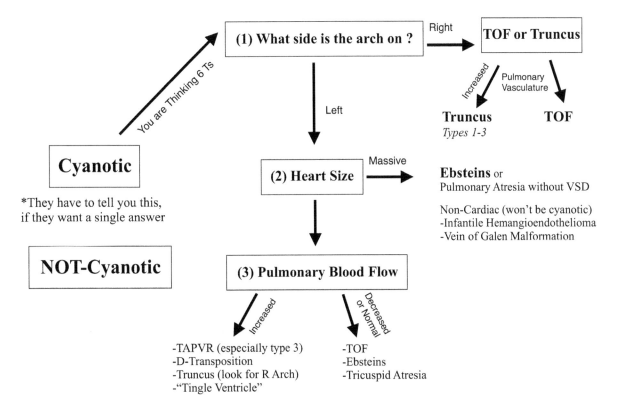

Walking through this outline. First ask yourself is it cyanotic or not? **They will have to tell you this in the stem.** Look for this in the stem every time, then cross out answers that are not cyanotic.

Cyanotic	Not Cyanotic
TOF	ASD
TAPVR	VSD
Transposition	PDA
Truncus	PAPVR
Tricuspid Atresia	Aortic Coarctation (adult type – post ductal)

Example: *Patient "X" is a newborn cyanotic, what is the most likely Dx?*

A - VSD

B- ASD

C- Demonic Possession

D - TOF

Without even looking at a picture (which they will probably show), you know the answer is D, because that is the only cyanotic one listed. If you were wondering about C - I did a google scholar search for *"Demonic Possession causing cyanosis"*, and although there were a few case reports none come down hard on cyanosis.

Battle Tactics: Neonatal Chest

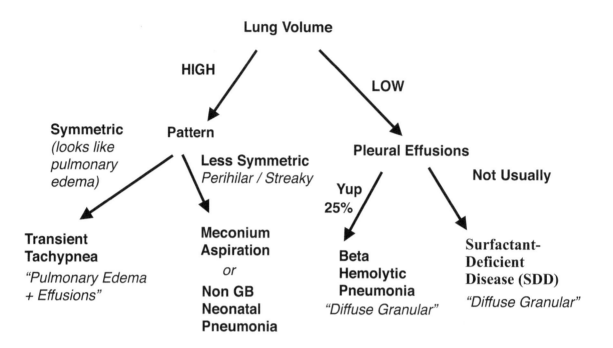

THIS vs **THAT:** *Meconium Aspiration or Non Group B Strep Pneumonia*

This is super tough without any history, and because of that I feel like the test writer has two options: (1) Stop being an asshole and give you some history, (2) not include both as answer choices - assuming only one is correct. Now, along those lines if you saw both as choices and the question header gives you no history you could eliminate them both as distractors - because they both can't be correct.

Example: What color is this box

A - Blue ✔

B - Looks Red

C - It has a Red Appearance

BUT
Prometheus !?

I Don't See a BOX!
How can I answer the question?!?

There can be situations where the picture is not necessary to get the question right. They could show you a picture of a grilled cheese sandwich and call it a chest x-ray. It could still be possible to get the question right by eliminating all but one possible choice. The question header can help you disqualify (as we discussed with cyanotic heart disease) or you can try and find choices that cannot be distinguished from each other. Both answers can't be right - so they must both be wrong.

Battle Tactics: Peds Chest & Misc

Prematurity — Guessing that the kid is premature can be helpful for eliminating choices (Meconium Aspiration is more of a post term thing), and raising your pretest probability (SDD, or NEC in a belly film). There are two main clues:

(1) *Humeral Head Ossification* - This tends to occur closer to term. If the humeral head is NOT ossified you can assume (in the world of multiple choice) that the kid is likely premature.

(2) *Lack of Subcutaneous Fat* - Premature kids tend to be very skinny, although I think of this more of a soft sign that is useful when absent more than present. I'll just say that if the kid appears chubby he is probably NOT premature.

The Thing in the Lung:

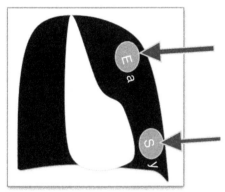

Left Upper Lobe:

Think **Congenital Lobar Emphysema (CLE)** first. But, remember CCAM has no lobar prevalence, so it can be anywhere

Left Lower Lobe:

Think **Sequestration** First. Congenital Diaphragmatic Hernia (CDHs) favors this side too

Case 1. Newborn with congenital heart disease

A. Intralobar Sequestration
B. Extralobar Sequestration
C. Congenital Lobar Emphysema

Case 2. 10 year old with recurrent pneumonia

A. Intralobar Sequestration
B. Extralobar Sequestration
C. Congenital Lobar Emphysema

*Intralobar is seen older kids,
**Extralobar is seen in infants with co-morbids
** CLE is in the upper lobe

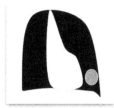

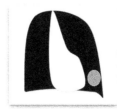

541

NG Tube Tricks: The presence of an NG tube (especially if not placed correctly) should alert you to some form of trickery.

The NG tube stops in the upper thoracic esophagus: Think esophageal atresia (probably in the setting of VACTERL).

The NG tube curling into the chest – it's either (1) in the lung, or (2) it's in a congenital diaphragmatic hernia. If I had to pick between the two (and it wasn't obvious), I'd say left side hernia, right side lung – just because those are the more common sides.

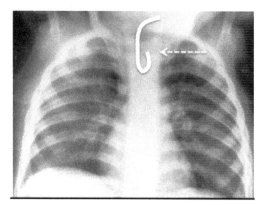

NG Tube Curls in the upper thoracic esophagus. First think Esophageal Atresia. Then think VACTERL

The Classic Congenital Lobar Emphysema Trick: They can show you a series of CXRs. The first one has an opacity in the lung (the affected lung is fluid filled). The next x-ray will show the opacity resolved. The following x-ray will show it getting more lucent, and more lucent. Until it's actually pushing the heart over. This is the classic way to show it in case conference, or case books

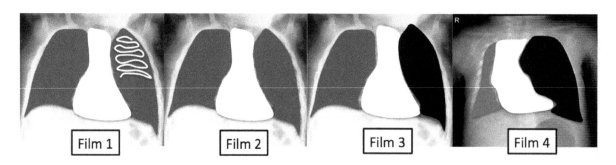

The School Aged CXR: *Things to look for:*

- **Big Heart** - Probably showing you a sickle cell case. Look for bone infarcts in shoulders.
- **Lucent Lung** - Think foreign Body (air trapping). Remember you put the affected side down (if it remains lucent- that confirms it).

THIS vs **THAT:** Cystic Fibrosis vs Primary Ciliary Dyskinesia

CF	PCD
Abnormal Mucus – Cilia can't clear it	Normal Mucus – Cilia don't work
Bronchiectasis (upper lobes)	Bronchiectasis (lower lobes)
Normal sperm, obliterated vas deferens	Normal vas deferens, sperm cannot swim normally

Battle Tactics: Peds Misc

The Mandible: There are only a few things that a mandible will be shown for with regards to Peds. Think Caffeys first - especially if the picture looks blurry and old (there hasn't been a case of this in 50 years). If it's osteonecrosis think about O.I. on bisphosphonates. If it's a dwarf case, think wide angled mandible with Pycnodysostosis. A "floating tooth" could be EG.

The Abdominal Plain Film - on a newborn - *Problem Solving Bubbles:*

Pattern	Path	Next Step
Single Bubble:	In a newborn this is Gastric (antral or pyloric atresia). In an older child think gastric volvulus	
Double Bubble	Duodenal Atresia	
Triple Bubble	Jejunal Atresia	
Single Bubble + Distal Gas + "Bilious Vomiting	Concern for Mid Gut Volvulus	Next Step = Upper GI
Multiple Dilated Loops	Concern for lower obstruction	Next Step = Contrast Enema

THIS vs THAT: Duodenal Atresia vs Jejunal Atresia:

Duodenal Atresia	Jejunal Atresia
Double Bubble	Triple Bubble
Failure to Canalize (often isolated atresia)	Vascular Insult * More likely associated with other atresias
Associated with Downs	

THIS vs **THAT**: Intralobar vs Extralobar Sequestration

Intralobar	Extralobar
No pleural covering	Has its own pleural covering
More Common	Less Common
Presents later with recurrent infection	Presents early with other bad congenital things (heart, etc...)

Heterotaxia: This can be inferred or asked several ways.

Heterotaxia Syndromes	
Right Sided	**Left Sided**
Two Fissures in Left Lung	One Fissure in Right Lung
Asplenia	Polysplenia
Increased Cardiac Malformations	Less Cardiac Malformations
Reversed Aorta/IVC	Azygous Continuation of the IVC

Orbital Calcifications:

Less than 3	Older than 3
Retinoblastoma	Toxo
CMV	Retinal Astrocytoma
Colobomatous Cyst	

Battle Tactics: Abdominal Masses / Diffuse Pathology

Peds Liver Masses				
Infantile Hepatic Hemangioma	Age 0-3	Endothelial growth factor is elevated	Progressively Calcify - as they involute	Associated: High Output CHF Skin Hemangiomas
Hepatoblastoma	Age 0-3	AFP is elevated	Calcifications are Common	Risk Factor = Prematurity Many Association: Wilms, Beckwith-Weidemann	may cause precocious puberty
Mesenchymal Hamartoma	Age 0-3	AFP is <u>negative</u>	Calcification are RARE CYSTIC MASS Favors Right Lobe	"Developmental anomaly"
HCC	Age > 5	AFP is elevated		Kids with cirrhosis (biliary atresia, Fanconi syndrome, glycogen storage disease)
Fibrolamellar Subtype HCC	Age > 5	AFP is <u>negative</u>	Calcifies more often than conventional HCC	No Cirrhosis Central Scar (scar does NOT enhance, and is T2 dark)
Undifferentiated Embryonal Sarcoma	Age > 5	AFP is <u>negative</u>	Cystic / Heterogeneously Solid Mass	Known to rupture
Mets (Neuroblastoma, Wilms)	Fetus - 4 6 - Early Teens	Multiple Masses in the Setting of Known Primary		

Adult Benign Liver Masses					
	Ultrasound	CT	MR	Trivia	
Hemangioma	Hyperechoic	Peripheral Nodular Discontinuous Enhancement	T2 Bright	Rare in Cirrhotics	
FNH	Spoke Wheel	Homogenous Arterial Enhancement	"Stealth Lesion - Iso on T1 and T2"	Central Scar	Bright on Delayed Eovist (Gd-EOB-DTPA)
Hepatic Adenoma	Variable	Variable	Fat Containing on In/Out Phase	OCP use, Glycogen Storage Disease	Can explode and bleed
Hepatic Angiomyolipoma	Hyperechoic	Gross Fat	T1/T2 Bright	Unlike renal AML, 50% don't have fat	Tuberous Sclerosis

Sulfur Colloid HOT or COLD		
Hepatic Adenoma	COLD	
FNH	40% HOT, 30% COLD, 30% Warm	
Cavernous Hemangioma	COLD	RBC Scan HOT
HCC	COLD	Gallium HOT
Cholangiocarcinoma	COLD	
Mets	COLD	
Abscess	COLD	Gallium HOT
Focal Fat	COLD	Xenon HOT

Regenerative Nodules	Dysplastic Nodules	HCC
Contains Iron	Contains Fat, Glycoprotein	
T1 Dark, T2 Dark	T1 Bright, T2 Dark	T2 Bright
Does NOT Enhance	Usually Does NOT Enhance	Does Enhance

This vs That: HCC vs Fibrolamellar Subtype HCC	
HCC	**FL HCC**
Cirrhosis	No Cirrhosis
Older (50s-60s)	Young (30s)
Rarely Calcifies	Calcifies Sometimes
Elevated AFP	Normal AFP

This vs That: Central Scars of FNH and Fibrolamellar HCC	
FNH	**FL HCC**
T2 Bright	T2 Dark (usually)
Enhances on Delays	Does NOT enhance
Mass is Sulfur Colloid Avid (sometimes)	Mass is Gallium Avid

Multiple Low Density (NOT Cystic) Liver Lesions	
Mets	Think Colon First - unless they have a known primary
HCC	Does the Liver look Cirrhotic?
Regeneratice Nodules	Does the Liver look Cirrhotic ?
Infections	Low Density Nodes - Think Mycobacterium Hyperenhancing Nodes - Think Bartonella
Sarcoid	Spleen Should be Involved Also Gamesmanship - Probably gets some hints in the form of a CXR, or Labs (elevated ACE)

Multiple Cystic Liver Lesions	
AD Polycystic Kidney	Different Size Cysts (small and big) Renal Cystic Disease
Von Meyenburg Complex (Hamatromas)	Small (< 1.5 cm) Will NOT connect with Ducts Uniform distribution
Choledochal Cysts (Caroli)	WILL communicate with duct Central "dot" Sign
Abscess	Bacterial and Fungal = Multiple, R > L Amoebic = Single and Sub-diaphragmatic Peripheral Enhancement Necrotic center will not enhance

Infection Buzzwords	
Viral Hepatitis	Starry Sky (US)
Pyogenic Abscess	Double Target (CT)
Candida	Bull's Eye (US) ●
Amoebic Abscess	"Extra Hepatic Extension"
Hydatid Disease	Water Lily, Sand Storm
Schistosomiasis	Tortoise Shell

Primary Hemochromatosis	Secondary Hemochromatosis
Genetic - increased absorption	Acquired - chronic illness, and multiple transfusions
Liver, **P**ancreas	Liver, **S**pleen
Heart, Thyroid, Pituitary	

This vs That: AIDS Cholangiopathy vs Primary Sclerosing Cholangitis	
AIDS	**PSC**
Focal Strictures of the extrahepatic duct > 2cm	Extrahepatic strictures rarely > 5mm
Absent saccular deformities of the ducts	Has saccular deformities of the ducts
Associated Papillary Stenosis	

Biliary Dilation	
Intrahepatic	**Extrahepatic ONLY**
Primary Sclerosing Cholangitis	Post Cholecystectomy
Infectious Cholangitis	Sphincter of Oddi Dysfunction
Pancreatic Head Mass	Type 1 Choledochocyst
CBD Stone — Late	CBD Stone - Early
Biliary Stricture	

THIS vs THAT: Chronic Pancreatitis Duct Dilation vs Pancreatic Malignancy Duct Dilation	
CP	**Cancer**
Dilation is Irregular	Dilation is uniform *(usually)*
Duct is < 50% of the AP gland diameter	Duct is > 50% of the AP gland diameter *(obstructive atrophy)*

Primary Hemochromatosis	Secondary Hemochromatosis
Genetic - increased absorption	Acquired - chronic illness, and multiple transfusions
Liver, **P**ancreas	Liver, **S**pleen
Heart, Thyroid, Pituitary	

This vs That: AIDS Cholangiopathy vs Primary Sclerosing Cholangitis	
AIDS	**PSC**
Focal Strictures of the extrahepatic duct > 2cm	Extrahepatic strictures rarely > 5mm
Absent saccular deformities of the ducts	Has saccular deformities of the ducts
Associated Papillary Stenosis	

Biliary Dilation	
Intrahepatic	**Extrahepatic ONLY**
Primary Sclerosing Cholangitis	Post Cholecystectomy
Infectious Cholangitis	Sphincter of Oddi Dysfunction
Pancreatic Head Mass	Type 1 Choledochocyst
CBD Stone — Late	CBD Stone - Early
Biliary Stricture	

THIS vs THAT: Chronic Pancreatitis Duct Dilation vs Pancreatic Malignancy Duct Dilation	
CP	**Cancer**
Dilation is Irregular	Dilation is uniform *(usually)*
Duct is < 50% of the AP gland diameter	Duct is > 50% of the AP gland diameter *(obstructive atrophy)*

Uncommon Types and Causes of Pancreatitis

Autoimmune Pancreatitis	Associated with elevated IgG4	Absence of Attack Symptoms	Responds to steroids	Sausage Shaped Pancreas, capsule like delayed rim enhancement around gland (like a scar). **No duct dilation. No calcifications.**
Groove Pancreatitis	Looks like a pancreatic head Cancer - but with little or no biliary obstruction.	Less likely to cause obstructive jaundice (relative to pancreatic CA)	Duodenal stenosis and /or strictures of the CBD in 50% of the cases	Soft tissue within the pancreaticoduodenal groove, with or without delayed enhancement
Tropic Pancreatitis	Young Age at onset, associated with malnutrition	Increased risk of adenocarcinoma		Multiple large calculi within a dilated pancreatic duct
Hereditary Pancreatitis	Young Age at Onset	Increased risk of adenocarcinoma	SPINK-1 gene	Similar to Tropic Pancreatitis
Ascaris Induced	Most commonly implicated parasite in pancreatitis			Worm may be seen within the bile ducts

When I Say - Autoimmune Pancreatitis

I Say Autoimmune Pancreatitis	You Say IgG4
I Say IgG4	Autoimmune Pancreatitis Retroperitoneal Fibrosis Sclerosing Cholangitis Inflammatory Pseudotumor Riedel's Thyroiditis

THIS vs THAT:
Autoimmune Pancreatitis vs Chronic Pancreatitis

Autoimmune Pancreatitis	Chronic Pancreatitis
No ductal dilation	Ductal Dilation
No calcifications	Ductal Calcifications

Cystic Pancreatic Lesions			
Main Branch IPMN	40s - 50s	Main Duct	High Malignant Potential (60%)
Side Branch IPMN	50s - 60s	Favor Head, Uncinate	Typically Benign (maybe 5% will develop malignancy) <u>Communicates with duct</u>
Serous Cystic	Grandma F > M > 60	Favor Head	Does NOT Communicate with Main Duct <u>Central</u> Calcifications "Micro-Cystic" - "Honeycomb" Benign Glycogen Rich Associated with von Hippel Lindau
Mucinous Cystic	Mother F > M 40s	Favor Body / Tail	Does NOT Communicate with Main Duct Peripheral Calcifications Larger Cysts (sometimes uni-locular) Premalignant
Solid Pseudo-Papillary	Daughter F > M 20s	Favor Tail	Large (5-10 cms) Solid with Cystic Parts Enhances like a Hemangioma Has a Capsule Asian or Black Female

Malignant Ulcer	Benign Ulcer
Width > Depth	Depth > Width
Located within Lumen	Project behind the expected lumen
Nodular, Irregular Edges	Sharp Contour
Folds adjacent to ulcer	Folds radiate to ulcer
Aunt Minnie: Carmen Meniscus Sign	Aunt Minnie: Hampton's Line

Direct Hernia	Indirect Hernia
Less common	More Common
Medial to inferior Epigastric	Lateral to inferior epigastric
Defect in Hesselbach triangle	Failure of processus vaginalis to close
NOT covered by internal spermatic fascia	Covered by internal spermatic fascia

Sigmoid Volvulus	Cecal Volvulus
Old Person (Constipated)	Younger Person (mass, prior surgery, or 3rd Trimester Pregnancy)
Points to the RUQ	Points to the LUQ

Crohns vs Ulcerative Colitis	
Crohns	**UC**
Slightly less common in the USA	Slightly more common in the USA
Discontinuous "Skips"	Continuous
Terminal Ileum – *String Sign*	Rectum
Ileocecal Valve "Stenosed"	Ileocecal Valve "Open"
Mesenteric Fat Increased *"creeping fat"*	Perirectal fat Increased
Lymph nodes are usually enlarged	Lymph nodes are NOT usually enlarged
Makes Fistulae	Doesn't Usually Make Fistulae

More Common In : Crohns vs UC	
Path	**More Common With**
Gallstones	Crohns
Primary Sclerosing Cholangitis	Ulcerative Coliits
Hepatic Abscess	Crohns
Pancreatitis	Crohns

This Could Be Useful

Cholangio:	CEA ↑	CA 19-9 ↑
Pancreatic CA:	CEA	CA 19-9 ↑↑
Colon CA:	CEA ↑	CA 19-9

Peds Cystic Renal Mass

 Unilateral

 Bilateral

Multicystic Dysplastic Kidney
- Neonate, No Renal Function (MAG 3)
- Associated with congenital UPJ obstruction
- Associated with reflux (VUR) -

AR- Polycystic Kidney Disease
- Enlarged, Hyperechoic
- Microcystic

Multilocular Cystic Nephroma
- "Micheal Jackson - Young Boy, Older Woman"
- Multiple Cysts - Herniates into the Renal Pelvis"

Cystic Wilms

Peds Tumor / Mass	Rapid Review Trivia
Mesoblastic Nephroma	*"Solid Tumor of Infancy"* (you can be born with it)
Nephroblastomatosis	"Nephrogenic Rests" - left over embryologic crap that didn't go away Might turn into wilms (bilateral wilms especially) "Next Step" - f/u ultrasound till 7-8 years old Variable appearance
Wilms	90% + Renal Tumors *"Solid Tumor of Childhood"* - **Never born with it** Grows like a solid ball (will invade rather than incase) Met to the lung (most common)
Clear Cell - Wilms	Met to Bone
Rhabdoid - Wilms	Brain Tumors It fucks you up, it takes the money (it believes in nothing Lebowski)
Multi-Cystic Nephroma	Micheal Jackson Tumor (Young Boys, Middle Age Women) Big cysts that don't communicate Septal Enhancement Can't Tell it is not Cystic Wilms (next step = resection)
RCC	*"Solid Tumor of Adolescent"* Syndromes - VHL, TS
Renal Lymphoma	Non-Hodgkin Multifocal

Neuroblastoma	Wilms
Age: usually less than 2 (can occur in utero)	Age: Usually around age 4 **(never before 2 months)**
Calcifies 90%	Calcifies Rarely (<10%)
Encases Vessels (doesn't invade)	Invades Vessels (doesn't encase)
Poorly Marginated	Well Circumscribed
Mets to Bones	Doesn't usually met to bones (unless clear cell Wilms variant). Prefers lung.

Neuroblastoma	Adrenal Hemorrhage
Heterogenous and vascular	Centrally Hypoechoic and Avascular
High on T2 , Iso-Low on T1	High on T1 (7 days - 7 weeks)
Will grow on followup	Should shrink on followup

Adult RCC Associations	
Subtype	**Syndrome / Association**
Clear Cell	Von Hippel-Lindau
Papillary	Hereditary papillary renal carcinoma
Chromophobe	Birt Hogg Dube
Medullary	Sickle Cell Trait

Renal Cyst Associations		
ADPCKD	Cysts in Liver	Kidneys are BIG
VHL	Cysts in Pancreas	
Acquired (uremic)		Kidneys are small

Bladder Cancer	
Transitional Cell CA	The "normal" kind Bladder CA >>> Ureter CA
Squamous Cell CA	Calcifications Chronic Catheter Schistosomiasis (worm)
Adeno-Carcinoma	Midline Urachus Association Bladder Exstrophy
Urethra	
Prostatic Urethra	Transitional Cell
Bulbar / Penile Urethra	Squamous Cell
Urethral Diverticulum	Adenocarcinoma

You See That	Think This
Big Kidney with Lots of Cysts Liver Cysts	AD Polycystic Kidney
Normal Sized Kidneys with Lots of Cysts Solid Renal Masses (RCCs) Pancreatic Cysts (simple and serous cystic) Pancreatic Masses Adrenal Masses (paragangliomas)	von Hippel - Lindau
Renal Cysts Multiple Fat Containing Renal Masses (AMLs) - maybe bleeding Lungs Cysts (LAM)	Tuberous Sclerosis
Small / Calcified Spleen Gallstones (or absent GB) Bone Infarcts	Sickle Cell
Severe Pancreatic Fatty Atrophy Small bowel stool Fatty Liver	Cystic Fibrosis
Big Liver, Big Spleen Bone Infarcts Extramedullary Hematopoiesis	Gaucher
Bilateral Adrenal Masses (Pheochromocytoma - not adenoma) Thyroid Cancer	MEN 2
Islet Cell Tumors Pituitary Adenoma	MEN 1
Renal Masses (Wilms, AML) Adrenal Masses (Pheochromocytoma) Skin Nodules Scoliosis	NF-1
Vascular Malformation in the Liver Bowel Angiodysplasia Enlarged Hepatic Artery Pulmonary AVM Brain Abscess	Osler Weber Rendu (Hereditary Hemorrhagic Telangiectasia)

Cyst Morphology Trivia:

- ADPCKD - Round and Distributed Throughout Kidney

- ARPCKD - Tubular Cysts which Spare Cortex

Battle Tactics: Schematic Thoracic Pathology

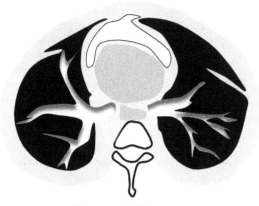

Normal Thymus
- Age < 10
- Homogenous
- No Mass Effect

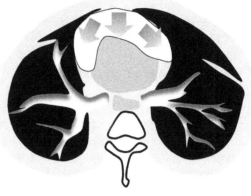

Lymphoma
- Age > 10
- Mass Effect
- SVC Compression
- Lymph Nodes
- Hodgkin > NHL

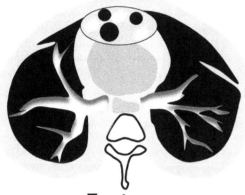

Teratoma
- Fat
- Cystic
- Calcifications

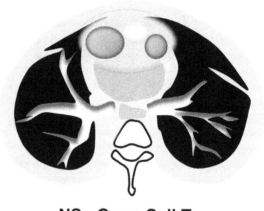

NS - Germ Cell Tumor
- Big
- Hemorrhage
- Necrosis
- Aggressive
- Klinefelter

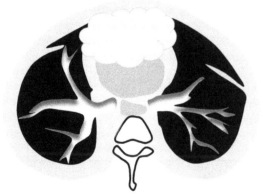

Seminoma
- Straddle Midline
- Bulky
- Lobulated

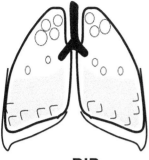

DIP

- Apical Emphysema (smoking related)
- Basilar Ground Glass
- Peripheral Basilar Reticulation
- Smoker - Severe end of RB-ILD

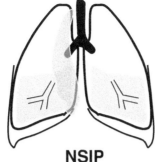

NSIP

- Basilar Ground Glass (sub-pleural sparing)
- Traction Bronchiectasis
- Scleroderma Association (dilated esophagus)

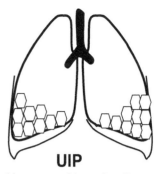

UIP

- Honeycombing - basilar predominant

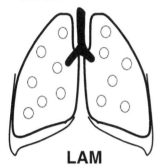

LAM

- Thin walled cysts - distributed evenly
- Tuberous sclerosis

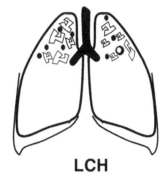

LCH

- Nodules with cavitation (early)
- Apical - "Bizarre" Cysts (late)
- Smoker -20s-30s
- Sparing of the costophrenic recesses

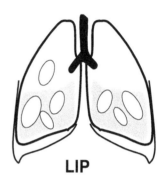

LIP

- Thin walled cysts (less than LAM)
- Ground Glass - clears with treatment
- Sjogrens, RA, HIV

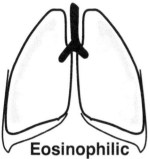

Eosinophilic Pneumonia

- Reverse Pulmonary Edema Pattern (peripheral)
- Ground glass and consolidation

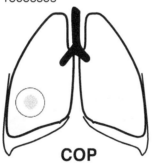

COP

- Atoll / Reverse Halo Sign - Consolidation around Ground Glass
- Patchy, Peripheral Consolidation

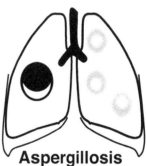

Aspergillosis

- Halo Sign - Ground Glass around consolidation
- Air Crescent - "invasive"

Upper Lobe Predominant	Lower Lobe Predominant
Most inhaled stuff (not asbestosis). Coal Workers, and Silicosis. This includes progressive massive fibrosis.	Asbestosis
CF	Primary Ciliary Dsykinesia
RB-ILD	Most Interstitial Lung Diseases (UIP, NSIP, DIP)
Centrilobular Emphysema	Panlobular Emphysema (Alpha 1)
Ankylosing Spondylitis	Rheumatoid Lung
Sarcoid	Scleroderma (associated with NSIP)

Collagen Vascular Disease Pulmonary Manifestations		
Lupus	More **pleural effusions and pericardial effusions** than with other connective tissue disease	Fibrosis is uncommon. Can get a "shrinking lung."
Rheumatoid Arthritis	Looks like UIP and COP. Lower lobes are favored.	Reticulations with or without honeycombing, and consolidative opacities which are organizing pneumonia
Scleroderma	**NSIP** > UIP; lower lobe predominant findings.	Look for the dilated fluid filled esophagus.
Sjogrens	**LIP**	Extensive ground glass attenuation with scattered thin walled cysts.
Ankylosing Spondylitis	<u>Upper lobe</u> **fibrobullous disease**	Usually unilateral first, then progresses to bilateral.

Infections in AIDS by CD4	
> 200	Bacterial Infections, TB
< 200	PCP, Atypical Mycobacterial
< 100	CMV, Disseminated Fungal, Mycobacterial

ACR Appropriateness Criteria:

- First Line for Suspected Metastatic Disease = CXR
- Recommendation for patients on mechanical ventilation = Daily CXR
- First Line for Chest Pain and High Suspicion for Aortic Dissection = CXR

Cardiac Trivia:

Pathology	Which Sequence(s) most useful?
Cardiac Myxoma	Low T1, High T2 (high myxoid content)
Acute vs Chronic MI	Look at T2 – Bright on Acute ; Dark on Chronic (fibrous scar)
Arrhythmogenic Right Ventricular Dysplasia (ARVD)	T1 Bright
Microvascular Obstruction	First Pass Perfusion (25 seconds post Gad)
Infarct	Delayed Enhancement (10-12 mins post Gad)

Cardiac MRI Enhancement Patterns:

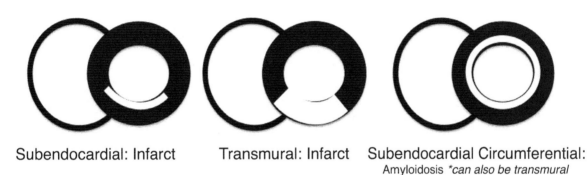

Subendocardial: Infarct   Transmural: Infarct   Subendocardial Circumferential:
                                                              Amyloidosis *can also be transmural

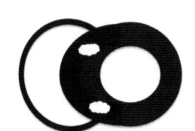

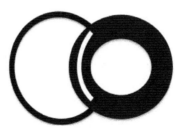

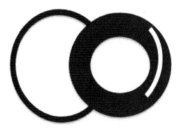

Midwall:
HCM

Midwall:
Myocarditis, Idiopathic Dilated CM

Midwall:
Myocarditis, Sarcoidosis

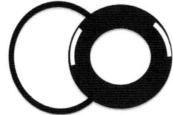

Epicardial:
Myocarditis, Sarcoidosis

Cardiac Surgery Types / Indications

Pulmonary Artery Banding	CHF in Infancy, Single Ventricle
Arterial Switch (Senning and Mustard)	Transposition of the Great Arteries
Rastelli (RV Baffle)	Transposition, Pulmonary Outflow Obstruction
Jatene (a type of arterial switch)	Transposition
Ross	Diseased Aortic Valves in Children
Bentall	Aortic Root / Valve Replacement in Marfan

Additional Cardiac Surgery Pearls

Glenn	Blalock Taussig	Fontan
Vein to Artery *(SVC to Pulmonary Artery)*	Artery to Artery *(Subclavian Artery to Pulmonary Artery)*	*It's complicated with multiple versions - steps are unlikely to be tested*
Primary Purpose: Take systemic blood directly to the pulmonary circulation (it bypasses the right heart).	Primary Purpose: Increase pulmonary blood flow	Primary Purpose: Bypass the right ventricle / direct systemic circulation into the PAs.
Most Testable Complications: -SVC Syndrome **-PA Aneurysms**	Most Testable Complications: -Stenosis at the shunt's pulmonary insertion site	Most Testable Complications: -Enlarged Right Artium causing arrhythmia **-Plastic Bronchitis**

Vasculitis:

Large Vessel	
Takayasu	Young Asian Female – thickened aneurysmal aorta
Giant Cell	Old Person with involvement of the "crutches" / armpit region (Subclavian, axillary, brachial).
Cogan Syndrome	Kid with eye and ear symptoms + Aortitis
Medium Vessel	
PAN	PAN is more common in a MAN (M > F). Renal Microaneurysm (similar to speed kidney). Associated with Hep B.
Kawasaki	Coronary Artery Aneurysm
Small Vessel (ANCA +)	
Wegeners	Nasal Septum Erosions, Cavitary Lung Lesions
Churg Strauss	Transient peripheral lung consolidations.
Microscopic Polyangiitis	Diffuse pulmonary hemorrhage
Small Vessel (ANCA -)	
HSP	Kids. Intussusception. Massive scrotal edema.
Behcets	Pulmonary artery aneurysm
Buergers	Male smoker. Hand angiogram shows finger occlusions.

Nukes Trivia:

Tracer	Analog	Energy	Physical Half Life
Tc – 99m		"Low" – 140	6 hours
Iodine -123	Iodine	"Low" – 159	13 hours
Xenon - 133		"Low" – 81	125 hours *(biologic t1/2 30 seconds)*
Thallium - 201	Potassium	"Low" – 135 (2%), 167 (8%), *use 71 ^{201}Hg daughter x-rays*	73 hours
Indium -111		"Medium" – 173 (89%), 247 (94%)	67 hours
Gallium - 67	Iron	Multiple; 93 (40%), 184 (20%), 300 (20%), 393 (5%)	78 hours
Iodine -131	Iodine	"High" - 365	8 days
Fluorine -18	Sugar	"High" - 511	110 mins
Strontium 89			50.5 DAYS (14 days in bone)
Samarium 153			46 Hours
Radium			11 Days
Yttrium 90			64 Hours
Rubidium 82			75 seconds
Nitrogen 13			10 mins

Probable Critical Organ *(depending on who you ask)*	
Tc - MDP	Bladder *(some sources say bone)*
Tc - Sulfur Colloid (IV)	Liver
Tc - Sulfur Colloid (Oral)	Proximal Colon
Tc - Pertechnetate	Stomach > Thyroid *(some sources say colon)*
Tc - Sestamibi	Proximal Colon
Tc - Heat Treated RBC	Spleen > Heart
Tagged RBC - MUGA	Heart
Tc - MAA	Lung
Tc - DMSA	Renal Cortex
Tc - MAG 3	Bladder
DTPA	Bladder
I-123 MIBG	Bladder *(some sources say adrenal medulla)*
I-131 MIBG	Liver *(some sources say adrenal medulla)*
I-131, I-123	Thyroid
In-111 WBC	Spleen
In-111 ProstaScint	Liver
In-111 Octreoscan	Spleen
Thallium 201	Renal Cortex
F18 FDG	Bladder
Gallium	Distal Colon
HIDA	Gallbladder Wall

	Mechanism of Localization	
Tc - Sestamibi	Passive Diffusion	Cross the cell membrane via lipophilic diffusion
Tc - Tetrofosmin	Passive Diffusion	Cross the cell membrane via lipophilic diffusion
Tc - HMPAO	Passive Diffusion	Delivery is flow related - then diffuse into brain
Tc - ECD	Passive Diffusion	Delivery is flow related - then diffuse into brain
DTPA	Filtration	
F18 - FDG	Facilitated Diffusion	Carrier mediated transport across membrane via GLUT
I-123, I-131	Active Transport	Use ATP to move AGAINST concentration gradient
Thallium	Active Transport (Na/K Pump)	
Rubidium	Active Transport (Na/K Pump)	
MIBG	Active Transport (Na facilitated norepinephrine uptake system)	
DMSA	Active Transport	
Pertechnatate	Secretion	Active transport OUT of a gland or tissue
MAG - 3	Secretion	Secreted by peritubular capillaries
Tc-99m IDA	Secretion	Secreted by hepatocytes
Sulfur Colloid	Phagocytosis	RES eats the colloid particles
Heat Treated RBCs	Sequestration	
MAA	Capillary Blockade	Lung Perfusion
MDP	Chemisorption	Chemical Covalent + Hydrogen Bonding
SM -153	Chemisorption	
Indium WBC	Cellular Migration	Cells migrate to the response of stimuli
Octreotide	Receptor Binding	
DAT Scan (I-123 Isoflupane)	Receptor Binding	

Tumors that are PET COLD	Not Cancer but PET HOT
BAC (Adeno In Situ) - Lung Cancer	Infection
Carcinoid	Inflammation
RCC	Ovaries in Follicular Phase
Peritoneal Bowel/Liver Implants	Muscles
Anything Mucinous	Brown Fat
Prostate	Thymus

FDG PET - Brain		
Alzheimer	Low posterior temporoparietal cortical activity	Identical to Parkinson Dementia
Multi Infarct	Scattered areas of decreased activity	
Dementia with Lewy Bodies	Low in lateral occipital cortex	Preservation of the mid posterior cingulate gyrus (**Cingulate Island Sign**)
Picks / Frontotemporal	Low frontal lobe	
Huntingtons	Low activity in caudate nucleus and putamen	

Tc DTPA	Tc MAG 3	Tc GH
Filtered (**GFR**)	Secreted (**ERPF**)	Filtered
Good For Native Kidneys with **Normal Renal Function**	Concentrated better by kidneys with **poor renal function**	Good for dynamic and cortical imaging.
Critical Organ Bladder	Critical Organ Bladder	Critical Organ Bladder

ATN	Immediate Post OP (3-4 days post op)	Perfusion Normal	Excretion Delayed
Cyclosporin Toxicity	**Long Standing**	Perfusion Normal	Excretion Delayed
Acute Rejection	Immediate Post OP	**Poor Perfusion**	Excretion Delayed

Tc WBC	In WBC	Agent	Localization	Tc WBC 4 Hours	Tc WBC 24 Hours
Renal	**NO** Renal	Indium WBC	Spleen	Lung	Lung Clear
		Indium WBC Damaged	Liver and Bone Marrow		
GI	**NO** GI	RBC Tagged	Heart		Bowel Starting
		RBC Damaged	Spleen		

Indium is BETTER than Gallium for Evaluating	Gallium is BETTER than Indium for Evaluating
• Suspected abdominal-pelvic abscess due to the lack of a normal bowel excretory pathway	• Spine • Diffuse Pulmonary Processes: Gallium is probably the agent of choice for the evaluation of pulmonary inflammatory abnormalities. • Lymphocyte mediated infection

Tc HMPAO is BETTER than In WBC for Evaluating	In WBC is BETTER than Tc HMPAO for Evaluating
• Children (lower Dose) • Inflammatory Bowel - *but you have to image early – like around an hour (*or 30 mins – depending on who you ask*). • Osteomyelitis in Extremity	• Fever of Unknown Origin

Neuro Trivia:

Toxo	Lymphoma
Ring Enhancing	Ring Enhancing
Hemorrhage more common after treatment	Hemorrhage less common after treatment
Thallium Cold	**Thallium HOT**
PET Cold	PET Hot
MR Perfusion: Decreased CBV	MR Perfusion: Increased (or Decreased) CBV

AIDS Encephalitis	PML	CMV	Toxo	Cryptococcus
Symmetric T2 Bright	Asymmetric T2 Bright	Periventricular T2 Bright	Ring Enhancement	Dilated Perivascular Spaces
	T1 dark	Ependymal Enhancement	Thallium Cold	Basilar Meningitis

NF-1	Optic Nerve Gliomas
NF-2	MSME; Multiple Schwannomas, Meningiomas, Ependymomas
VHL	Hemangioblastoma (brain and retina)
TS	Subependymal Giant Cell Astrocytoma, Cortical Tubers
Nevoid Basal Cell Syndrome (Gorlin)	Medulloblastoma
Turcot	GBM, Medulloblastoma
Cowdens	Lhermitte-Dulcos (Dysplastic cerebellar gangliocytoma)

Maximum Bleeding – Aneurysm Location	
ACOM	Interhemispheric Fissure
PCOM	Ipsilateral Basal Cistern
MCA Trifurcation	Sylvian Fissure
Basilar Tip	Interpeduncular Cistern, or Intraventricular
PICA	Posterior Fossa or Intraventricular

Path	Demographics	Typical Location	Trivia	Imaging Characteristics
Inverting Papilloma	40-70 M>F (4:1)	Lateral nasal wall centered at the middle meatus, with occasional extension into the antrum	40% show "entrapped bone" *Cerebriform Pattern* **10% Harbor a Squamous Cell CA**	Cerebriform Pattern May have focal hyperostosis on CT
Esthesioneuroblastoma	Bimodal 20s & 60s	Dumbbell shaped with waist at the cribiform plate		**AVID homogeneous enhancement**
SNUC	Broad Range (30s-90s)	Ethmoid origin more common than maxillary	<u>Large,</u> typically > 4cm on presentation	**Fungating and Poorly defined** Heterogeneous enhancement with necrosis
Squamous Cell CA	95% > 40 years old	Maxillary Antrum is involved in 80%	**Most Common Malignancy of Sino-Nasal track**	Aggressive Antral Soft Tissue Mass, with destruction of sinus walls **Low signal on T2 (highly cellular)** Enhances less than some other sinus malignancies
JNA *(Juvenile Nasopharyngeal Angiofibroma)*	**Nearly Exclusively Male Rare < 8 or > 25**	**Origin in the Spenopalantine Foramen (SPF)**	Radiation alone cures in 80%	**Enhancing mass arising from the SPF in adolescent male** Dark Flow Voids on T1 **Avidly Enhances**
Sinonasal Lymphoma	Usually older, peak is 60s	Nasal Cavity > Sinuses	Highly variable appearance	Homogeneous mass in nasal cavity with bony destruction **Low Signal on T2 (highly cellular)**

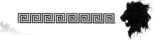

- When I say "Subglottic Hemangioma," You Say PHACES Syndrome
- When I say "PHACES Syndrome," You say Cutaneous Hemangioma
- When I say "Ropy Appearance," You say Meconium Aspiration
- When I say "Post Term Delivery," You Say Meconium Aspiration
- When I say "Fluid in the Fissures," You say Transient Tachypnea
- When I say "History of c-section", You say Transient Tachypnea
- When I say "Maternal sedation", You say Transient Tachypnea
- When I say "Granular Opacities + Premature", You say RDS
- When I say "Granular Opacities + Term + High Lung Volume," You say Pneumonia
- When I say "Granular Opacities + Term + Low Lung Volume," You say B-Hemolytic Strep
- When I say "Band Like Opacities", You say Chronic Lung Disease (BPD)
- When I say "Linear Lucencies" , You say Pulmonary Interstitial Emphysema
- When I say "Pulmonary Hypoplasia," You say diaphragmatic hernia
- When I say "Lung Cysts and Nodules," You Say LCH or Papillomatosis
- When I say "Lower lobe bronchiectasis," You Say Primary Ciliary Dyskinesia
- When I say "Upper lobe bronchiectasis," You Say CF
- When I say "Posterior mediastinal mass (under 2)," You Say Neuroblastoma
- When I say "No air in the stomach", You say Esophageal Atresia
- When I say "Excessive air in the stomach", You say "H" Type TE fistula
- When I say "Anterior Esophageal Impression," You say pulmonary sling
- When I say "Pulmonary Sling," You say tracheal stenosis.
- When I say "Single Bubble," You say Gastric (antral or pyloric) atresia
- When I say "Double Bubble," You say duodenal atresia
- When I say "Duodenal Atresia", You say Downs
- When I say "Single Bubble with Distal Gas," You say maybe Mid Gut Volvulus
- When I say "Non-bilious vomiting", You say Hypertrophic Pyloric Stenosis
- When I say "Paradoxial aciduria" You say Hypertrophic Pyloric Stenosis
- When I say "Bilious vomiting - in an infant", You say Mid Gut Volvulus
- When I say "Corkscrew Duodenum" You say Mid Gut Volvulus
- When I say "Reversed SMA and SMV" You say Malrotation
- When I say "Absent Gallbladder" You say biliary atresia
- When I say "Triangle Cord Sign" You say biliary atresia
- When I say "Asplenia" , You say "cyanotic heart disease"
- When I say "Infarcted Spleen," You say Sickle Cell
- When I say "Gall Stones," You say Sickle Cell
- When I say "Short Microcolon," You say Colonic Atresia
- When I say "Long Microcolon," You say Meconium ileus or distal ileal atresia
- When I say "Saw tooth colon," You say Hirschsprung
- When I say "Calcified mass in the mid abdomen of a newborn", you say Meconium Peritonitis
- When I say "Meconium ileus equivalent," you say Distal Intestinal Obstruction Syndrome (CF).
- When I say "Abrupt caliber change of the aorta below the celiac axis" , You say Hepatic Hemangioendothelioma.
- When I say "Cystic mass in the liver of a newborn," you say Mesenchymal Hamartoma

- When I say "Elevated AFP, with mass in the liver of a newborn," you say Hepatoblastoma
- When I say "Common Bile Duct measures more than 10 mm", You say Choledochal Cyst
- When I say "Lipomatous pseudohypertrophy of the pancreas," You say CF
- When I say "Unilateral Renal Agenesis" You say unicornuate uterus
- When I say "Neonatal Renal Vein Thrombosis," You say maternal diabetes
- When I say "Neonatal Renal Artery Thrombosis," You say Misplaced Umbilical Artery Catheter
- When I say "Hydro on Fetal MRI," You say Posterior Urethral Valve
- When I say "Urachus," You say bladder Adenocarcinoma
- When I say "Nephroblastomatosis with Necrosis," you say Wilms
- When I say "Solid Renal Tumor of Infancy," you say Mesoblastic Nephroma
- When I say "Solid Renal Tumor of Childhood," you say Wilms
- When I say "Midline pelvic mass, in a female," you say Hydrometrocolpos
- When I say "Right sided varicocele," you say abdominal pathology
- When I say "Blue Dot Sign," you say Torsion of the Testicular Appendage
- When I say "Hand or Foot Pain / Swelling in an Infant", You say - sickle cell with hand foot syndrome.
- When I say Extratesticular scrotal mass, you say embryonal rhabdomyosarcoma
- When I say "Narrowing of the interpedicular distance," you say Achondroplasia
- When I say "Platyspondyly (flat vertebral bodies)," you say Thanatophoric
- When I say "Absent Tonsils after 6 months" You say "Immune Deficiency"
- When I say "Enlarged Tonsils well after childhood (like 12-15)" You say "Cancer"… probably lymphatic
- When I say "Mystery Liver Abscess in Kid, "You say "Chronic Granulomatous Disease"
- When I say "narrowed B Ring," You say Schatzki (Schat"B"ki Ring)
- When I say "esophageal concentric rings," You say Eosinophilic Esophagitis
- When I say "shaggy" or "plaque like" esophagus, You say Candidiasis
- When I say "looks like candida, but an asymptomatic old lady," you say Glycogen Acanthosis
- When I say "reticular mucosal pattern," you say Barretts
- When I say "high stricture with an associated hiatal hernia," you say Barretts
- When I say "abrupt shoulders," you say cancer
- When I say "Killian Dehiscence," you say Zenker Diverticulum
- When I say "transient, fine transverse folds across the esophagus," you say Feline Esophagus.
- When I say "bird's beak," you say Achalasia
- When I say "solitary esophageal ulcer," you say CMV or AIDS
- When I say "ulcers at the level of the arch or distal esophagus," you say Medication induced
- When I say "Breast Cancer + Bowel Hamartomas," you say Cowdens
- When I say "Desmoid Tumors + Bowel Polyps," you say Gardners
- When I say "Brain Tumors + Bowel Polyps," you say Turcots
- When I say "enlarged left supraclavicular node," you say Virchow Node (GI Cancer)
- When I say "crosses the pylorus," you say Gastric Lymphoma
- When I say "isolated gastric varices," you say splenic vein thrombus
- When I say "multiple gastric ulcers," you say Chronic Aspirin Therapy.
- When I say "multiple duodenal (or jejunal) ulcers," you say Zollinger-Ellsion
- When I say "pancreatitis after Billroth 2," you say Afferent Loop Syndrome
- When I say "Weight gain years after Roux-en-Y," you say Gastro-Gastro Fistula
- When I say "Clover Leaf Sign - Duodenum," you say healed peptic ulcer.
- When I say "Sand Like Nodules in the Jejunum," you say Whipples

- When I say "Sand Like Nodules in the Jejunum + CD4 <100," you say MAI
- When I say "Ribbon-like bowel," you say Graft vs Host
- When I say "Ribbon like Jejunum," you say Long Standing Celiac
- When I say "Moulage Pattern," you say Celiac *(moulage = loss of jejunal folds)*
- When I say "Fold Reversal - of jejunum and ileum," you say Celiac
- When I say "Cavitary (low density) Lymph nodes," you say Celiac
- When I say "hide bound" or "Stack or coins," you say Scleroderma
- When I say "Megaduodenum," you say Scleroderma
- When I say "Duodenal obstruction, with recent weight loss," you say SMA Syndrome
- When I say "Coned shaped cecum," you say Amebiasis
- When I say "Lead Pipe," you say Ulcerative Colitis
- When I say "String Sign," you say Crohns
- When I say "Massive circumferential thickening, without obstruction," you say Lymphoma
- When I say "Multiple small bowel target signs," you say Melanoma
- When I say "Obstructing Old Lady Hernia," you say Femoral Hernia
- When I say "sac of bowel," you say Paraduodenal hernia.
- When I say "scalloped appearance of the liver," you say Pseudomyxoma Peritonei
- When I say "HCC without cirrhosis," you say Hepatitis B (or Fibrolamellar HCC)
- When I say "Capsular retraction," you say Cholangiocarcinoma
- When I say "Periportal hypoechoic infiltration + AIDS," you say Kaposi's
- When I say "sparing of the caudate lobe," you say Budd Chiari
- When I say "large T2 bright nodes + Budd Chiari," you say Hyperplastic nodules
- When I say "liver high signal in phase, low signal out phase," you say fatty liver
- When I say "liver low signal in phase, and high signal out phase," you say hemochromatosis
- When I say "multifocal intrahepatic and extrahepatic biliary stricture," you say PSC
- When I say "multifocal intrahepatic and extrahepatic biliary strictures + papillary stenosis," you say AIDS Cholangiopathy.
- When I say "bile ducts full of stones," you say Recurrent Pyogenic Cholangitis
- When I say "Gallbladder Comet Tail Artifact," you say Adenomyomatosis
- When I say "lipomatous pseudohypertrophy of the pancreas," you say CF
- When I say "sausage shaped pancreas," you say autoimmune pancreatitis
- When I say "autoimmune pancreatitis," you say IgG4
- When I say "IgG4" you say RP Fibrosis, Sclerosing Cholangitis, Fibrosing Mediastinitis, Inflammatory Pseudotumor
- When I say "Wide duodenal sweep," you say Pancreatic Cancer
- When I say "Grandmother Pancreatic Cyst" you say Serous Cystadenoma
- When I say "Mother Pancreatic Cyst" you say Mucinous
- When I say "Daughter Pancreatic Cyst," you say Solid Pseudopapillary
- When I say "bladder stones," you say neurogenic bladder
- When I say "pine cone appearance," you say neurogenic bladder
- When I say "urethra cancer," you say squamous cell CA
- When I say "urethra cancer - prostatic portion," you say transitional cell CA
- When I say "urethra cancer - in a diverticulum," you say adenocarcinoma
- When I say "long term supra-pubic catheter," you say squamous Bladder CA
- When I say "e-coli infection," you say Malakoplakia
- When I say "vas deferens calcifications," you say diabetes

- When I say "calcifications in a fatty renal mass," you say RCC
- When I say "protrude into the renal pelvis," you say Multilocular cystic nephroma
- When I say "no functional renal tissue," you say Multicystic Dysplastic Kidney
- When I say "Multicystic Dysplastic Kidney," you say contralateral renal issues (50%)
- When I say "Emphysematous Pyelonephritis," you say diabetic
- When I say "Xanthogranulomatous Pyelonephritis," you say staghorn stone
- When I say "Papillary Necrosis," you say diabetes
- When I say "shrunken calcified kidney," you say TB ("putty kidney")
- When I say "bilateral medulla nephrocalcinosis," you say Medullary Sponge Kidney
- When I say "big bright kidney with decreased renal function," you say HIV
- When I say "history of lithotripsy," you say Page Kidney
- When I say "cortical rim sign," you say subacute renal infarct
- When I say "history of renal biopsy," you say AVF
- When I say "reversed diastolic flow," you say renal vein thrombosis
- When I say "sickle cell trait," you say medullary RCC
- When I say "Young Adult, Renal Mass, + Severe HTN," you say Juxtaglomerular Cell Tumor
- When I say "squamous cell bladder CA," you say Schistosomiasis
- When I say "entire bladder calcified," you say Schistosomiasis
- When I say "urachus," you say adenocarcinoma of the bladder
- When I say "long stricture in urethra," you say Gonococcal
- When I say "short stricture in urethra," you say Straddle Injury
- When I say "Unicornuate Uterus," you say Look at the kidneys
- When I say "T-Shaped Uterus," you say DES related or Vaginal Clear Cell CA
- When I say "Marked enlargement of the uterus," you say Adenomyosis
- When I say "Adenomyosis," you say thickening of the junctional zone (> 12 mm)
- When I say "Wolffian duct remnant," you say Gartner Duct Cyst
- When I say "Theca Lutein Cysts," you say moles and multiple gestations
- When I say "Theca Lutein Cysts + Pleural Effusions," you say - Hyperstimulation Syndrome (patient on fertility meds).
- When I say "Low level internal echoes," you say Endometrioma
- When I say "T2 Shortening," you say - Endometrioma - "Shading Sign"
- When I say "Fishnet appearance," you say Hemorrhagic Cyst
- When I say "Ovarian Fibroma + Pleural Effusion," you say Meigs Syndrome
- When I say "Snow Storm Uterus, " you say Complete Mole - 1st Trimester
- When I say "Serum β-hCG levels that rise in the 8 to 10 weeks following evacuation of molar pregnancy," you say Choriocarcinoma
- When I say "midline cystic structure near the back of the bladder of a man," you say Prostatic Utricle
- When I say "lateral cystic structure near the back of the bladder of a man," you say Seminal Vesicle Cyst
- When I say "isolated orchitis," you say mumps
- When I say "onion skin appearance," you say epidermoid cyst
- When I say "multiple hypoechoic masses in the testicle," you say lymphoma
- When I say "cystic elements and macro-calcifications in the testicle," you say Mixed Germ Cell Tumor
- When I say "homogenous and microcalcifications," you say seminoma
- When I say "gynecomastia + testicular tumor," you say Sertoli Leydig
- When I say "fetal macrosomia," you say Maternal Diabetes
- When I say "one artery adjacent to the bladder," you say two vessel cord

- When I say "painless vaginal bleeding in the third trimester," you say placenta previa
- When I say "mom doing cocaine," you say placenta abruption
- When I say "thinning of the myometrium - with turbulent doppler," you say placenta creta
- When I say "mass near the cord insertion, with flow pulsating at the fetal heart rate," you say placenta chorioangioma
- When I say "Cystic mass in the posterior neck -antenatal period," you say cystic hygroma.
- When I say "Pleural effusions, and Ascites on prenatal US," you say hydrops.
- When I say "Massively enlarged bilateral kidneys," you say ARPKD
- When I say "Twin peak sign," you say dichorionic diamniotic
- When I say "obliteration of Raider's Triangle," you say aberrant right subclavian
- When I say "flat waist sign," you say left lower lobe collapse
- When I say "terrorist + mediastinal widening," you say Anthrax
- When I say "bulging fissure," you say Klebsiella
- When I say "dental procedure gone bad, now with jaw osteo and pneumonia," you say Actinomycosis.
- When I say "culture negative pleural effusion, 3 months later with airspace opacity," you say TB
- When I say "hot-tub," you say Hypersensitivity Pneumonitis
- When I say "halo sign," you say Fungal Pneumonia - Invasive Aspergillus
- When I say "reverse halo or atoll sign," you say COP
- When I say "finger in glove," you say ABPA
- When I say "ABPA," you say Asthma
- When I say "septic emboli + jugular vein thrombus," you say Lemierre
- When I say "Lemierre," you say Fusobacterium Necrophorum
- When I say "Paraneoplatic syndrome with SIADH," you say Small Cell Lung CA
- When I say "Paraneoplatic syndrome with PTH," you say Squamous Cell CA
- When I say "Small Cell Lung CA + Proximal Weakness," you say Lambert Eaton
- When I say "Cavity fills with air, post pneumonectomy," you say Bronchopleural Fistula
- When I say "malignant bronchial tumor," you say carcinoid
- When I say "malignant tracheal tumor," you say Adenoid Cystic
- When I say "AIDS patient with lung nodules, pleural effusion, and lymphadenopathy," you say Lymphoma
- When I say "Gallium Negative," you say Kaposi
- When I say "Thallium Negative," you say PCP
- When I say "Macroscopic fat and popcorn calcifications," you say Hamartoma
- When I say "Bizarre shaped cysts," you say LCH
- When I say "Lung Cysts in a TS patient," you say LAM
- When I say "Panlobular Emphysema - NOT Alpha 1," you say Ritalin Lung
- When I say "Honeycombing," you say UIP
- When I say "The histology was heterogeneous," you say UIP
- When I say "Ground Glass with Sub pleural Sparing," you say NSIP
- When I say "UIP Lungs + Parietal Pleural Thickening," you say Asbestosis
- When I say "Cavitation in the setting of silicosis," you say TB
- When I say "Air trapping seen 6 months after lung transplant," you say Chronic Rejection / Bronchiolitis Obliterans Syndrome
- When I say "Crazy Paving," you say PAP
- When I say "History of constipation," you say Lipoid Pneumonia - inferring mineral oil use / aspiration.
- When I say "UIP + Air trapping," you say Chronic Hypersensitivity Pneumonitis
- When I say "Dilated Esophagus + ILD," = Scleroderma (with NSIP)
- When I say "Shortness of breath when sitting up," you say Hepatopulmonary syndrome
- When I say "Episodic hypoglycemia," you say solitary fibrous tumor of the pleura
- When I say "Pulmonary HTN with Normal Wedge Pressure," you say Pulmonary Veno-occlusive disease.
- When I say "Yellow Nails" you say Edema and Chylous Pleural Effusions (Yellow Nail Syndrome).
- When I say "persistent fluid collection after pleural drain/tube placement," you say Extrapleural Hematoma.
- When I say "Displaced extrapleural fat," you say Extrapleural Hematoma.
- When I say "Massive air leak, in the setting of trauma," you say bronchial or tracheal injury
- When I say "Hot on PET – around the periphery," you say pulmonary infarct

- When I say "Multi-lobar collapse," you say sarcoid
- When I say "Classic bronchial infection," you say TB
- When I say "Panbronchiolitis," you say tree in bud (not centrilobular or random nodules)
- When I say "Bronchorrhea," you say Mucinous BAC
- When I say "ALCAPA," you say Steal Syndrome
- When I say "Supra-valvular Aortic Stenosis" you say Williams Syndrome
- When I say "Bicuspid Aortic Valve and Coarctation" you say Turners Syndrome
- When I say "Isolated right upper lobe edema," you say Mitral Regurgitation
- When I say "Peripheral pulmonary stenosis," you say Alagille Syndrome
- When I say "Box shaped heart", you say Ebsteins
- When I say "Right Arch with Mirror Branching," you say congenital heart.
- When I say "hand/thumb defects + ASD," you say Holt Oram
- When I say "ostium primum ASD (or endocardial cushion defect)," you say Downs
- When I say "Right Sided PAPVR," you say Sinus Venosus ASD
- When I say "Calcification in the left atrium wall," you say Rheumatic Heart Disease
- When I say "difficult to suppress myocardium," you say Amyloid
- When I say "blood pool suppression on delayed enhancement," you say Amyloid
- When I say "septal bounce," you say constrictive pericarditis
- When I say "ventricular interdependence," you say constrictive pericarditis
- When I say "focal thickening of the septum - but not Hypertrophic Cardiomyopathy," you say Sarcoid.
- When I say "ballooning of the left ventricular apex," you say Tako-Tsubo
- When I say "fat in the wall of a dilated right ventricle," you say Arrhythmogenic Right Ventricular Cardiomyopathy (ARVC)
- When I say "kid with dilated heart and mid wall enhancement," you say Muscular Dystrophy
- When I say "Cardiac Rhabdomyoma," you say Tuberous Sclerosis
- When I say "Bilateral Ventricular Thrombus," you say Eosinophilic Cardiomyopathy
- When I say "Diffuse LV Subendocardial enhancement not restricted to a vascular distribution," you say Cardiac Amyloid.
- When I say "Glenn Procedure," you say acquired pulmonary AVMs
- When I say "Pulmonary Vein Stenosis," you say Ablation for A-Fib
- When I say "Multiple Cardiac Myxomas," you say Carney's Complex
- When I say "vessel in the fissure of the ligamentum venosum," you say replaced left hepatic artery.
- When I say "vessel coursing on the pelvic brim," you say Corona Mortis
- When I say "ascending aorta calcifications," you say Syphilis and Takayasu
- When I say "tulip bulb aorta," you say Marfans
- When I say "really shitty Marfan's variant," you say Loeys-Dietz
- When I say "tortuous vessels," you say Loeys-Dietz
- When I say "renal artery stenosis with HTN in a child," you say NF-1
- When I say "nasty looking saccular aneurysm, without intimal calcifications" you say Mycotic.
- When I say "tree bark intimal calcification," you say Syphilitic (Luetic) aneurysm
- When I say "painful aneurysm in smoker, sparing the posterior wall," you say Inflammatory aneurysm.
- When I say "Turkish guy with pulmonary artery aneurysm," you say Behcets
- When I say "GI bleed with early opacification of a dilated draining vein," you say Colonic Angiodysplasia
- When I say "spider web appearance of hepatic veins on angiogram," you say Budd Chiari
- When I say "non-decompressible varicocele," you say look in the belly for badness
- When I say "right sided varicocele," you say look in the belly for badness
- When I say "swollen left leg," you say May Thurner
- When I say "popliteal aneurysm," you say look for the AAA (and the other leg)
- When I say "most dreaded complication of popliteal aneurysm," you say distal emboli
- When I say "Great saphenous vein on the wrong side of the calf - lateral side," you say Marginal Vein of Servelle - which is supposedly pathognomonic for Klippel-Trenaunay Syndrome
- When I say "Asian," you say Takayasu
- When I say "Involves the aorta," you say Takayasu
- When I say "Kids with vertigo and aortitis," you say Cogan Syndrome
- When I say "Nasal perforation + Cavitary Lung Lesions," you say Wegeners
- When I say "diffuse pulmonary hemorrhage," you say Microscopic Polyangitis
- When I say "Smoker + Hand Angiogram," you say Buergers
- When I say "Construction worker + Hand Angiogram," you say Hypothenar Hammer

- When I say "Unilateral tardus parvus in the carotid," you say stenosis of the innominate
- When I say "Bilateral tardus parvus in the carotids," you say aortic stenosis
- When I say "Bilateral reversal of flow in carotids," you say aortic regurg
- When I say "Lack of diastolic flow on carotid US," you say Brain Death
- When I say IVC greater than 28 mm, you sat Mega Cava
- When I say Mega Cava, you say Birds Nest Filter
- When I say "Hairpin turn - during bronchial angiography," you say anterior medullary (spinal cord) artery
- When I say "Fever, WBC, Nausea, and Vomiting after Uterine Artery Embolization," you say Post Embolization Syndrome (obviously could also be infection)
- When I say "Most medial vessel in the leg," you say posterior tibial artery
- When I say "the source of 85% of upper GI bleeds," you say left gastric artery
- When I say "the source of bleeding from a duodenal ulcer," you say GDA
- When I say "Pulmonary AVM," you say HHT
- When I say "most feared complication of bronchial artery embolization," you say spinal cord infarct
- When I say "high risk of bleeding for liver transplant," you say transjugular approach
- When I say "most feared complication of brachial arterial access," you say compartment syndrome
- When I say "cold painful fingers during dialysis," you say "Steal syndrome"
- When I say "ulcer on medial ankle," you say venous stasis
- When I say "ulcer on dorsum of foot," you say ischemia or infected ulcer
- When I say "ulcer on plantar surface of foot," you say neutropenic ulcer\
- When I say "pulsatile lower limb venous doppler," you say right heart failure.
- When I say "hot clumps of signal in the lungs on Liver Spleen sulfur colloid," you say too much Al in the Tc.
- When I say "HOT spleen," you say WBC scan or Octreotide (sulfur colloid will be a warm spleen.
- When I say "Bone Scan with Hot Skull Sutures," you say renal osteodystrophy
- When I say "Bone Scan with Focal Breast Uptake," you say breast CA
- When I say "Bone Scan with Renal Cortex Activity," you say hemochromatosis
- When I say "Bone Scan with Liver Activity," you say either too much Al, Amyloid, Hepatoma, or Liver Necrosis
- When I say "Bone Scan with Sternal Lesion," you say breast CA.
- When I say "Bone Scan with Diffusely Decreased Bone Uptake," you say (1) Free Tc, or (2) Bisphosphonate Therapy.
- When I say "Tramline along periosteum of long bones," you say lung CA
- When I say "Super Hot Mandible in Adult," you say Fibrous Dysplasia
- When I say "Super Hot Mandible in Child," you say Caffeys
- When I say "Periarticular uptake on delayed scan," you say RSD
- When I say "Focal uptake along the lesser trochanter," you say Prosthesis loosening
- When I say "Tracer in the brain on a VQ study," you say Shunt
- When I say "Tracer over the liver on Ventilation with Xenon," you say Fatty Liver
- When I say "Gallium Negative, Thallium Positive," you say Kaposi
- When I say "High T3, High T4, low TSH, - low thyroid uptake," you say Quervains (Granulomatous thyroiditis).
- When I say "persistent tracer in the lateral ventricles > 24 hours," you say NPH
- When I say "Renal uptake on sulfur colloid," you say CHF
- When I say "Renal transplant uptake on sulfur colloid", you say Rejection
- When I say "Filtered Renal Agent," you say DTPA (or GH)
- When I say "Secreted Renal Agent," you say MAG-3
- When I say "PET with increased muscle uptake," you say insulin
- When I say "Diffuse FDG uptake in the thyroid on PET," you say Hashimoto
- When I say "I see the skeleton on MIBG," you say diffuse neuroblastoma bone mets
- When I say "Cardiac tissue taking up FDG more intense than normal myocaridum," you say hibernating myocardium

- I say "made with a generator", you say Tc99 and Rubidium
- When I say "cervical kyphosis", you say NF-1
- When I say "lateral thoracic meningocele," you say NF-1
- When I say "bilateral optic nerve gliomas," you say NF-1
- When I say "bilateral vestibular schwannoma," you say NF-2
- When I say "retinal hamartoma," you say TS
- When I say "retinal angioma," you say VHL
- When I say "brain tumor with restricted diffusion," you say lymphoma
- When I say "brain tumor crossing the midline," you say GBM (or lymphoma)
- When I say "Cyst and Nodule in Child," you say Pilocystic Astrocytoma
- When I say "Cyst and Nodule in Adult," you say Hemangioblastoma
- When I say "multiple hemangioblastoma," you say Von Hippel Lindau
- When I say "Swiss cheese tumor in ventricle," you say central neurocytoma
- When I say "CN3 Palsy," you say posterior communicating artery aneurysm
- When I say "CN6 Palsy," you say increased ICP
- When I say "Ventricles out of size to atrophy," you say NPH
- When I say "Hemorrhagic putamen," you say Methanol
- When I say "Decreased FDG uptake in the lateral occipital cortex," you say Lewy Body Dementia
- When I say "TORCH with Periventricular Calcification," you say CMV
- When I say "TORCH with hydrocephalus," you say Toxoplasmosis
- When I say "TORCH with hemorrhagic infarction," you say HSV
- When I say "Neonatal infection with frontal lobe atrophy," you say HIV
- When I say "Rapidly progressing dementia + Rapidly progressing atrophy," you say CJD
- When I say "Expanding the cortex," Oligodendroglioma
- When I say "Tumor acquired after trauma (LP)," you say Epidermoid
- When I say "The Palate Separated from the Maxilla / Floating Palate," you say LeFort 1
- When I say "The Maxilla Separated from the Face" or "Pyramidal" you say LeFort 2
- When I say "The Face Separated from the Cranium," you say LeFort 3
- When I say "Airless expanded sinus," you say mucocele
- When I say "DVA," you say cavernous malformation nearby
- When I say "Single vascular lesion in the pons," you say Capillary Telangiectasia
- When I say "Elevated NAA peak," you say Canavans
- When I say "Tigroid appearance," you say Metachromatic Leukodystrophy
- When I say "Endolymphatic Sac Tumor," you say VHL
- When I say "T1 Bright in the petrous apex," you say Cholesterol Granuloma
- When I say "Restricted diffusion in the petrous apex," you say Cholesteatoma
- When I say "Lateral rectus palsy + otomastoiditis," you say Grandenigo Syndrome
- When I say "Cochlear and semicircular canal enhancement," you say Labyrinthitis
- When I say "Conductive hearing loss in an adult," you say Otosclerosis
- When I say "Noise induced vertigo," you say Superior Semicircular Canal dehiscence
- When I say "Widening of the maxillary ostium," you say Antrochonal Polyp
- When I say "Inverting papilloma," you say squamous cell CA (10%)
- When I say "Adenoid cystic," you say perineural spread
- When I say "Left sided vocal cord paralysis," you say look in the AP window
  When I say "Bilateral coloboma," you say CHARGE syndrome
- When I say "Retinal Detachment + Small Eye" you say PHPV
- When I say "Bilateral Small Eye," you say Retinopathy of Prematurity
- When I say "Calcification in the globe of a child," you say Retinoblastoma
- When I say "Fluid-Fluid levels in the orbit," you say Lymphangioma
- When I say "Orbital lesion, worse with Valsalva," you say Varix
- When I say "Pulsatile Exophthalmos," you say NF-1 and CC Fistula
- When I say "Sphenoid wing dysplasia," you say NF-1
- When I say "Scimitar Sacrum," you Currarino Triad
- When I say "bilateral symmetrically increased T2 signal in dorsal columns," you say B12 (or HIV)
- When I say "Owl eye appearance of spinal cord," you say spinal cord infarct
- When I say "Enhancement of the nerve roots of the cauda equina," you say Guillain Barre
- When I say "Subligamentous spread of infection," you say TB
- When I say, "Posterior elbow dislocation," you say Capitellum fracture

- When I say "Chondroblastoma in an adult", you say "Clear Cell Chondrosarcoma"
- When I say "Malignant epiphyseal lesion", you say "Clear Cell Chondrosarcoma"
- When I say "Permeative lesion in the diaphysis of a child" , you say "Ewings"
- When I say "T2 bright lesion in the sacrum" , you say "Chordoma"
- When I say "Lytic T2 DARK lesion" , you say "Fibrosarcoma"
- When I say "Sarcomatous transformation of an infarct", you say "MFH"
- When I say, "Epiphyseal Lesion that is NOT T2 Bright" , You say Chondroblastoma
- When I say, "short 4th metacarpal," You say pseudopseudohypoparathyroidism and Turner Syndrome
- When I say, "band like acro-osteolysis," You say Hajdu-Cheney
- When I say "fat containing tumor in the retroperitoneum," you say liposarcoma
- When I say "sarcoma in the foot" you say synovial sarcoma.
- When I say "avulsion of the lesser trochanter," you say pathologic fracture
- When I say "cross over sign," you say pincher type Femoroacetabular Impingement
- When I say "Segond Fracture," you say ACL tear
- When I say "Reverse Segond Fracture," you say PCL
- When I say "Arcuate Sign," you say fibular head avulsion or PCL tear
- When I say "Deep Intercondylar Notch," you say ACL tear
- When I say "Bilateral Patellar Tendon Ruptures," you say chronic steroids
- When I say "Wide ankle mortise," you say show me the proximal fibula (Maisonneuve).
- When I say "Bilateral calcaneal fractures," you say associated spinal compression fx ("lover's leap")
- When I say "Dancer with lateral foot pain," you say avulsion of 5th MT
- When I say "Old lady with sudden knee pain with standing," you say SONK
- When I say "Looser's Zones," you say osteomalacia or rickets (vitamin D)
- When I say "Unilateral RA with preserved joint spaces," you say RSD
- When I say "T2 bright tumor in finger," you say Glomus
- When I say "Blooming in tumor in finger," you say Giant Cell Tumor of Tendon Sheath (PVNS)
- When I say "Atrophy of teres minor," you say Quadrilateral Space syndrome
- When I say "Subluxation of the Biceps Tendon," you say Subscapularis tear
- When I say "Too many bow ties," you say Discoid Meniscus
- When I say "Celery Stalk ACL - T2" you say Mucoid Degeneration
- When I say "Drumstick ACL - T1" you say Mucoid Degeneration
- When I say "Acute Flat foot," you say Posterior Tibial Tendon Tear
- When I say "Boomerang shaped peroneus brevis," you say tear - or split tear
- When I say "Meniscoid mass in the lateral ankle," you say Anteriolateral Impingement Syndrome
- When I say "Scar between 3rd and 4th metatarsals," you say Morton's neuroma
- When I say "Osteomyelitis in the spine," you say IV drug user
- When I say "Osteomyelitis in the spine with Kyphosis," you say TB (Gibbus Deformity)
- When I say "Unilateral SI joint lysis," you say IV Drug User
- When I say "Psoas muscle abscess," you say TB
- When I say "Rice bodies in joint," you say TB - sloughed synovium
- When I say "Calcification along the periphery," you say myositis ossificans
- When I say "Calcifications more dense in the center," you say Osteosarcoma - reverse zoning
- When I say "Permeative lesion in the diaphysis of a child," you say Ewings
- When I say "Long lesion in a long bone," you say Fibrous Dysplasia
- When I say "Large amount of edema for the size of the lesion," you say Osteoid Osteoma
- When I say "Cystic bone lesion, that is NOT T2 bright," you say Chondroblastoma
- When I say "Lesion in the finger of a kid," you say Periosteal chondroma
- When I say "looks like NOF in the anterior tibia with anterior bowing," you say Osteofibrous Dysplasia.
- When I say " RA + Pneumoconiosis," you say Caplan Syndrome

- When I say " RA + Big Spleen + Neutropenia," you say Felty Syndrome
- When I say "Epiphyseal Overgrowth," you say JRA (or hemophilia).
- When I say "Reducible deformity of joints - in hand," you say Lupus.
- When I say "destructive mass in a bone of a leukemia patient," you say Chloroma
- When I say "shrinking breast," you say ILC
- When I say "thick Coopers ligaments," you say edema (CHF)
- When I say "thick fuzzy coopers ligaments - with normal skin," you say blur
- When I say "dashes but no dots," you say Secretory Calcifications
- When I say "cigar shaped calcifications," you say Secretory Calcifications
- When I say "popcorn calcifications," you say degenerated fibroadenoma
- When I say "breast within a breast," you say hamartoma
- When I say "fat-fluid level," you say galactocele
- When I say "rapid growing fibroadenoma," you say Phyllodes
- When I say "swollen red breast, not responding to antibiotics," you say Inflammatory breast CA
- When I say "lines radiating to a single point," you say Architectural distortion.
- When I say "Architectural distortion + Calcifications," you say IDC + DCIS
- When I say "Architectural distortion without Calcifications," you say ILC
- When I say "Stepladder Sign," you say Intracapsular rupture on US
- When I say "Linguine Sign," you say Intracapsular rupture on MRI
- When I say "Residual Calcs in the Lumpectomy Bed," you say local recurrence
- When I say "No Calcs in the core," you say milk of calcium (requires polarized light to be seen).

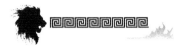
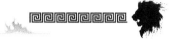
- Pulmonary Interstitial Emphysema (PIE) - put the bad side down
- Bronchial Foreign Body - put the lucency side down (if it stays that way, it's positive)
- Papillomatosis has a small (2%) risk of squamous cell CA
- Pulmonary sling is the only variant that goes between the esophagus and the trachea. This is associated with trachea stenosis.
- Thymic Rebound – Seen after stress (chemotherapy) – Can be PET-Avid
- Lymphoma – Most common mediastinal mass in child (over 10)
- Anterior Mediastinal Mass with Calcification – Either treated lymphoma, or Thymic Lesion (lymphoma doesn't calcify unless treated).
- Neuroblastoma is the most common posterior mediastinal mass in child under 2 (primary thoracic does better than abd).
- Hypertrophic Pyloric Stenosis - NOT at birth, NOT after 3 months (3 weeks to 3 months)
- Criteria for HPS - 4 mm and 14 mm (4mm single wall, 14mm length).
- Annular Pancreas presents as duodenal obstruction in children and pancreatitis in adults.
- Most common cause of bowel obstruction in child over 4 = Appendicitis
- Intussusception - 3 months to 3 years is ok, earlier or younger think lead point
- Gastroschisis is ALWAYS on the right side
- Omphalocele has associated anomalies (gastroschisis does not).
- Physiologic Gut Hernia normal at 6-8 weeks
- AFP is elevated with Hepatoblastoma
- Endothelial growth factor is elevated with Hemangioendothelioma
- Most Common cause of pancreatitis in a kid = Trauma (seatbelt)
- Weigert Meyer Rule - Duplicated ureter on top inserts inferior and medial
- Most common tumor of the fetus or infant - Sacrococcygeal Teratoma
- Most common cause of idiopathic scrotal edema - HSP
- Most common cause of acute scrotal pain age 7-14 - Torsion of Testicular Appendages
- Bell Clapper Deformity is the etiology for testicular torsion.
- SCFE is a Salter Harris Type 1
- Physiologic Periostitis of the Newborn doesn't occur in a newborn - seen around 3 months
- Acetabular Angle should be < 30, and Alpha angle should be more than 60.
- Most Common benign mucosal lesion of the esophagus = Papilloma
- Esophageal Webs have increased risk for cancer, and Plummer-Vinson Syndrome (anemia + web)
- Dysphagia Lusoria is from compression by a right subclavian artery (most patients with aberrant rights don't have symptoms).
- Achalasia has an increased risk of squamous cell cancer (20 years later)
- Most common mesenchymal tumor of the GI tract = GIST
- Most common location for GIST = Stomach
- Abscesses are almost exclusively seen in Crohns (rather than UC)
- Nodes + UC = Common in the setting of active disease
- Nodes (larger than 1cm) + Crohns = Cancer

- Diverticulosis + Nodes = Cancer (maybe) -> next step endoscopy.
- Krukenberg Tumor = Stomach (GI) met to the ovary
- Menetrier's involves fundus and spares the antrum
- The stomach is the most common location for sarcoid (in the GI tract)
- Gastric Remnants have an increased risk of cancer years after Billroth
- Most common internal hernia = Left sided paraduodenal
- Most common site of peritoneal carcinomatosis = retrovesical space
- An injury to the bare area of the liver can cause a retroperitoneal bleed
- Primary Sclerosing Cholangitis associated with Ulcerative Colitis
- Extrahepatic ducts are normal with Primary Biliary Cirrhosis
- Anti-mitochondrial Antibodies - positive with primary biliary cirrhosis
- Mirizzi Syndrome - the stone in the cystic duct obstructs the CBD
- Mirizzi has a 5x increased risk of GB cancer.
- Dorsal pancreatic agenesis - associated with diabetes and polysplenia
- Hereditary and Tropical Pancreatitis - early age of onset, increased risk of cancer
- Felty's Syndrome - Big Spleen, RA, and Neutropenia
- Splenic Artery Aneurysm - more common in women, and more likely to rupture in pregnant women.
- Insulinoma is the most common islet cell tumor
- Gastrinoma is the most common islet cell tumor with MEN
- Ulcerative Colitis has an increased risk of colon cancer (if it involves colon past the splenic flexure). UC involving the rectum only does not increase risk of CA.
- Calcifications in a renal CA - are associated with an improved survival
- RCC bone mets are "always" lytic
- There is an increased risk of malignancy with dialysis
- Horseshoe kidneys are more susceptible to trauma
- Most common location for TCC is the bladder
- Second most common location for TCC is the upper urinary tract
- Upper Tract TCC is more commonly multifocal (12%) - as opposed to bladder (4%)
- The cysts in acquired renal cystic disease improve after renal transplant, although the risk of renal CA in the native kidney remains elevated. In fact, the cancers tend to be more aggressive because of the immunosuppressive therapy needed to not reject a transplant.
- Weigert Meyer Rule - Upper Pole inserts medial and inferior
- Ectopic Ureters are associated with incontinence in women (not men)
- Leukoplakia is pre-malignant; Malakoplakia is not pre-malignant
- Extraperitoneal bladder rupture is more common, and managed medically
- Intraperitoneal bladder rupture is less common, and managed surgically
- Indinavir (HIV medication) stones are the only ones not seen on CT.
- Uric Acid stones are not seen on plain film
- Endometrial tissue in a rudimentary horn (even one that does NOT communicate) increases the risk of miscarriage
- Arcuate Uterus does NOT have an increased risk of infertility (it's a normal variant)
- Fibroids with higher T2 signal respond better to UAE
- Hyaline Fibroid Degeneration is the most common subtype
- Adenomyosis - favors the posterior wall, spares the cervix

- Hereditary Non-Polyposis Colon Cancer (HNPCC) – have a 30-50x increased risk of endometrial cancer
- Tamoxifen increases the risk of endometrial cancer, and endometrial polyps
- Cervical Cancer that has parametrial involvement (2B) - is treated with chemo/radiation. Cervical Cancer without parametrial involvement (2A) - is treated with surgery
- Vaginal cancer in adults is usually squamous cell
- Vaginal Rhabdomyosarcoma occurs in children / teenagers
- Premenopausal ovaries can be hot on PET (depending on the phase of cycle). Post menopausal ovaries should Never be hot on PET.
- Transformation subtypes: Endometrioma = Clear Cell, Dermoid = Squamous
- Postpartum fever can be from ovarian vein thrombophlebitis
- Fractured penis = rupture of the corpus cavernosum and the surrounding tunica albuginea.
- Prostate Cancer is most commonly in the peripheral zone, - ADC dark
- BPH nodules are in the central zone
- Hypospadias is the most common association with prostatic utricle
- Seminal Vesicle cysts are associated with renal agenesis, and ectopic ureters
- Cryptorchidism increases the risk of cancer (in both testicles), and the risk is not reduced by orchiopexy
- Immunosuppressed patients can get testicular lymphoma -hiding behind blood testes barrier
- Most common cause of correctable infertility in a man is a varicocele.
- Undescended testicles are more common in premature kids.
- Membranes disrupted before 10 weeks, increased risk for amniotic bands
- The earliest visualization of the embryo is the "double bleb sign"
- Hematoma greater than 2/3 the circumference of the chorion has a 2x increased risk of abortion.
- Biparietal Diameter - Recorded at the level of the thalamus from the outermost edge of the near skull to the inner table of the far skull.
- Abdominal Circumference - does not include the subcutaneous soft tissues
- Abdominal Circumference is recorded at the the level of the junction of the umbilical vein and left portal vein
- Abdominal Circumference is the parameter classically involved with asymmetric IUGR
- Femur Length does NOT include the epiphysis
- Umbilical Artery Systolic / Diastolic Ratio should NOT exceed 3 at 34 weeks - makes you think pre-eclampsia and IUGR
- A full bladder can mimic a placenta previa
- Nuchal lucency is measured between 9-12 weeks, and should be < 3 mm. More than 3mm is associated with Downs.
- Lemon sign will disappear after 24 weeks
- Aquaductal Stenosis is the most common cause of non-communicating hydrocephalus in a neonate
- The tricuspid valve is the most anterior
- The pulmonic valve is the most superior
- There are 10 lung segments on the right, and 8 lung segments on the left
- If it goes above the clavicles, it's in the posterior mediastinum (cervicothoracic sign)
- Azygos Lobe has 4 layers of pleura
- Most common pulmonary vein variant is a separate vein draining the right middle lobe
- Most common cause of pneumonia in AIDS patient is Strep Pneumonia
- Most common opportunistic infection in AIDS = PCP.

- Aspergilloma is seen in a normal immune patient
- Invasive Aspergillus is seen in an immune compromised patient
- Fleischner Society Recommendations do NOT apply to patient's with known cancers
- Eccentric calcifications in a solitary pulmonary nodule pattern is considered the most suspicious.
- A part solid nodule with a ground glass component is the most suspicious morphology you can have
- Most common early presentation of lung CA is a solitary nodule (right upper lobe)
- Lung Fibrosis patients (UIP, etc…) more commonly have lower lobe CA
- Stage 3B lung CA is unresectable (contralateral nodal involvement ; ipsilateral or contralateral scalene or supraclavicular nodal involvement, tumor in different lobes).
- The most common cause of unilateral lymphangitic carcinomatosis is bronchogenic carcinoma lung cancer invading the lymphatics
- There is a 20 year latency between initial exposure and development of lung cancer or pleural mesothelioma
- Pleural effusion is the earliest and most common finding with asbestosis exposure.
- Silicosis actually raises your risk of TB by about 3 fold.
- Nitrogen Dioxide exposure is "Silo Filler's Disease," gives you a pulmonary edema pattern.
- Reticular pattern in the posterior costophrenic angle is supposedly the first finding of UIP on CXR
- Sarcoidosis is the most common recurrent primary disease after lung transplant
- Pleural plaque of asbestosis typically spares the costophrenic angles.
- Pleural effusion is the most common manifestation of mets to the pleura.
- There is an association with mature teratomas and Klinefelter Syndrome.
- Injury close to the carina is going to cause a pneumomediastinum rather than a pneumothorax
- Hodgkin Lymphoma spreads in a contiguous fashion from the mediastinum and is most often unilateral.
- Non-Hodgkin Lymphoma is typically bilateral with associated abdominal lymphadenopathy
- MRI is superior for assessing superior sulcus tumors because you need to look at the brachial plexus.
- Leiomyoma is the most common benign esophageal tumor (most common in the distal third).
- Esophageal Leiomyomatosis may be associated with Alport's Syndrome
- Bronchial / Tracheal injury must be evaluated with bronchoscopy
- If you say COP also say Eosinophilic Pneumonia
- If you say BAC also say lymphoma
- Bronchial Atresia is classically in the LUL
- Pericardial cysts MUST be simple, Bronchogenic cysts don't have to be simple
- PAP follows a rule of 1/3s post treatment; 1/3 gets better, 1/3 doesn't, 1/3 progresses to fibrosis
- Dysphagia Lusoria presents later in life as atherosclerosis develops
- Carcinoid is COLD on PET
- Wegener's is now called Granulomatosis with Polyangiitis – Wegener was a Nazi. Apparently he was not just a Nazi, he was a real asshole. I heard the guy used to take up two parking spots at the grocery store on Sunday afternoons.
- The right atrium is defined by the IVC.
- The right ventricle is defined by the moderator band.
- The tricuspid papillary muscles insert on the septum (mitral ones do not).
- Lipomatous Hypertrophy of the Intra-Atrial Septum - can be PET Avid (it's brown fat)
- LAD gives off diagonals
- RCA gives off acute marginals
- LCX gives off obtuse marginals
- RCA perfuses SA and AV nodes (most of the time)
- Dominance is decided by which vessel gives off the posterior descending - it's the right 85%
- LCA from the Right Coronary Cusp - always gets repaired
- RCA from the Left Coronary Cusp - repaired if symptoms
- Most common location of myocardial bridging is in the mid portion of the LAD.
- Coronary Artery Aneurysm - most common cause in adult = Atherosclerosis
- Coronary Artery Aneurysm - most common cause in child = Kawasaki
- Left Sided SVC empties into the coronary sinus

- Rheumatic heart disease is the most common cause of mitral stenosis
- Pulmonary Arterial Hypertension is the most common cause of tricuspid atresia.
- Most common vascular ring is the double aortic arch
- Most common congenital heart disease is a VSD
- Most common ASD is the Secundum
- Infracardiac TAPVR classically shown with pulmonary edema in a newborn
- "L" Transposition type is congenitally corrected (they are "L"ucky).
- "D" Transposition type is doomed.
- Truncus is associated with CATCH-22 (DiGeorge)
- Rib Notching from coarctation spares the 1st and 2nd Ribs
- Infarct with > 50% involvement is unlikely to recover function
- Microvascular Obstruction is NOT seen in chronic infarct
- Amyloid is the most common cause of restricted cardiomyopathy
- Primary amyloid can be seen in multiple myeloma
- Most common neoplasm to involve the cardiac valves = Fibroelastoma
- Most commonly the congenital absence of the pericardium is partial and involves the pericardium over the left atrium and adjacent pulmonary artery (*the left atrial appendage is the most at risk to become strangulated*).
- Glenn shunt - SVC to pulmonary artery (vein to artery)
- Blalock-Taussig Shunt - Subclavian Artery to Pulmonary Artery (artery - artery)
- Ross Procedure - Replaces aortic valve with pulmonic, and pulmonic with a graft (done for kids).
- Aliasing is common with Cardiac MRI. You can fix it by: (1) opening your FOV, (2) oversampling the frequency encoding direction, or (3) switching phase and frequency encoding directions.
- Giant Coronary Artery Aneurysms (> 8mm) don't regress, and are associated with MIs.
- Wet Beriberi (thiamine def) can cause a dilated cardiomyopathy.
- Most common primary cardiac tumor in children = Rhabdomyoma.
- 2nd most common primary cardiac tumor in children = Fibroma
- Most common complication of MI is myocardial remodeling.
- Unroofed coronary sinus is associated with Persistent left SVC.
- Most common source of cardiac mets = Lung Cancer (lymphoma #2).
- A-Fib is most commonly associated with left atrial enlargement
- Most common cause of tricuspid insufficiency is RVH (usually from pulmonary HTN / cor pulmonale).
- Artery of Adamkiewicz comes off on the left side (70%) between T8-L1 (90%)
- Arch of Riolan - middle colic branch of the SMA with the left colic of the IMA.
- Most common hepatic vascular variant = right hepatic artery replaced off the SMA
- The proper right hepatic artery is anterior the right portal vein, whereas the replaced right hepatic artery is posterior to the main portal vein.
- Accessory right inferior hepatic vein - most common hepatic venous variant.
- Anterior tibialis is the first branch off the popliteal
- Common Femoral Artery (CFA): Begins at the level of inguinal ligament
- Superficial Femoral Artery (SFA): Begins once the CFA gives off the profunda femoris
- Popliteal Artery: Begins as the SFA exits the adductor canal
- Popliteal Artery terminates as the anterior tibial artery and the tibioperoneal trunk
- Axillary Artery: Begins at the first rib
- Brachial Artery: Begins as it crosses the teres major
- Brachial Artery: Bifurcates to the ulnar and radial artery
- Intraosseous Branch: Typically arises from the ulnar artery
- Superficial Arch = From the Ulna, Deep Arch = From the Radius
- The "coronary vein," is the left gastric vein
- Enlarged splenorenal shunts are associated with hepatic encephalopathy.
- Aortic Dissection, and intramural hematoma are caused by HTN (70%)
- Penetrating Ulcer is from atherosclerosis.

- Strongest predictor of progression of dissection in intramural hematoma = Maximum aortic diameter > 5cm.
- Leriche Syndrome Triad: Claudication, Absent/ Decreased femoral pulses, Impotence.
- Most common associated defect with aortic coarctation = bicuspid aorta (80%)
- Neurogenic compression is the most common subtype of thoracic outlet syndrome
- Splenic artery aneurysm - More common in pregnancy, more likely to rupture in pregnancy.
- Median Arcuate Compression - worse with expiration
- Colonic Angiodysplasia is associated with aortic stenosis
- Popliteal Aneurysm; 30-50% have AAA, 10% of patient with AAA have popliteal aneurysm, 50-70% of popliteal aneurysms are bilateral.
- Medial deviation of the popliteal artery by the medial head of the gastrocnemius = Popliteal Entrapment
- Type 3 Takayasu is the most common (arch + abdominal aorta).
- Most common vasculitis in a kid = HSP (Henoch-Schonlein Purpura)
- Tardus Parvus infers stenosis proximal to that vessel
- ICA Peak Systolic Velocity < 125 = "No Significant Stenosis" or < 50%
- ICA Peak Systolic Velocity 125-230 = 50-69% Stenosis or "Moderate"
- ICA Peak Systolic Velocity > 230 = >70% Stenosis or "Severe"
- 18G needle will accept a 0.038 inch guidewire,
- 19G needle will allow a 0.035 inch guidewire.
- Notice that 0.039, 0.035, 0.018 wires are in INCHES
- 3 French = 1 mm
- French size is the OUTSIDE of a catheter and the INSIDE of a sheath
- End Hole Only Catheters = Hand Injection Only
- Side Hole + End Hole = Power Injection OK, Coils NOT ok
- Double Flush Technique = For Neuro IR — no bubbles ever
- "Significant lesion" = A systolic pressure gradient > 10 mm Hg at rest
- Things to NOT stick a drain in: Tumors, Acute Hematoma, and those associated with acute bowel rupture and peritonitis
- Renal Artery Stenting for renal failure - tends to not work if the Cr is > 3.
- Persistent sciatic artery is prone to aneurysm
- Even if the cholecystostomy tube instantly resolves all symptoms, you need to leave the tube in for 2-6 weeks (until the tract matures), otherwise you are going to get a bile leak.
- MELD scores greater than 24 are at risk of early death with TIPS
- The target gradient post TIPS (for esophageal bleeding) is between 9 and 11.
- Absolute contraindication for TIPS - Heart Failure, Severe Hepatic Failure
- Most common side effect of BRTO is gross hematuria
- Sensitivity = GI Bleed Scan = 0.1mL/min , Angiography = 1.0 mL/min
- For GI Bleed - after performing an embolization of the GDA (for duodenal ulcer), you need to do a run of the SMA to look at the inferior pancreaticoduodenal
- Most common cause of lower GI bleed is diverticulosis
- TACE will prolong survival better than systemic chemo
- TACE: Portal Vein Thrombosis is considered a contraindication (sometimes) because of the risk of infarcting the liver.
- Go above the rib for Thora
- Left Bundle Branch Block needs a pacer before a Thoracic Angiogram
- Never inject contrast through a Swan Ganz catheter for a thoracic angiogram
- You treat pulmonary AVMs at 3mm
- Hemoptysis - Active extravasation is NOT typically seen with the active bleed.
- UAE - Gonadotropin-releasing medications (often prescribed for fibroids) should be stopped for 3 months prior to the case
- The general rule for transgluteal is to avoid the sciatic nerves and gluteal arteries by access through the sacrospinous ligament medially (close to the sacrum, inferior to the piriformis).
- When to pull an abscess catheter; As a general rule – when the patient is better (no fever, WBC normal), and output is < 20 cc over 24 hours.

- If the thyroid biopsy is non-diagnostic, you have to wait 3 months before you re-biopsy.
- Posterior lateral approach is the move for percutaneous nephrostomy
- You can typically pull a sheath with an ACT < 150-180
- Artery calcifications (common in diabetics) make compression difficult, and can lead to a false elevation of the ABI.
- Type 2 endoleaks are the most common
- Type 1 and Type 3 endoleaks are high pressure and need to be fixed stat
- Venous rupture during a fistula intervention can ofter be treated with prolonged angioplasty (always leave the balloon on the wire).
- Phlegmasia alba = massive DVT, without ischemia and preserved collateral veins.
- Phlegmasia cerulea dolens = massive DVT, complete thrombosis of the deep venous system, including the collateral circulation.
- You are more likely to develop Venous Thromboembolism if you are paraplegic vs tetraplegic.
- Circumaortic left renal vein: the anterior one is superior, the posterior one is inferior, and the filter should be below the lowest one.
- Risk of DVT is increased with IVC filters
- Filter with clot > 1cm³ of clot = Filter Stays In
- Acute Budd Chiari with fulminant liver failure = Needs a TIPS
- Pseudoaneurysm of the pancreaticoduodenal artery = "Sandwich technique" - distal and proximal segments of the artery feeding off the artery must be embolized
- Median Arcuate Ligament Syndrome - First line is surgical release of the ligament
- Massive Hemoptysis = Bronchial artery - Particles bigger than 325 micrometers
- Acalculous Cholecystitis = Percutaneous Cholecystostomy
- Hepatic encephalopathy after TIPS = You can either (1) place a new covered stent constricted in the middle by a loop of suture - deployed in the pre-existing TIPS, (2) place two new stents - parallel to each other (one covered self expandable, one uncovered balloon expandable).
- Recurrent variceal bleeding after placement of a constricted stent - balloon dilation of the constricted stent
- Appendiceal Abscess - Drain placement * just remember that a drain should be used for a mature (walled off) abscess and no frank pertioneal symptoms
- Inadvertent catheterization of the colon (after trying to place a drain in an abscess) - wait 4 weeks for the tract to mature - verify by over the wire tractogram, and then remove tube.
- DVT with severe symptoms and no response to systemic anticoagulation = Catheter Directed Thrombolysis
- Geiger Mueller - maximum dose it can handle is about 100mR/h
- Activity level greater than 100 mCi of Tc-99m is considered a major spill.
- Activity level greater than 100 mCi of Tl-201 is considered a major spill.
- Activity level greater than 10 mCi of In-111, is considered to represent a major spill.
- Activity level greater than 10 mCi of Ga-67, is considered to represent a major spill.
- An activity level greater than 1 mCi of I-131 is considered to constitute a major spill.
- Annual Dose limit of 100 mrem to the public
- Not greater than 2 mrem per hour – in an "unrestricted area"
- Total Body Dose per Year = 5 rem
- Total equivalent organ dose (skin is also an organ) per year = 50 rem
- Total equivalent extremity dose per year = 50 rem (500mSv)
- Total Dose to Embryo/fetus over entire 9 months – 0.5rem
- NRC allows no more than 0.15 micro Ci of Mo per 1 mili Ci of Tc, at the time of administration.
- Chemical purity (Al in Tc) is done with pH paper
- The allowable amount of Al is < 10 micrograms
- Radiochemical purity (looking for Free Tc) is done with thin layer chromatography
- Free Tc occurs from - lack of stannous ions or accidental air injection (which oxidizes)

- Prostate Cancer bone mets are uncommon with a PSA less than 10 mg/ml
- Flair Phenomenon occurs 2 weeks - 3 months after therapy
- Skeletal Survey is superior (more sensitive) for lytic mets
- AVN - Early and Late is COLD, Middle (repairing) is Hot.
- Particle size for VQ scan is 10-100 micrometers
- Xenon is done first during the VQ scan
- Amiodarone - classic thyroid uptake blocker
- Hashimotos increases risk for lymphoma
- Hot nodule on Tc, shouldn't be considered benign until you show that it's also hot on I[123]. This is the concept of the discordant nodule.
- History of methimazole treatment (even years prior) makes I-131 treatment more difficult
- Methimazole side effect is neutropenia
- In pregnancy PTU is the blocker of choice
- Sestamibi in the parathyroid depends on blood flow and mitochondria
- You want to image with PET - following therapy at interval of 2-3 weeks for chemotherapy, and 8-12 weeks for radiation is the way to go. This avoids "stunning" – false negatives, and inflammatory induced false positive.
- [111]In Pentetreotide is the most commonly used agent for somatostatin receptor imaging. The classic use is for carcinoid tumors
- Meningiomas take up octreotide
- In 111 binds to neutrophils, lymphocytes, monocytes and even RBCs and platelets
- Tc99m HMPAO binds to neutrophils
- WBCs may accumulate at post op surgical sites for 2-3 weeks
- Prior to MIBG you should block the thyroid with Lugols Iodine or Perchlorate
- Scrotal Scintigraphy: The typical agent is Tc-99m Pertechnetate. This agent is used as both a flow agent and a pool agent.
- Left bundle branch block can cause a false positive defect in the ventricular septum (spares the apex)
- Pulmonary uptake of Thallium is an indication of LV dysfunction
- MIBG mechanism is that of an Analog of Norepinephrine - actively transported and stored in the neurosecretory granules
- MDP mechanism is that of a Phosphate analog - which works via Chemisorption
- Sulfur Colloid mechanism = Particles are Phagocytized by RES
- The order of tumor prevalence in NF2 is the same as the mnemonic MSME (schwannoma > meningioma > ependymoma).
- Maldeveloped draining veins is the etiology of Sturge Weber
- All phakomatosis (NF 1, NF -2, TS, and VHL) EXCEPT Sturge Weber are autosomal dominant - family screening is a good idea.
- Most Common Primary Brain Tumor in Adult = Astrocytoma
- "Calcifies 90% of the time" = Oligodendroglioma
- Restricted Diffusion in Ventricle = Watch out for Choroid Plexus Xanthogranuloma (not a brain tumor, a benign normal variant)
- Pituitary - T1 Big and Bright = Pituitary Apoplexy
- Pituitary - Normal T1 Bright = Posterior Part (because of storage of Vasopressin , and other storage proteins)
- Pituitary - T2 Bright = Rathke Cleft Cyst
- Pituitary – Calcified = Craniopharyngioma
- CP Angle – Invades Internal Auditory Canal = Schwannoma
- CP Angle - Invades Both Internal Auditory Canals = Schwannoma with NF2
- CP Angle – Restricts on Diffusion = Epidermoid
- Peds – Arising from Vermis = Medulloblastoma
- Peds - "tooth paste" out of 4th ventricle = Ependymoma
- Adult myelination pattern: T1 at 1 year, T2 at 2 years
- Brainstem and posterior limb of the internal capsule are myelinated at birth.
- CN2 and CNV3 are not in the cavernous sinus

- Persistent trigeminal artery (basilar to carotid) increases the risk of aneurysm
- Subfalcine herniation can lead to ACA infarct
- ADEM lesions will NOT involve the calloso-septal interface.
- Marchiafava-Bignami progresses from body -> genu -> splenium
- Post Radiation changes don't start for 2 months (there is a latent period).
- Hippocampal atrophy is first with Alzheimer Dementia
- Beaked Tectum = Chiari 2
- Beaker Anterior Inferior L1 = Hurlers
- Sometimes Beaked Pons = Multi-System Atrophy
- Most common TORCH is CMV
- Toxo abscess does NOT restrict diffusion
- Small cortical tumors can be occult without IV contrast
- JPA and Ganglioglioma can enhance and are low grade
- Nasal Bone is the most common fracture
- Zygomaticomaxillary Complex Fracture (Tripod) is the most common fracture pattern and involves the zygoma, inferior orbit, and lateral orbit.
- Supplemental oxygen can mimic SAH on FLAIR
- Putamen is the most common location for hypertensive hemorrhage
- Restricted diffusion without bright signal on FLAIR should make you think hyperacute (< 6 hours) stroke.
- Enhancement of a stroke: Rule of 3s - starts at day 3, peaks at 3 weeks, gone at 3 months
- PAN is the Most Common systemic vasculitis to involve the CNS
- Scaphocephaly is the most common type of craniosynostosis
- Piriform aperture stenosis is associated with hypothalamic pituitary adrenal axis issues.
- Cholesterol Granuloma is the most common primary petrous apex lesion
- Large vestibular aqueduct syndrome has absence of the bony modiolus in 90% of cases
- Octreotide scan will be positive for esthesioneuroblastoma
- The main vascular supply to the posterior nose is the sphenopalatine artery (terminal internal maxillary artery).
- Warthins tumors take up pertechnetate
- Sjogrens gets salivary gland lymphoma
- Most common intra-occular lesion in an adult = Melanoma
- Enhancement of nerve roots for 6 weeks after spine surgery is normal. After that it's arachnoiditis
- Hemorrhage in the cord is the most important factor for outcome in a traumatic cord injury.
- Currarino Triad: Anterior Sacral Meningocele, Anorectal malformation, Sarcococcygeal osseous defect
- Type 1 Spinal AVF (dural AVF) is by far the more common.
- Herpes spares the basal ganglia (MCA infarcts do not)
- Most common malignant lacrimal gland tumor = adenoid cystic adenocarcinoma
- Arthritis at the radioscaphoid compartment is the first sign of a SNAC or SLAC wrist
- SLAC wrist has a DISI deformity
- Pull of the Abductor pollucis longus tendon is what causes the dorsolateral dislocation in the Bennett Fx
- Carpal tunnel syndrome has an association with dialysis
- Degree of femoral head displacement predicts risk of AVN
- Proximal pole of the scaphoid is at risk for AVN with fracture
- Most common cause of sacral insufficiency fracture is osteoporosis in old lady
- Patella dislocation is nearly always lateral
- Tibial plateau fracture is way more common laterally
- SONK favors the medial knee (area of maximum weight bearing)
- Normal SI joints excludes Ank Spon
- Looser Zones are a type of insufficiency fracture

- T score of -2.5 marks osteoporosis
- First extensor compartment = de Quervains
- First and Second compartment = intersection syndrome
- Sixth extensor compartment = early RA
- Flexor pollicis longus goes through the carpal tunnel, flexor pollicis brevis does not
- The pisiform recess and radiocarpal joint normally communicate
- The periosteum is intact with both Perthes and ALPSA lesions. In a true bankart it is disrupted.
- Absent anterior/superior labrum, + thickened middle glenohumeral ligament is a Buford complex.
- Medial meniscus is thicker posteriorly.
- Anterior talofibular ligament is the most commonly torn ankle ligament
- TB in the spine - spares the disc space (so can brucellosis).
- Scoliosis curvature points away from the osteoid osteoma
- Osteochondroma is the only benign skeletal tumor associated with radiation.
- Mixed Connective Tissue Disease requires serology (Ribonucleoprotein) for Dx
- Medullary Bone Infarct will have fat in the middle
- Bucket Handle Meniscal tears are longitudinal tears
- Anterior Drawer Sign = ACL
- Posterior Drawer Sign = PCL
- "McMurray" = MCL
- No grid on mag views.
- BR-3 = < 2% chance of cancer
- BR-5 = > 95% chance of cancer
- Nipple enhancement can be normal on post contrast MRI - don't call it Pagets.
- Upper outer quadrant has the highest density of breast tissue, and therefore the most breast cancers.
- Majority of blood (60%) is via the internal mammary
- Majority of lymph (97%) is to the axilla
- The sternalis muscle can only be seen on CC view
- Most common location for ectopic breast tissue is in the axilla
- The follicular phase (day 7-14) is the best time to have a mammogram (and MRI).
- Breast Tenderness is max around day 27-30.
- Tyrer Cuzick is the most comprehensive risk model, but does not include breast density.
- If you had more than 20Gy of chest radiation as a child, you can get a screening MRI
- BRCA 2 (more than 1) is seen with male breast cancer
- BRCA 1 is more in younger patients, BRCA 2 is more in post menopausal
- BRCA 1 is more often a triple negative CA
- Use the LMO for kyphosis, pectus excavatum, and to avoid a pacemaker / line
- Use the ML to help catch milk of calcium layering
- Fine pleomorphic morphology to calcification has the highest suspicion for malignancy
- Intramammary lymph nodes are NOT in the fibroglandular tissue
- Surgical scars should get lighter, if they get denser - think about recurrent cancer.
- You CAN have isolated intracapsular rupture.
- You CAN NOT have isolated extra (it's always with intra).
- If you see silicone in a lymph node, you need to recommend MRI to evaluate for extracapsular rupture
- The number one risk factor for implant rupture is the age of the implant
- Tamoxifen causes a decrease in parenchymal uptake, then a rebound.
- T2 Bright things - these are usually benign. Don't forget colloid cancer is T2 bright.

CPSIA information can be obtained
at www.ICGtesting.com
Printed in the USA
LVHW100728120920
665423LV00006B/1